The Loss of Self

Revised and Updated Edition

The Loss of Self

A Family Resource for the Care of
Alzheimer's Disease and Related Disorders

Revised and Updated Edition

Donna Cohen, Ph.D.

Carl Eisdorfer, Ph.D., M.D.

W.W. Norton & Company • *New York* • *London*

page 25: "Faded Glory." By Jeanetta Dean. Reprinted by permission of author.
page 131: "Stand by Me." By Jerry Leiber, Mike Stoller, Ben E. King. © 1961 Jerry Leiber
Music & Mike Stoller Music. Copyright renewed. All rights reserved. Used by permission.

For information about permission to reproduce selections from this book, write to Permissions,
W.W. Norton & Company, Inc., 500 Fifth Avenue, New York, NY 10110

The text of this book is composed in Bembo
with the display set in Bembo and Base Nine B
Composition by Matrix Publishing Services
Manufacturing by The Maple-Vail Book Manufacturing Group
Book design by Chris Welch

Library of Congress Cataloging-in-Publication Data

Cohen, Donna.
  The loss of self : a family resource for the care of Alzheimer's disease and related
disorders / Donna Cohen, Carl Eisdorfer.—Rev. and updated ed.
    p. cm.
  Includes bibliographical references and index.
  ISBN 0-393-05016-5
  1. Alzheimer's disease—Patients—Rehabilitation. 2. Alzheimer's
disease—Patients—Home care. 3. Alzheimer's disease—Patients—Family relationships. I.
Eisdorfer, Carl. II. Title.

RC523 .C65 2001
618.97'683—dc21

                                                                00-046077

W. W. Norton & Company, Inc., 500 Fifth Avenue, New York, N.Y. 10110
www.wwnorton.com

W. W. Norton & Company Ltd., 10 Coptic Street, London WC1A 1PU

1 2 3 4 5 6 7 8 9 0

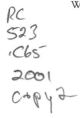

Throughout this book we tell the stories of patients and families who shared their pains and triumphs, their frustrations and hopes. In order to protect their privacy, we have changed their names and any identifying details. Dialogues, interviews, letters, and communications have also been altered to preserve anonymity.

To our families

Who are infinitely precious to us.
They gave us the love and knowledge
To sustain a sense of self
And treat others as our own.

Contents

Contents

Preface

One of our patients with Alzheimer's disease once made a haunting request: "Write a book for those of us who tried. It's not important that we failed—that the doctors can't cure us, that this brain disease destroys us, and that ultimately our families can't take care of us. What matters is that we all tried." We took up the gauntlet and wrote the first edition of *The Loss of Self* as a testament to the courage of the millions of patients and families who live each day with dignity and who refuse to be dehumanized by the disease. At the request of our publisher and as a response to our readers, we have revised the first edition to provide the latest scientific advances on causes, early detection, diagnosis, treatment, and family caregiving and to continue to share the personal thoughts and experiences of many of our patients and their families, who showed us not only how to live with their burden but also how to prevail.

This book offers practical information about how to recognize when memory problems are serious; how to get a comprehensive diagnosis; what to do after the diagnosis; where to go for help; how to understand the patient's subjective experience of the illness; how to work effectively with the patient and other family members, even when relationships are not loving; how to develop a plan of care for the family; how to cope with emotions; how to develop financial and legal plans; how to deal with a range of family and marital issues, including sexual difficulties; how to handle psychiatric problems using behavioral interventions and drugs; and how to cope with violence, suicidal and homicidal ideation, and end-of-life care. We have also increased the repertoire of practical as well as compassionate strategies to balance the many competing needs of patients and family members, to resolve family conflict, and to interact effectively with physicians and other health professionals. When we refer to physicians throughout the book we are referring to the patient's physician.

The Loss of Self tries to help families organize themselves to explore options for long-term care such as at home, in the community, at assisted living residences, and in nursing homes. It provides information about the history and the financing of health care in this country, including managed care, and explains why services are not more available to support the family. The challenge to the family is to meet the many needs of the patient, to find resources in the community, and to be able to deal with the financial and emotional costs of caring.

Alzheimer's disease has become one of biomedical science's most glamorous topics since the first edition of *The Loss of Self* was published in 1986. Research discoveries have brought an era of early detection, antidementia drugs, genetic interventions including possible immunization, and therapeutic interventions to empower patients and families to cope more effectively. The media coverage of new research findings has excited the public's imagination, fueling optimism about treating the disease as well as preventing it.

Over the next millennium, there will be an unprecedented increase in life expectancy due to advances in science and medicine. As a result, society will face many challenges in dealing with the aging population, and Alzheimer's disease is one of the most serious. The prevalence of Alzheimer's disease and other dementias of later life has created an urgent public health agenda because the number of affected persons is growing and because people with the disease are living longer than ever before. Alzheimer's disease affects more than four million middle-aged and older Americans, and at least fifteen million are estimated to be affected throughout the world. More than thirty-four million people worldwide will develop Alzheimer's disease by 2025.

Although people still stumble when pronouncing the name of the psychiatrist, Alois Alzheimer, who first reported the disease in 1907, most know about the condition named after him: a progressive brain disorder involving a slow but progressive deterioration of the mind, sometimes lasting five, ten, or fifteen years or more. Alzheimer's disease is the most common cause of progressive and irreversible dementia in later life, but it is not the only cause. More than fifty other nonreversible dementias also impair cognitive abilities. In addition, many medical conditions mimic the symptoms, and they are treatable and therefore reversible.

Alzheimer's disease is more than a disease of the brain. It is an illness, a personal journey, subjectively experienced by the person with the diagnosis. It gradually robs the individual of everything that defines a sense of self, and it disrupts that individual's life as well as the lives of family members and others close to him or her. One gentleman told us, "It's not just that this disease keeps me from taking care of myself, it prevents me from being a husband, father, and friend! I have always been one who has given to others, and now I am compelled to receive! Woe unto me!"

Although people with dementia lose their memory and other cognitive abilities, not all skills and abilities deteriorate at the same rate, and personal insight varies widely. Indeed, nonverbal skills are maintained, even into the later phases, meaning that patients can perceive and react with emotional intelligence when other cognitive skills are impaired. As a consequence, individuals with the disease often manifest behavioral problems and act strangely, showing anger, fear, and sometimes violence, because they are unable to communicate feelings and emotions.

Patients are people—first, last, and always. They have wishes, desires, beliefs, and preferences that need to be expressed and understood. Not to understand individuals-turned-patients is to prevent them from working in a partnership with others to deal effectively with the impact of the disease. The subjective experiences of patients and family members and of living with hope and tempered optimism remain powerful themes of this revised book.

When we wrote the first edition of *The Loss of Self*, most people suffering from the disease and their families struggled alone, leading what one husband called "lives of quiet desperation in a world of 36 hour days," trying to cope with the impact of the disease. Families had nowhere to go for help and little if any information to read. In one of a series of films we helped produce between 1975 and 1979, called *The Thirty-Six Hour Day*, a daughter whose mother had Alzheimer's disease declared emotionally, "Everywhere we went no one could tell us anything about it. Everything we learned about Alzheimer's disease we learned from living with it!" The title of our medical education film was later adopted for the book by Peter Rabins and Nancy Mace.

Today, patients and their families have more help available to them. The Alzheimer's Association, founded in Chicago in 1979 as the Alzheimer's Disease and Related Disorders Association (ADRDA) by seven groups throughout the United States, has grown to be a prominent effective national organization. Alzheimer's Disease International (ADI) has existed since 1985, serving as an umbrella organization for countries around the world who have national associations. The mission of these groups is to raise money for research, support family groups, disseminate information, and organize public advocacy efforts.

Alzheimer's disease research and clinical centers have developed throughout the country and the world. Many books have been published, and several Web sites exist on the Internet. Features in newspapers and magazines as well as on television and radio continue to report scientific advances about the causes of the disorder, early detection, and new drugs that may help many patients to function better. Discoveries will continue throughout the new millennium, and there is optimism about the future. At the same time, the burden of caring is better understood, and we have increased our knowledge about the cost of caring on the health and well-being of those who are devoted to someone with Alzheimer's disease.

Scientific advances in the detection, diagnosis, management, and treatment of Alzheimer's disease will make caring for affected relatives more challenging for families as well as society in the future. With the anticipated ability to detect Alzheimer's disease in very early stages and to slow dementia with neuroprotective drugs, there will likely be greater numbers of patients to treat. With decreasing mortality from physical diseases, there also will be increasing numbers of patients living longer with severe dementia and medical comorbidities. Caring for a growing population of mildly as well as severely impaired persons will present social, clinical, and ethical challenges. We will be challenged to do our best!

The word *care* means many things. According to the dictionary it means to protect, provide for, watch over, love, like, cherish, treasure, and respect, to provide only a few definitions. In this context, all who provide care for a person with dementia, whether at home or in a nursing home, face constant challenges to sustain the patient and themselves. Our research and that of many others has clearly shown that caregiving is stressful and associated with a high risk for emotional and physical dysfunction as well as mortality. We know a great deal more about therapeutic interventions to reduce the burden of caregiving and strengthen the principal caregiver and others in the family.

Caring and the value of human life are a part of society's moral fabric. Given the increasing incidence of irreversible disease in our older population, already considered by many to be a drain on the productive capacity of society, the pressure to rethink our moral contract with the aged is an issue of international concern. The challenge is to find effective and affordable ways to help those who need help and ease the burden on the caring family. It is to these caregiving families and friends that we dedicate this work.

Ethical and moral issues cannot be ignored in caring for cognitively impaired and terminally ill patients. Our philosophy recognizes that caring is costly in time as well as emotions and finances. It also generates a reward—one perhaps more implicit than explicit—but there is no personal human growth without stress and strain. Overwhelming stress can lead to collapse, but finding helpful interventions such as information and education can make the difference between becoming overwhelmed and dealing successfully with crises.

Working with our patients and families over the years has been a special privilege for us. Despite the pathos of a tragic illness, many of our patients and families achieve enormous growth and develop a special intimacy we have been privileged to share. They have taught us to appreciate life and its inalienable dignity. They have touched our lives forever.

D.C. & C.E.

Acknowledgments

The Loss of Self is a book of hope and an affirmation of life. It reflects the influences of many people who have inspired us as well as many circumstances that have challenged us. Composing the acknowledgments has created a window for personal reflection and appreciation on many levels:

> To confess that this book would not have been possible without the contributions of thousands of patients and families, living and dead, whose identities must be disguised but whose lives have touched us forever;
>
> To recognize that scientific discoveries and sociopolitical changes in health care will have made parts of this book outdated upon publication, but that the voices of our patients and families will still convey universal truths about caring and the value of life;
>
> To recognize the enduring contributions of the families and professionals who were the founders of the national Alzheimer's Association, friends and associates with whom we shared the birthing pains of what is now the most prominent organization dedicated to Alzheimer's disease and related dementias, as well as the accomplishments of those who are part of the Alzheimer's Association now and in the future;
>
> To appreciate the humanity and courage of President Ronald Reagan, his wife and caregiver, Nancy, and the family who carry the torch, giving others the strength to endure and prevail; and

To acknowledge and thank many people who are inscribed in our souls, who may not be named here but who are not forgotten.

Those who have contributed to our efforts over the years are legion. Our feelings about confidentiality, in some instances, and our concern that we omit any of you have led to the difficult decision that recognition of you as a group is most fitting. Our deeply felt thanks for your help. There are a few we wish to offer a special acknowledgment:

Tabitha Griffin, our gifted editor at W. W. Norton, who came into our lives with grace, energy, and confidence in what our book offered to families.

Wayne Hill, a talented and energetic assistant, who adopted us and our book as a personal mission, doing research as well as retyping the manuscript through many iterations, and who shared our joys and tensions in this labor of love. We know that you are a candidate for double eyeball and wrist replacements from sitting at the computer!

Dee Keiser, a dear friend, who also helped in the final preparations of our book and who shared the tears and laughter of caring for her own mother with Alzheimer's disease.

Joyce Johnson, a long time assistance and friend who has worked with us on other books, for caring so deeply about the work and for helping in many ways.

Bill Lester, whose computer and technical knowledge are magical, as well as Judy Perry and Tiffany Vergon for always being there to check the details.

The community of friends, colleagues, and collaborators in our research, clinical, educational, and advocacy activities in many academic homes—Duke University, the University of Washington, the Albert Einstein College of Medicine, the University of Illinois at Chicago, the University of Miami, and the University of South Florida.

With *The Loss of Self*, we hope that we have been able to do more than write a technical resource. The stories of our patients and families describe human beings who have refused to be dehumanized by the devastation of disease. We hope that their pain and their triumphs will inspire all of us to have the courage to meet the challenge of caring for ourselves and one another.

The Loss of Self

Revised and Updated Edition

1

The Loss of Self

I am hungry for the life that is being taken away from me. I am a human being. I still exist. I have a family. I hunger for friendship, happiness, and the touch of a loved hand. What I ask for is that what is left of my life shall have some meaning. Give me something to die for! Help me to be strong and free until my self no longer exists. —J.T.

James Thomas, the man who wrote these lines in his diary, died at the age of seventy, having lived with Alzheimer's disease for more than eight years. Mr. Thomas began a daily journal shortly after he was diagnosed, in an effort to come to terms with what he called "God's cruel joke." Many of the entries in the early phases of the dementia reveal courage, energy, and a sense of purpose as he, his wife Jean, and his family struggled together to overcome his losses. Approximately a year after the diagnosis he wrote:

No theory of medicine can explain what is happening to me. Every few months I sense that another piece of me is missing. My life . . . my self . . . are falling apart. I can only think half thoughts now. Someday I may wake up and not think at all . . . not know who I am. Most people expect to die someday, but who ever expected to lose their self first.

James kept the journal daily with his wife's assistance. He named it "Song of Myself," after one of his favorite poems by Walt Whitman.

James knew that everything would soon be lost from his memory. He wanted to record his granddaughter's childhood, his son's struggle to build a business, as well as the daily events that had meaning for Jean and him. As long as he could write or dictate to his wife, he felt a sense of worth. It also gave him great pleasure to read through the entries, knowing that he could still hold on to some of his memories. Long after James could neither write nor talk, Jean would sit with her husband and write in his journal. Although he could not actively participate, the ritual remained part of their life until he died.

Alzheimer's disease is a cruel disorder. However, no matter how devastating it is, the essential humanity of the "person-turned-patient" remains. Lewis Mumford, who wrote many books and was the father of city planning in the United States, had Alzheimer's disease. His wife cared for him at home well into the later stages, when he was incontinent and incapacitated. Mrs. Mumford reported that her husband retained his essential quality, dignity, throughout the course of dementia: "My Lewis was always dignified, even when he did undignified things!"

As the disease progresses, even with the few antidementia medications currently available, there is little or no hope of recovery of memory. But people do not consist of memory alone. People have needs as well as feelings, imagination, desires, drives, will, and moral being. It is in these realms that there are ways to touch patients and let them touch us.* The millions of people who suffer from dementia, like James Thomas, have much to teach us about living and how to enjoy being alive even with a catastrophic illness.

Increasingly over the past twenty-five years, the brain disorders of later life have become a personal tragedy in millions of lives throughout the world. Both the person with the illness and the family suffer with the inexorable dissolution of self. Loss of sight, hearing, an arm, or a leg challenges a person to cope with significant change. However, the individual with Alzheimer's disease must eventually come to terms with a far more frightening prospect—the complete loss of self. And for the family, according to one daughter, "The death of the mind is the worst death imaginable." Family members share a life of emotional turmoil as they witness the disintegration of someone they love.

*See O. Sacks, p. 334.

A great deal can be done for patients and for their families to ease the burden of Alzheimer's disease and related disorders. And even with the discovery of new agents to hopefully halt, retard, or prevent the dementia, we will still need to care for millions of human beings. Almost everyone who is willing can take an active role in treatment throughout the course of the illness. Resources and therapeutic strategies including psychotherapy, group and family therapies, exist to meet many of the needs of the families and help members cope with the changes in their lives.

Family caregiving can be a satisfying experience, but caregiving also creates a range of physical, emotional, and financial demands that place family members at risk for negative outcomes, for example, physical and mental health problems and disruptions in work and family life. Without assistance, the chronicle of care often unnecessarily carries family members to the limits of physical and mental exhaustion.

After the diagnosis is made, an individual may live five, ten, or fifteen years or more. These are long human years. Therefore, it is important to set realistic goals, involve appropriate family members to make plans together, find appropriate professional help, and prepare for the future and all the changes it will bring. If the patient and family as well as fictive kin and close friends are able to prepare themselves to deal with the future, there is time to live and love, despite the ravages of a progressive brain disease.

Jean Thomas described a moving incident with her husband, James, and one of their grandchildren that occurred several months after James had been diagnosed as having Alzheimer's disease.

It was a Saturday morning, and I was working upstairs in my sewing room making a dress for Evelyn, the oldest grandchild, to wear in the school play. Evelyn sat in the yard rehearsing her lines as Juliet, with James reading the part of Romeo. Even though James read slowly and had trouble pronouncing several words, he and Evelyn were very good together. I was proud of Ev for involving him. It was her idea for James to help her practice, and he enjoyed it thoroughly.

I remember calling down to Evelyn to take a break and try on the dress for me. While we were pinning the hem, there was a funny sound outside. I walked over to the window to be greeted by James climbing up a ladder. He placed his arms around me and spoke softly: "I wish I were the young Romeo, strong of body and mind, for I love you so." We both smiled, and then I began to cry, remembering that those were the exact words James spoke years ago on our first date when he climbed up a ladder to my window!

That night during dinner, James and I talked about what had happened that morning. It was a turning point in the way I thought about his diagnosis. Up until that time both of us had been upset and irritable. I was frightened and unable to talk with James. However, seeing him on the ladder and caught in the warmth of his embrace, I understood for the first time that my husband was still someone I could touch and love. And just as important, he could still love me, even with the Alzheimer's. The disease would change him, but we still shared a life together and we had a future.

Throughout this book we tell the stories of many individuals with dementia and of their families who have struggled with their fears, anxieties, and hopes. Many stories are heartbreaking, but many more are moving and profound testaments to the ability of people to transcend suffering and find meaning in their lives. Elizabeth Gold, whose husband had Alzheimer's disease, called the disease "life's last battleground." She went on to say,

I cannot believe that God let my husband survive Hitler to get this disease. He was the only one in his family not to be killed by Hitler's army. My Joe was a good man who lived for me, his children, and his congregation.

Now, even with the Alzheimer's disease, he still goes to worship each day. I do not know how many of the prayers he still understands, but of one thing I am sure. Joe finds inner peace and comfort there. One Saturday he came home and sat down with me for dinner. I prepared to say the blessing when he reached for my hand and kissed it: "My lips cannot say the words, but you know my spirit fights to speak. I must fight to worship in a silence that goes beyond words."

Our patients and families have taught us that there is a life that transcends Alzheimer's disease and related disorders. It is important to see individuals with dementia in the context of their family as well as their personal needs and aspirations. Every patient has a history, complete with accomplishments and failures, relationships with other people, as well as dreams and ambitions for the future, however limited. Furthermore, patients and families, including teenagers and children, need and respond to each other in very human ways, even in the later stages of dementia.

Jeanetta Dean wrote a poem when she was eighteen about her great uncle, Lloyd Copeland, who was diagnosed with Alzheimer's disease at age ninety and died eight years later. He had been a prominent, beloved leader in his community for years, serving in many elected capacities, including on the city council and as mayor. Jeanetta wrote "Faded Glory" after seeing him for several months in the same restaurant every Sunday with his wife.

FADED GLORY
Thinning skin with violent ripples
Loosely hung on dated bones,
He shuffles along, his silver crown fallen;
His eyes are dim, his mind . . . scrambled.
Words escape his frame in whispers;
Digging in his pocket with an uncertain pride,
Retrieves his wallet worn, ragged, and
Carefully unfolds his kin for display.

Jeanetta had to introduce herself to him every Sunday, and he seemed to behave as if he should know who she was. He always pulled out his wallet and showed her old tattered pictures of his family as if she had never seen them before. Jeanetta wrote,

It saddened me to think that someone so accomplished could be reduced to the confused old man that stood before me who was now living in the past. He had done so much in his lifetime— only to have it erased in his own mind. "Faded Glory" is my attempt to immortalize this pathetic image, lest I should forget.

Ironically, Alzheimer's disease forces people to deal with each other in a smaller time frame. The anticipated enjoyment and freedom of the later years are changed. However, our patients and families have taken the challenge valiantly, finding time to love and care for each other, even when relationships have been strained or torn asunder. John Hauge published an illustrated book, *Heavy Snow: My Father's Disappearance into Alzheimer's*, which is the moving story of a son caring for his father. It is also a story that shows how reconciliation between an estranged father and son is possible because of the disease. The introduction sets the stage for evolving growth and personal sharing between father and son:

> One winter morning I was walking with my father outside his nursing home. It was snowing heavily. I glanced back at our trail and noticed that his tracks had almost vanished, while mine were still defined. I joked with him about this and asked what he thought it meant. He replied, "I'm not surprised. I often feel like I'm disappearing."

The Myth of "Senility"

Alzheimer's disease and other forms of dementia afflict an estimated four million or more middle-aged and older persons in the United States alone and affect the lives of at least fifteen million family members. Perhaps 10 percent or more of the world's population over the age of sixty-five has Alzheimer's disease or a related form of dementia. However, Alzheimer's disease and similar disorders are not normal consequences of aging.

We all know of individuals in the later decades of life who continue to be creative, productive, and in full command of their mental faculties. It is no longer rare to find college students in their sixties or individuals working productively at a job in their seventies. The list of older artists, writers, political figures, scientists, and other prominent persons is virtually endless. Thomas Jefferson founded the University of Virginia at the age of sixty-five. Goethe finished *Faust* in his middle seventies. George Bernard Shaw began writing his first novel after the age of sixty. Verdi was nearly eighty when he composed *Falstaff*, one of his best operas. James Michener wrote forty-nine books before his death at age eighty-nine, and Martha Graham choreographed scores of dances until her death at age ninety-eight.

As we improve our ability to deal with the diseases of later life, more and more individuals will be able to remain productive. One advantage of the growing number and proportion of older persons in our society is that all of us are getting firsthand experience with older persons who remain vital, effective, and involved with their world. Simply stated, people do not lose their minds as they age. When we see profound losses in older persons, these are in every sense the result of some identifiable problem or disease.

A large number of diseases cause memory loss in middle-aged and older people. Among the very old, these conditions are seen so frequently that for many years they were confused with aging itself. The term *senile* was used to refer to older persons who were unable to function intelligently and care for themselves. If younger persons were affected with these conditions, they were identified as "prematurely senile" or "presenile."

The terms *senile* and *senility* are misleading. They have as much professional status as the word *crazy*. Unfortunately, the idea that aging and senility go together has been a part of the mythology of our culture and literature for centuries. Shakespeare's "seven ages of man" relates the last part of life to "second childishness and mere oblivion, sans teeth, sans eyes, sans taste, sans everything." Toynbee in his book *Mankind and Mother Earth* proposes that mankind has a choice between death and senility. What sad nonsense! Advancing age is accompanied by a greater risk for disease and frailty, but aging itself is not a disease, and it does not cause dementia.

Growing older does carry a risk that dementia may develop, and the risk increases with age. Alzheimer's disease is rare in persons under age sixty, and approximately $1^1/_2$–2 percent of persons sixty to sixty-five years old are affected. The percentage doubles every five years, so that by age ninety the risks are about fifty-fifty. *Dementia* is defined in the dictionary as "a condition of being out of one's mind." It also is a medical term referring to decreased mental performance. Dementia is a "syndrome," not a disease. A *syndrome* refers to a group of symptoms, in this case the loss of many aspects of cognition such as language, learning, memory, thinking, and reasoning. A dementia syndrome may be temporary or permanent, but the symptoms occur as a result of a disease or an abnormal condition. The term *dementia* is valuable because it alerts us to look for the underlying cause of the mental disturbance, and it implies the existence of medical and psychological procedures to diagnose and care for individuals who exhibit such losses.

Forms of Dementia

Since dementia is a group of symptoms, it should not be surprising that some of the conditions that lead to symptoms of cognitive impairment may be reversible. In such situations, if the patient is diagnosed and treated promptly, the dementia may clear without any long-term effects. Indeed, the conditions of as many as 25 to 30 percent of the individuals complaining of memory problems have a treatable cause.

A wide variety of conditions can cause dementia. They are thoroughly reviewed in the next chapter. Infections, diabetes, poor nutrition, heart disease, pulmonary diseases, depression, anxiety, and the use of alcohol and many types of drugs can cause transient periods of delirium, a condition often confused with dementia as well as more persistent memory problems. However, many other factors besides poor health have a significant impact on a person's behavior. Lack of motivation to perform, feelings of inadequacy about one's self worth and competence, financial insecurity, social isolation, recent losses like the death of a friend or family member, or any major life change can cause a reaction that may appear as a significant dementia. Although these issues usually are considered when younger patients are examined, unfortunately they may be ignored when an older person is the patient.

Not all of the disorders that lead to intellectual loss are reversible. These diseases include cerebrovascular diseases also known as vascular dementias, Pick's disease, Huntington's chorea, Korsakoff's syndrome, Creutzfeldt-Jakob disease, some forms of Parkinson's disease, and the most prevalent of all dementias, Alzheimer's disease. Over the past few years, with improved diagnostic procedures, other conditions have emerged that are variants of Alzheimer's disease and non-Alzheimer dementias caused by changes in specific brain areas. It is important to recognize that although these diseases may not be reversible as of this writing, there is nonetheless a great deal we can do for the patient and the family.

Recognizing Dementia

The early diagnosis of dementia is crucial for two reasons. First, if there is a treatable disease or condition, the problem may be reversed, if detected soon enough. If too much time passes before diagnosis, that chance may be lost. This is especially the case when older persons treated for medical problems in the hospital develop a delirium, usually from medications. If the delirium (e.g., the rapid appearance of confusion, disorientation, and hallucinations) is not recognized as such and treated, dementia can become permanent.

Second, even if the dementia is nonreversible and due to Alzheimer's disease or a related disorder, early detection and diagnosis lead to early intervention and treatment. When the diagnosis is made in the early stages of the disease, patients and families are in the best position to deal with the impact of the dementia on their future. If an accurate diagnosis is delayed too long, the consequences may include emotional distress, family upheaval, and even physical harm to the patient or others. There are new drugs that help slow the progression of the disease but do not reverse it. Thus, the earlier these medications are started, the better.

An early diagnosis is often hard to make because it can be extremely difficult to decide when something is seriously wrong. A progressive dementia may go unrecognized for months or even years because the individual may conceal it well or be protected by friends and family, or there is an unspoken conspiracy of denial about the mistakes the patient is making.

Men and women from all walks of life and all occupations have reported that they knew something was wrong but found ways to cope for a while. They delegated more work to other people, talked less, wrote notes to themselves, or limited their activities to ones they could manage. A government official reported to us that he could not remember conversations or questions well enough to make decisions. He survived in his job for more than a year by insisting that all questions be submitted to him in writing, ostensibly to have a "paper trail," so that he could give a more studied answer. A senior pilot (not flying a U.S. commercial airliner) told us that for more than six months he had worried about his judgment while flying, although his copilots and engineers never suspected a problem. On days "when he did not feel like himself," he allowed the copilot to fly the plane. He felt confident about continuing to fly most of the time, but at the same time he experienced anxiety about getting lost in airports, driving home, or finding his hotel in another city. One night, after getting lost for ninety minutes while driving home after a long flight, he finally decided to see a physician.

Often people who live and work with someone showing the early signs of dementia may consciously or unconsciously delay the recognition of a problem out of loyalty or denial. One president of a corporation functioned adequately for over a year with the help of his wife, secretary, chauffeur, and two assistants. It was only when he had a minor traffic accident one weekend that the disease became public. He forgot which direction to turn and stopped suddenly in the middle of an intersection, only to be struck in the rear by another car. The police thought he was drunk or hurt because he seemed so confused and disoriented. A medical evaluation led to a more comprehensive set of examinations, and ultimately the diagnosis of Alzheimer's disease.

After the diagnosis is made, it is always easy to look back and recognize that a serious problem was developing. Unfortunately, before the dementia is diagnosed, family members often feel something is wrong but cannot pinpoint the source of their discomfort. These feelings can become intense and often affect the family for a long time to come. It is not only a husband or a wife but also children who feel and react to the strain. In the following interview, Henry and Sandra Long describe the early frustration before they knew that Henry's dad had Alzheimer's disease, as well as their sadness that they cannot undo the past.

MR. L.: We first noticed that Dad had a problem finding the correct words for a situation. He always had a tendency toward this, in my opinion, but it began to get worse. It also became difficult to deal with him because he did not seem to listen. He would ask a question. We would respond to the question, and then he would ask it again a short time later.

This was even apparent in telephone calls. It was so frustrating, and we would ask ourselves, "Why isn't he listening to us? Why is he doing this?" We didn't know what it was at that time.

MRS. L.: We felt like he didn't care enough to listen. It was as if he really wasn't interested in me or in what I was doing. I realize now that was a faulty perception on my part. But that was the feeling then.

After we married, Henry and I moved away, and we had very little contact with his parents. However, we moved back five years ago, and it has been difficult to get close to Henry's dad.

DR.: Even though you were never close to him, he had a powerful effect on you?

MRS. L.: Yes, it has always bothered me, and now it's especially frustrating. I know why I was never able to get close to him. And now I never will. I can't go back and change anything, because he's not going to ever understand that.

DR.: Mr. Long, how did you feel?

MR. L.: Frustrated and irritated. Why wasn't the man listening to what we were saying? Why didn't he understand what we were saying? Was he too busy thinking about something else? Yes, I would get upset, and I would especially get angry because I didn't think he was listening to Sandra when I thought he should be. And I look back now and understand what's been happening. It's too bad. I wish I never got angry.

DR.: You seem to be self-critical as you look back on it now?

MRS. L.: Yes, a little bit. I lost my temper with my father when he had a problem that he couldn't do anything about. Now it's too late to say I'm sorry. He has deteriorated too much.

Husbands or wives often report communication problems or difficulties in the marriage at the beginning of the disease. Lois Neuman told us:

I thought my husband was having an affair. He seemed less interested in me for a while, but I thought it would pass. We had been married forty-five years, and you understand how people need space every once in a while.

But it didn't pass, and I began to get angry. We fought a great deal the year before the dementia was diagnosed. I didn't want to lose my husband to another woman. Now I have lost him to something much worse.

In the following interview, Greg and Tina Jenson describe some of the early marital discord before Greg was diagnosed with Alzheimer's disease three years prior to this interview.

MRS. J.: I think the first time it struck me that something was wrong was about five years ago. We began to bicker, and we couldn't understand each other. Our communication was breaking down. We even went to a psychiatrist. We had been married for over thirty years at the time, and our arguments were different from anything that had ever happened between us before. As I look back on it now, I understand, but at the time I was baffled. We thought it was because we had both retired the year before, and that we were both having difficulty adjusting to retirement. However, it wasn't that.

DR.: Greg, what are some of the difficulties that you experienced over the past few years?

MR. J.: We went through pretty much what Tina had told you . . . of not getting along after many good years. It just didn't seem right. We were getting on each other's nerves.

DR.: How did you feel you might be getting on your wife's nerves?

MR. J.: Oh, little things that previously wouldn't have bothered us.

DR.: Your wife had mentioned that you had both recently retired at the time the difficulty started.

MR. J.: Yes.

DR.: I also understand that you went to see a psychiatrist because you thought there might be some conflict in your relationship with each other?

MR. J.: Yes.

MRS. J.: And later we realized that the cause of our problem was Greg's memory losses. He would say, "Let's go with so and so to see such and such a place," and then forget what he had said. Then I would say, "You said we were going," and he would get angry. "You are putting words in my mouth. I never said that!" I couldn't understand what was happening. I didn't know anything about Alzheimer's disease, and I was completely baffled. Another problem was the double bind. He would urge me to go ahead and do something and then say that he would worry about me if I did it. I was damned if I did and damned if I didn't.

DR.: As time went by, did you seek other help?

MRS. J.: No. We seemed to adjudicate this between ourselves. We were determined that we were going to get along well, and we did for a while. One of the ways in which we did this was to each seek separate interests. I took courses at the community college. Greg did work around the place. We left more spaces between ourselves.

Later we came up against other problems that eventually led to the diagnosis of Alzheimer's disease. We switched doctors. A new general practitioner examined us, one right after the other.

I recall that Greg was seen first, and I went in second. The doctor said to me, "I'm amazed at your husband. He's younger than you, and yet he seems much older than you. He's aging very rapidly, and I must get to the cause of it." This was the first inkling I had that something was wrong. The doctor sent us to a neurologist.

DR.: And what were the results of the examination?

MRS. J.: I didn't get any written report, but the neurologist explained what was happening. I wanted to know the truth. He told me Greg probably had Alzheimer's disease.

It is not unusual for individuals to have difficulty communicating with each other. This is precisely what often makes the early recognition of dementia difficult. However, when these problems persist, losses in the ability to communicate with others weakens even the strongest relationships. When this disruption is accompanied by personality changes, temper tantrums, irritability, and suspiciousness, the situation usually becomes toxic. Angry outbursts may be directed at almost anyone and for no apparent reason. This is particularly troublesome since most persons involved do not understand why the outbursts have occurred or why the patients are not able to control their emotions.

In the following interview, a physician talked with Jane Dombrowski and her three young daughters about the early changes in Mr. Dombrowski and how the disease affected them as a family. Mrs. Dombrowski was forty, and her three daughters from youngest to oldest include Suzie, aged seven, Jean, fourteen, and Margo, seventeen.

DR.: Margo, when did you first begin to feel that something might be wrong with your dad?
MARGO: It's really hard for me to say. I didn't live at home, and I didn't seem him that often. I think one of the first times I noticed a problem was when I needed a ride to a job interview. It was far away, and my dad gave me a ride. We couldn't find the place, and he finally got so frustrated he said, "To hell with the job, to hell with the interview," and he took off. I don't think I've ever seen him madder. That was when I started noticing things were wrong.
DR.: How would you describe him before he got sick?
MARGO: Easygoing. He'd never get involved in arguments unless it got so bad he felt he had to stop it. He usually left the arguing to us.
DR.: What happened after he got sick?
MARGO: If he heard fighting, he would lose his temper and tell us to stop it.
DR.: Did he ever start them?
MARGO: With me, yes. I don't know about the other girls, but we got in some really terrible arguments. Once he got so mad we started hitting each other—which is something we had never done before. I had never hit my dad. I just got so mad at him because he started yelling at me and hitting me for no reason at all. I got fed up and hit him back.

Phases of Change

What must it feel like to be stricken with Alzheimer's disease or any of the other progressive brain disorders? The "individuals-turned-patients" have much to tell us if we watch and listen. To the extent possible, people need and want to be empowered and involved in their care. This preserves their dignity and enhances their well-being and comfort. Therefore, understanding a patient's perceptions, beliefs, emotions, thoughts, and desires is essential. This is true early in the illness when cognitive skills are not as impaired and we can involve them in discussions about a range of issues. It is just as true when individuals are profoundly impaired, and we are making decisions for them. Even in later phases, spending time and energy to understand and respond to personal needs will enhance their comfort and quality of life.

Coping with dementia is a process involving a series of psychological adaptations as the disease imposes significant limitations on the person. From our interviews we have learned how thousands of patients perceived and reacted to their losses before and during the diagnosis as well as in the later stages. We have categorized the subjective experience into six phases:

- Recognition and concern: "Something is wrong."
- Denial: "Not me."
- Anger, guilt, and sadness: "Why me?"
- Coping: "In order to go on, I must do . . ."
- Maturation: "Living each day 'til I die."
- Separation from self

Not every patient experiences these phases in the order described, but they provide a way to understand and respond to what patients need during the different stages of illness. Similar phases can be identified for other chronic, debilitating illnesses, but Alzheimer's disease, "the death of the mind," has special characteristics. In the rest of the book we describe specific strategies and tactics for working with patients throughout these phases. The insidious onset makes the period before diagnosis confusing to patients and families. After the diagnosis some patients deny the disease; others do not. Some become angry and depressed; some do not. Coping with the disease is difficult because dementia impairs the parts of the brain required to adjust and adapt. However, most patients in the early and middle phases are capable of learning to cope with the limitations of their deficits. It is important to ask people what they think and feel, and to have the patience to wait for the answer. Working with the patients helps to establish a sense of limited control.

The maturation phase may last for years. Patients may need a great deal of structure and supervision. They may be difficult to deal with, but they are still human beings with needs to feel worthwhile, to be intimate and accepted, as well as to be active and mobile. In the last hard-to-describe phase, the personality is all but gone. People react to sights and sounds but their behavior is reactive rather than active. The major needs are to be comfortable, secure, and active within their abilities.

Caring for the patient with Alzheimer's disease is not an insurmountable task. It is, however, a management challenge, especially to learn how the patient thinks and feels when comprehension and communication are difficult or impossible. In this book we describe many psychological, behavioral, social, and environmental strategies and tactics to guide the process of communicating, understanding, and interacting with the patient. We will help you learn how to speak the patient's language once you recognize that you are speaking Virgil and the patient is speaking Dante.

We wrote *The Loss of Self* not only to help families, and indeed anyone caring for individuals-turned-patients to cope with the ethical and practical challenges of caring, but also to enable them to understand the experience of dementia. Therein lies the knowledge and power to form an effective alliance with patients and to make decisions balancing their needs with those of other family members. However, the consequences of even optimal solutions to balancing the needs of patients and caregivers may be painful, as Mrs. Cross describes in this letter:

> Glenn and I planned a trip to Asia the summer my mother died. We both knew this absence would be difficult for her, and we debated long and hard about taking our trip. We finally decided to go.
>
> We asked several of our special friends to visit Mom each day, and we arranged a schedule. Our friends were so wonderful! They visited her daily and sometimes took her out of the home. However, I'm not sure my mother ever recognized me again. When we returned, another part of her had died. I can't help but wonder what her final days would have been like had we stayed home.

It is likely that Mrs. Cross's mother would have lost her ability to recognize her daughter even if they had not taken the trip.

The chapters of this book provide a framework for families to make many difficult decisions and to deal with the consequences. There are ways to transcend the tragedy of dementia. The information and stories that follow show how those with dementia and caring family members cope with the challenge to reaffirm their existence and redefine their lives.

The first challenge is to discern whether something is wrong and then to determine what is causing the symptoms. The next is to recognize not only that the future will be affected by what is wrong but also that early diagnosis can help in structuring a meaningful family life. The ensuing chapter describes how to obtain the most accurate medical diagnosis, because a correct diagnosis is the beginning of the caring process.

2

The Diagnosis of Dementia

I have always been successful at everything I have done. I am a senior part-
ner in a large accounting firm. I have always been on top of the office. I
have had a perfect memory, knowing every detail about my clients' accounts,
even the minutiae.

Now my memory is a problem. I forget the time of appointments. Some-
times I even forget who I am going to see and what we are going to talk
about. I read accounts, and then I can't remember what I read. My mind
goes blank!

Something has been happening that really scares me. This morning I
could not remember the entree I had at dinner last night, and this has hap-
pened several times over the past few months.

It is normal occasionally to forget names or facts at any age. "Where did I put my car keys?" "Where is the letter I left on the desk?" "I would have introduced you, but I couldn't remember her name." We have all had the experience of having a word at the tip of our tongue but being unable to get it out. Some of us have never been very good at remembering names, directions, or numbers, but we learn to live with the inconvenience, to rely on others, and often to joke about our lapses.

When do memory lapses signal dementia—the serious disturbance in mental ability indicating that a person has passed the boundaries of nor-mality and that the brain is not functioning adequately? To answer this question, it is helpful to know a few facts about memory and the other cognitive abilities that are necessary for people to function intelligently. The word *cognition* is derived from the Latin "cognoscere," which means "to know." When cognition is impaired to the point where individuals have difficulty knowing what, when, why, or how to do things in their life, an evaluation is necessary.

Memory is only one of many cognitive abilities controlled by the brain. The list of abilities is long and includes such skills as the recognition of words, objects, and people; thinking; speech and language; mathematical calculation; reasoning and judgment; attention; problem solving; and many others. Disturbances in any of these abilities make it more difficult for a person to remember and act intelligently. Furthermore, deficits in thinking, judgment, talking, remembering, or decision making are interrelated and affect each other.

In dementia, memory for recent life experiences may be impaired more than memories of the distant past. Learning new information may become a problem, while remembering people, places, and events from the past is not. As this happens, an individual in the early stages of dementia may begin to confuse the present and the past. If language disturbances are present, the individual may have difficulty expressing a thought, reading a sentence, or understanding what is said and responding. A change in the ability to concentrate and pay attention causes confusion, since the individual cannot pick up important clues from the environment. These clues are necessary to help a person act appropriately. There are also many "higher-order" mental abilities called *executive functions* that refer to the ability to organize information, to think and reason, to solve problems, and to make choices between alternatives. These also may change as dementia begins to reveal itself.

Cognitive losses are the result of brain failure. The phrase "brain failure" can be used like "heart failure" or "kidney failure" to mean that a bodily organ is not able to do its job. This incapacity may have many causes, some of which are treatable and reversible and some of which are not. Analogies are never ideal, but a comparison of brain failure to the breakdown of an automobile or any complex piece of machinery may be instructive. A car will not run well or will not run at all if the clutch is worn, the oil has leaked out, the fuel tank is empty, the carburetor is not adjusted properly, the electrical system is faulty, or any number of different parts fail.

The machinery of the human brain is exquisitely complex—certainly more complex than an automobile. When something is wrong, it affects not only the mind but also much of what the body does. The ability to walk, talk, eat, sleep, and make love may be disrupted by failure of the brain to function properly. The expression of emotions like anger, jealousy, happiness, and fear is often disturbed when a disease of the brain exists. Emotional control may be affected seriously, and strong feelings will be expressed for no apparent reasons, or the intensity may be totally out of proportion to the cause. Rage, anger, foul and abusive language, and even violent threats emerge where mild annoyance might once have been expressed. Emotions may shift quickly from one extreme to another for little apparent reason. Laughter or giggling will follow on the heels of crying or anger. Any or all of these may occur in association with a dementing illness.

Dementia evolves slowly but relentlessly. The changes may seem subtle until one day odd or atypical behaviors become distressing enough to upset or unsettle the family. An engineer or bookkeeper has serious trouble adding numbers at work. Grandmother asks to go out to lunch with Aunt Bessie, who has been dead for two years. A master's-level bridge player loses the ability to play no-trump. Individuals forget how to organize and complete work assignments or household chores, or have difficulty with shopping and dressing.

The skills individuals need to drive a car may be affected in the early stages. People with early Alzheimer's disease are distracted more easily by other vehicles and the scenery. They may forget where they are going or how to get somewhere, and as a result they may behave erratically behind the wheel. An excellent driver takes the wrong freeway exit five times before finding the way home. Sudden turns, driving in circles, traffic violations, and other problems related to the individual's confusion create dangerous situations and often lead to accidents. A gentleman left home one afternoon to drive to the neighborhood grocery, and he was found the next day in another state, confused as to how or why he went there.

The inability to adjust to new situations is a problem for many individuals, even early in the disease. Problems may become apparent on a vacation or immediately after a move into a different house or apartment. Travel may result in major family crises when the patient is unable to remember enough to orient himself or herself in a hotel or a new city. While on a vacation in Hawaii, a wife found her husband urinating in their hotel room closet. These startling and often heartbreaking examples are varied and numerous.

How to Judge When Cognitive Losses Are Serious

In many cases the initial changes in mental ability are more subtle and difficult to pin down. Then how does one know when forgetfulness or lapses in judgment become serious enough to require professional attention? The answer is that there is simply no clear line marking the boundary between normal and abnormal mental ability. The border is a zone rather than a line, and careful assessment is necessary to decide whether a problem exists. However, it is helpful to highlight several indications that should signal to the individual and the family a reason for concern.

1. Changes in mental ability that are unusual for a particular individual are worthy of attention. Some people who pride themselves on their memory for facts, names, faces, and places will get lost in the neighborhood or fail to recognize close friends or relatives. They may even refer to or ask to visit someone who is dead. The loss of an ability in an area of previous strength, as in the case of a bookkeeper who begins to make numerous mistakes in calculations, a mechanic who forgets the parts of an engine, or teachers and scholars who are unable to find the words to express themselves, is an important danger signal.
2. The mental changes persist. Although some days may be better than others, there is no improvement over weeks or months. It is human to have days when we feel sharp and on top of everything, as well as days when we feel less alert. Occasionally our words slip out inappropriately or we mispronounce common phrases. When word-finding problems, unusual behaviors, memory lapses, or other language disturbances continue over time, the index of suspicion should rise.
3. The decline is *progressive*. There may be good and bad days, but things are clearly getting worse with the passage of time. The lapses appear to be getting more severe and occur more often. It is the gradual na-

ture of the changes that usually delays judgment about the seriousness of the problem, since day-to-day differences may seem subtle. Over time, however, the magnitude of the losses becomes evident.

4. The changes disrupt the routine of life. They affect job performance, marital communication, sexual relations, and family and social life— indeed almost all facets of existence. Individuals may withdraw from friends and activities, not communicate, not answer questions, or not initiate conversations. Mannerisms may change, such as in the long-winded loquacious talker who begins to use short, terse words and phrases.

5. Unfamiliar or bizarre changes in emotional expression occur. Calm people may become irritable, excitable, edgy, or jumpy. Profanity erupts from people who seldom used foul language in the past. Angry and aggressive outbursts or sadness and crying are observed in individuals who rarely express emotions in public. Emotional outbursts are a particularly suspicious sign when they appear and fade rapidly for little or no obvious reason.

The presence of *any* of these signs is important enough to be taken seriously, and it should lead one to seek qualified professional help. Before going through a full diagnostic examination, the person who has suspicious problems may be given one of several brief screening tests of memory and other mental skills. The score on these tests will help determine the need for a full examination.

How Dementia Is Diagnosed

There are no medical laboratory tests that can positively diagnose Alzheimer's disease with complete certainty during the life of the individual, but there are clinical examinations and diagnostic criteria that make it possible for experienced clinicians to diagnose Alzheimer's disease with better than 90 percent accuracy. Physicians who do not specialize in geriatrics have a higher rate of diagnostic errors, so finding a capable doctor is critical.

The definitive diagnosis of Alzheimer's disease is based on an examination of brain tissue, almost always postmortem. Brain biopsies are occasionally done to obtain tissue samples, but they are not performed solely to confirm a diagnosis of Alzheimer's disease. Furthermore, the analysis of brain biopsy material does not always verify the diagnosis. The brain changes that characterize Alzheimer's disease do not occur uniformly throughout the brain. Thus, healthy specimens may be taken from the brain, and areas where neuronal destruction has occurred may be missed. The brain can be examined directly, but this is done only when there is another medical indication, such as a brain tumor or abscess. In practical terms, the definite diagnosis of Alzheimer's disease is established after the patient has died and a careful postmortem study of several areas of the brain has been performed.

At the time of the diagnosis, a series of medical and psychiatric evaluations must be undertaken to determine what type of dementia is present, whether it is treatable and therefore reversible, whether it has a cause that is not reversible, and if so, what the most probable condition is. The conclusion the physician reaches is known as a *clinical diagnosis.* On the basis of what is already known about others with the same or similar symptoms and of the clinical findings for the patient, the physician makes predictions about the reversibility of the disorder and the types of treatment needed.

A great deal rests on the clinical diagnosis, which should be determined as carefully as possible. Among individuals who are examined by a physician because of complaints of memory problems, there are many who have a condition that can be treated. If no reversible causes of dementia can be found (and these will be reviewed shortly), the diagnosing physician must decide which one of the nonreversible dementias is present.

Differential diagnosis is the process of making a clinical diagnosis by deciding which of a group of possible causes is most likely to be responsible for the patient's signs and symptoms. Laboratory tests are performed to determine which causes can be eliminated or found to exist. Ideally, clinicians from several disciplines should examine the individual. The differential diagnosis of Alzheimer's disease involves the knowledge of the characteristic features of the disease, conditions that may exacerbate the disease, and conditions that masquerade as features of the clinical pathological picture.

Research advances over the past fifteen years have improved physicians' accuracy in making a clinical diagnosis, replacing the old notion that the clinical diagnosis of Alzheimer's disease was rendered when they could not find any other basis for an individual's symptoms. It is no longer a diagnosis of exclusion—increasingly physicians are able to identify features that strengthen their clinical judgment. The two most commonly used sets of criteria to diagnose the disease are those from the American Psychiatric Association's *Diagnostic and Statistical Manual of Mental Disorders*, fourth revision (DSM-IV), and those established by a scientific task force of the National Institute of Neurological and Communicative Disorders and Stroke and the Alzheimer's Association (NINCDS/AA).

The examinations and laboratory tests involved in making the diagnosis of Alzheimer's disease and related dementias should include the following:

1. A complete *physical examination* is performed to identify all possible health conditions, including poor nutrition. Many physical diseases can cause disorientation, difficulty with concentration, confusion, and the memory problems associated with dementia, and these should be identified and treated.

2. *Laboratory tests* are done routinely in conjunction with the physical examination. They provide additional information to help the physician assess the state of health or disease. Blood and urine samples are needed to analyze the body's chemistry. The results reveal information about how well the various organs and glands of the body are functioning and about the presence of infections, vitamin deficiencies, lead poisoning, syphilis, and human immunodeficiency virus (HIV) infection. An electrocardiogram and X rays will also be taken as a general rule. A spinal tap may be done to obtain a sample of the cerebrospinal fluid, which bathes and supports the spinal cord and the brain. Examination of the sample can diagnose meningitis and encephalitis. If abnormalities are found in routine tests, special diagnostic tests may follow. If the physician recommends such special procedures, ask for an explanation about their value.

3. *Personal and family medical histories* are necessary for a good evaluation. The thorough physician will want to be familiar with an individual's previous illnesses, hospitalizations, and operations and will ask questions about a wide range of possible symptoms. The medical history of the family can provide extremely valuable information. The pres-

ence of dementia in other family members is an important part of the history, but it is not necessarily predictive of the identified patient having the diagnosis. Inquiries about previous work or even hobbies can help indicate whether an individual has been exposed to trauma, dangerous chemicals, or toxins that may have caused brain damage. Information about exercise and eating habits, use of caffeine, and fluid intake is also important.

4. *An accurate history of current and recent use of medications and alcohol or drugs* is essential for the physician to determine whether the individual is suffering from the effects of drug use or misuse. Older patients often take many different drugs. Too much medication, the wrong combination of drugs, or the side effects of a drug can cause dementia. It is important for the patient and family members to inform the physician about all medications. This includes drugs purchased over the counter at a pharmacy or store as well as prescription drugs.

5. *A neurological examination* is important to determine whether there is a specific disease in any part of the nervous system. The neurologist may repeat some questions about the medical history and even perform a short physical examination again. A routine neurological examination includes tests of mental status and alertness as well as assessments of muscle strength, reflexes, and the ability to feel such different sensations as a pinprick, vibration, or heat or cold in different parts of the body. The neurologist also pays special attention to the senses of smell, hearing, and vision and use of the muscles in the mouth and tongue. Language skills, posture, walking ability, and muscle coordination likewise are examined.

Neurological tests are fairly simple to perform, and any abnormalities found can help locate lesions in specific areas of the nervous system. This information is extremely useful for the diagnosis of brain disorders other than Alzheimer's disease. With the exception of an indication of cognitive impairment on the mental status test, the results of the neurological exam usually are normal in the early stages of Alzheimer's disease. Abnormal reflexes appear as the dementia progresses, indicating an increasing degree of brain involvement. A number of dementias such as those associated with Parkinson's disease and the recently described syndrome called frontotemporal dementia can be confused with Alzheimer's disease. However, the physician can make the differential diagnosis based on the results of careful neurological and psychiatric examinations.

6. A comprehensive *psychiatric examination* complements the neurological evaluation. The psychiatric interview is a carefully organized set of questions to determine not only whether the individual is suffering from a significant mental disorder but also what the nature of the disorder is. The answers are used to evaluate a wide range of thoughts and feelings as well as to weigh the effect of major life changes such as the death of a family member or friend, financial problems, or family conflict.

   A careful psychiatric interview with appropriate psychological testing can identify the type and severity of the mental disability as well as the presence of personality disorders, depression, anxiety, or other problems that can cause dementia or make it worse if the dementia is caused by other disorders. An examination of the patient's language skills, ability to control impulses, mood, and behavior, as well as the nature of memory and other cognitive deficits plays a critical role in establishing the diagnosis.

   Depression in late life can be confused with dementia. It may co-exist with dementia, particularly in early stages, or it may be a risk factor for future dementia. Research suggests that perhaps 30 percent of persons who have a first episode of clinical depression in later life are at risk to develop Alzheimer's disease.

7. *Psychological testing* is an important part of the diagnostic examination. A complete battery of psychological tests usually takes several hours. However, the information obtained can be used to document intellectual strengths and losses. After the diagnosis is made, the results of testing also provide essential information for developing a treatment plan, as well as advising the patient and family about the range of activities that are safe and manageable for the forseeable future. The results also establish a baseline for evaluating the effect of any treatment.

8. A systematic *functional assessment* provides critical information about what an affected person can and cannot do. Serious memory losses have a negative impact on daily activities. There are two general domains of functional assessment: activities of daily living (ADLs) and instrumental activities of daily living (IADLs). ADLs are personal care

functions necessary for independent living, such as eating, dressing, walking, toileting, bathing, and transferring, as from the bed to a chair. IADLs are more complex daily activities such as managing money, using the telephone, housekeeping, and taking drugs.

9. *Special diagnostic laboratory evaluations* are used to reach an accurate clinical diagnosis. The electroencephalogram (EEG) is a record of the brain's electrical activity, which is picked up by wires pasted on the scalp, amplified, and recorded on a machine. The EEG usually can provide a good index of the general state of the brain's activity. Abnormal electrical activity may be seen on the EEG if there is a brain tumor or seizure activity or if a stroke has occurred. The EEG cannot be used to specifically diagnose Alzheimer's disease but it helps to determine whether other diseases of the brain such as Creutzfeld-Jakob disease are present. In Alzheimer's disease there may be evidence on the EEG for what is called "diffuse slowing." The recordings of the brain's electrical activity show the presence of lower frequencies and slow electrical waves.

10. *Brain imaging* is another part of the diagnostic process. Computerized tomography (CT) studies are often a part of the dementia workup. The term *computerized axial tomography* (CAT) is also used. Thus, *CAT scans* and *CT scans* are equivalent terms. The CT machine is a special type of X-ray apparatus. It sends a series of X rays through the brain, and a computer analyzes them to create an image of the structures inside the brain. A CT scan is different from routine X rays, which distinguish denser bone tissue from soft tissue.

Magnetic resonance imaging (MRI) is a more sensitive technique to examine the brain. With the use of strong magnets and the injection of specialized fluids into the body, MRI shows the activity of the nerve cells in different parts of the brain. It also shows patterns of blood circulation. Thus, the presence of areas of poor circulation or vascular lesions can be detected as well as any loss of brain tissue in various regions.

The MRI results seen in severe Alzheimer's disease show that the *hippocampus*, a major center for memory, attention, and learning in the brain, has shrunk considerably from cell death. The images also show that there is almost no neuronal activity in a section of the hippocampus known as the *entorhinal cortex*. However, in people with mild memory losses associated with older age, the entorhinal cortex is active, but another region of the hippocampus, the subiculum, is affected. The entorhinal cortex is the first area of the hippocampus to be affected in Alzheimer's disease.

Imaging can be a valuable diagnostic tool. Some dementias such as Lewy body disease and frontal lobe dementias appear *clinically* similar to Alzheimer's disease, but they have different imaging characteristics. Lewy body dementia may occur in Parkinson's disease patients, but it may account for many as 25 percent of patients with dementia. Frontal lobe syndromes such as Pick's disease are associated with specific changes in the frontal areas of the brain, and a different pattern of behavior, psychiatric symptoms, and dementia emerges. Pick's disease is a less frequent form of dementia, often confused with Alzheimer's.

Imaging studies are useful to identify abnormal structural changes. Specific pathology like brain tumors or damage due to small strokes can be visualized. Several images taken over time can show brain changes that indicate Alzheimer's disease. If enough brain cells are lost, the amount of brain tissue shrinks and the size of the ventricles in the brain increases. The ventricles are the spaces inside the brain filled with cerebrospinal fluid.

Enlarged ventricles and decreased brain size alone are not diagnostic of Alzheimer's disease because they also are seen in the course of normal aging. However, when serial images show progressively larger ventricles, when cognitive losses are worsening, and when all testable causes of dementia have been eliminated, Alzheimer's disease is probably the correct diagnosis.

11. *New technologies to image the brain* are being used to diagnose dementia. The two described here are positron emission tomography (PET) and single-photon emission computerized tomography (SPECT). Although they are not used routinely to diagnose dementias, they are being employed experimentally to learn more about what happens to the brain in Alzheimer's disease. Perhaps someday brain disorders will be detectable much earlier.

PET is a diagnostic research technology based on nuclear physics and computer science. It provides a picture of the brain that shows how it metabolizes or burns up its source of energy, a sugar called glucose. One way to conceptualize the image derived from PET is to think about the pictures we get from infrared cameras. Supersensitive to heat rather than to light, they enable us to "see in the dark."

During a PET study, the individual lies on a padded table. His or her head is inserted into the doughnut-like hole of a large machine. Doctors then inject into the individual's arm radioactive glucose, which makes its way into the brain. The most active parts of the brain consume greater amounts of glucose, and therefore the concentration of radioactivity is greatest in these areas. Inside the machine are many detectors that absorb the radiation and carry signals to a computer. The computer gathers messages from all of the detectors and creates an image of activity in the brain. Bright spots show exactly where the radioactive glucose has accumulated.

PET is an experimental procedure. The experimental results to date reveal a significant reduction in sugar metabolism in different regions of the brain of patients with Alzheimer's disease. People in early stages show very decreased glucose metabolism in a part of the brain known as the *posterior temporoparietal region*. However, people with atherosclerosis of the brain show a similar pattern of glucose metabolic changes, so the diagnostic value awaits further research.

Someday PET may be a valued clinical diagnostic tool. At the moment it is an expensive experimental procedure. If PET research leads to diagnostic breakthroughs and becomes more available and affordable, it may revolutionize the diagnosis of Alzheimer's disease in the long run.

SPECT analyzes the brain's blood glucose flow and metabolism. SPECT results are not as precise as the results from PET, but the procedure is less expensive.

During the series of careful examinations needed to obtain an accurate diagnosis of Alzheimer's disease or a related disorder, it is important to ask questions about any tests the physician wants to conduct. The entire set of evaluations may cost $1,000 or more if done on an outpatient basis. Are all the tests necessary? The answer is usually yes. Up to 30 or 35 percent of all individuals who show symptoms of dementia have a condition that can be treated and is therefore potentially reversible. In many instances, prompt diagnosis and appropriate treatment will reverse the dementia entirely. Delay or failure to conduct a crucial test increases the chance that the patient may not fully recover from some reversible problem.

Helena Swanson argued with her children for six months before she and her husband, Oscar, visited a geriatric psychiatrist. She was embarrassed about his condition; furthermore, she did not see how a "shrink" could help. Oscar had already been diagnosed as having dementia for about eight months and had been growing increasingly despondent and withdrawn. After the examination, Oscar began a combined drug-psychotherapy program, and within six months not only had his depression cleared but his cognitive functioning improved dramatically as well. It soon became obvious that Oscar did not have Alzheimer's disease. His internist and neurologist had missed the depressive illness entirely. Obviously, not all visits to the psychiatrist yield dramatic results. However, depression is a frequent and unrecognized cause of memory problems.

Under the present regulations, not all diagnostic costs are reimbursed by Medicare. Perhaps 60 to 80 percent of the expenses are reimbursable if the examination is done on an outpatient basis. Almost all costs are reimbursed if patients are hospitalized for the diagnosis. In most cases, however, it is better to evaluate patients out of the hospital. For patients who are already mildly impaired, the hospital stay itself can be stressful, causing them to become more confused and disoriented. Hospitalization is usually necessary only for patients who, in addition to having memory loss, are very frail and sick and for patients who are abusive and difficult to deal with at home. Some managed health care organizations are reluctant to refer individuals to specialists for the diagnosis of dementia. It is important for family members to be firm and aggressive about the need for a comprehensive diagnostic examination.

Reversible Causes of Dementia

Since an accurate diagnosis is so important to the future life of the patient, great care must be exercised during the initial evaluation. Awareness of some of the common causes of dementia that are treatable, if discovered, can contribute toward this goal.

Infections

Infectious disorders are frequent causes of dementia. A major illness accompanied by a fever, regardless of the cause, can precipitate problems in memory and thinking in persons of any age. Infectious diseases change the body's metabolism, cause pain, and often affect the way people behave. Older individuals with even modest infections can become confused and lethargic, eat sparingly, and find little pleasure in social activities. As a result of the withdrawal, they may ignore requests to do many things, refuse to answer questions, and generally communicate less effectively. This behavior gives the false appearance of progressive dementia when in reality the difficulties are a result of the infection.

A special note about fevers in older persons is worthy of mention. Some older persons show little rise in temperature, even when they have a serious infection. Special attention should be paid to other symptoms such as headaches, loss of appetite, unusual lethargy, and pain.

Metabolic and Nutritional Disorders

A number of physical disorders are the result of disturbances in the body's metabolism. Many of these diseases are capable of causing intellectual problems as well as physical symptoms. The cells and tissues of the body contain many substances, and innumerable chemical reactions must occur between them to sustain life. *Metabolism* refers to the chemical reactions by which the materials necessary for life are synthesized, utilized by the body, and broken down as waste products or for reuse. Many factors such as a shortage of needed enzymes and minerals, dehydration, and poor diet can disrupt metabolism. An individual with thyroid problems may feel run-down, have difficulty concentrating, and become forgetful. A disturbance in the body's electrolytes, such as sodium and potassium, can result from dehydration or too much fluid consumption, kidney problems, or the use of drugs like diuretics. Too much sodium or potassium, as well as too little, can cause a change in mental state.

Uncontrolled diabetes also can lead to behavioral disturbances and mimic dementia. Levels of glucose and insulin can fluctuate as a result of changes in diet, in exercise patterns, or in body weight. While this may seem obvious, subtle changes in exercise and nutrition occur in older people over time. Often neither the family doctor nor the individual will stop to consider the effect of these changes. For example, the diabetic patient who retires, travels, or changes lifestyle and physical activity will need to adjust his or her nutrition and insulin use.

Malnutrition over time can lead to significant metabolic changes that are often first observed as memory loss or other cognitive problems. It is important to find out what the older person is actually consuming rather than to accept what is reported. Vitamin deficiencies are common in older persons. It is estimated that at least 10 percent of all persons over the age of sixty-five are deficient in thiamine, riboflavin, ascorbic acid (vitamin C), and vitamin A.

The diet of older persons may vary as a function of economic circumstances or social isolation, or because of problems with their teeth or mouth. Many older people have difficulty purchasing or preparing food because of poor access to transportation, limited mobility, or physical frailty. Eating is also a social activity. The same meals eaten night after night following the loss of a spouse or the death of close friends are lonely occasions. It is difficult and simply less enjoyable to prepare balanced meals for one person, and eating habits generally deteriorate. A significant change in eating habits is also an important sign of depression.

Cardiovascular and Pulmonary Diseases

Diseases of the heart and lungs also can contribute to cognitive losses, depression, and other behavioral changes. The cardiovascular system acts as a slave to the other organs of the body. It not only delivers nutrients and other substances in the blood to all parts of the body but also circulates blood cells and helps maintain a constant temperature in the body as well. A decrease in the working performance of the heart and blood vessels or impaired oxygen exchange in the lungs can affect the amount of oxygen and other nutrients that reach the brain.

Many vascular problems like high blood pressure, arrhythmias, severe heart disease, and arteriosclerosis in the blood vessels of the brain affect memory and learning. Although it is clear that not everyone with cardiovascular disease has intellectual deficits, the potential vascular basis for a change in mental status deserves a careful evaluation. Some of these conditions can be treated successfully, thereby partially or completely reversing the cognitive changes.

Medications

Drug-related problems are probably the most common cause of cognitive impairment. If they are identified early and corrected, the disturbances usually can be corrected. What are some of the drugs that frequently have serious side effects? Diuretics used in the treatment of high blood pressure can cause an electrolyte imbalance and subsequent cognitive difficulties. Long-term use of certain medications like digitalis as well as hormones such as thyroid and insulin can lead to problems in later life because they have side effects that cause losses in cognitive abilities in some persons.

It is not unusual for older people to be taking more than one drug. Estimates are that persons over sixty-five living in the community are taking an average of five drugs each day and that those in nursing homes may take more than ten. Drug combinations can be dangerous because many drugs interact with each other, causing a wide range of physical problems as well as sedation, agitation, drowsiness, or memory loss.

The time invested to understand drug and alcohol use will pay off. What drugs is the individual taking? How old are they? Where did they come from—the doctor, the drugstore, the grocery store, or a neighbor? Are they being taken at the proper intervals? With or without food? Are they dangerous when used with alcohol? How many doctors does the patient have? Does each physician know what the other is doing or prescribing? Is the dosage too high or too low? Are the drugs really necessary?

As we will review in Chapter 5, changes in the nervous system that occur with age affect drug actions. Older persons are generally more sensitive to drugs. Smaller doses, perhaps 20 to 50 percent of the doses used for a young adult, are generally recommended. Large doses may actually cause a full-blown, dementia-like syndrome.

Structural Damage in the Brain

The brain is surrounded by several membranes and encased in the skull for protection. Although well protected, it can be damaged by changes inside the skull as well as by external events such as a blow to the head, an automobile accident, a fall, and other types of trauma. A thorough psychiatric and neurological examination, including a CT scan, should determine whether structural damage is causing the dementia observed in a patient.

Brain tumors and subdural hematomas are two common causes of structural damage. Brain tumors may not be detected for a long time, and the first sign of one in older persons—or in younger persons, for that matter—may be subtle cognitive losses and changes in emotions or behavior. A subdural hematoma is a blood clot underneath one of the membranes surrounding the brain, called the *dura mater*. The clot causes increasing pressure inside the bony structure of the head, and this affects the brain itself. Subdural hematomas can be caused by a blow to the head resulting from a fall or by anything else that ruptures blood vessels. A CT scan shows a subdural hematoma and should be done, since patients may have forgotten about the fall and family members may not have observed it.

Hydrocephalus is the name of an important structural disorder that deserves special discussion. It is not a common problem. However, it has received a great deal of attention because it is sometimes reversible. There are two major forms of hydrocephalus—primary and secondary. In the condition called *secondary hydrocephalus*, the pressure of the cerebrospinal fluid within the ventricles of the brain is increased. Cerebrospinal fluid is produced in the brain and circulates throughout the tissues of the brain and the spinal cord. A number of conditions inside the skull cavity, such as a brain hemorrhage (bleeding), head trauma, or meningitis (an infection), can block the natural flow of the cerebrospinal fluid and thereby increase the pressure. The pressure sometimes can be relieved by a procedure called *shunting*. This is a neurosurgical operation in which a tube is placed in the brain to allow the fluid to drain into other areas of the body such as the gut, where it may be absorbed without harm.

Primary hydrocephalus, also called *normal-pressure hydrocephalus*, is difficult to diagnose, and its cause is unknown. (The use of the word *primary* before the name of any disease indicates that its cause is unknown.) The spinal fluid pressure appears normal, but the CT scan shows that the ventricles on both sides of the brain are very wide. Patients with primary hydrocephalus also usually show three very specific symptoms. First, they walk with difficulty, appearing to have forgotten how to do so and exerting great effort to move their arms, legs, and feet. Second, they are incontinent. Third, they give evidence of intellectual deterioration. When a patient shows these three signs at the beginning of an illness, a careful neurological workup is necessary before a decision about placing a shunt is made. Normal-pressure hydrocephalus is rare, with only about 5,000 cases reported each year in the United States. Although it is almost never seen in persons over age sixty-five, it occurs in 5 to 6 percent of those under age sixty-five who have dementia.

Neurosurgery to transfer cerebrospinal fluid from the brain area into a body cavity, such as the gut, is effective in about 65 percent of patients with secondary hydrocephalus. Only 40 percent of patients with primary, normal-pressure hydrocephalus show some improvement. However, the mortality rate associated with this procedure ranges between 6 and 10 percent. Furthermore, surgical complications and infections reportedly occur in more than 40 percent of patients. In these instances, another operation must be done and a new shunt inserted.

The use of shunting as an "exploratory diagnostic procedure" in the patient with a clinical diagnosis of Alzheimer's disease is not justified. The neurosurgical procedure is not without substantial risk, and the patient becomes vulnerable to a variety of complications associated with the operation. These, in turn, often make the patient's mental condition worse, and the emotional toll on the family can be profound. Thus, the risk-benefit ratio of the procedure should be considered very carefully.

Visual and Hearing Losses

Impaired sight and hearing have a significant impact on the ability of individuals to understand questions posed by an examiner. Older persons with sensory impairments, especially the very old and frail, can appear to be unable to answer questions. It is unfortunate that many people, including physicians, underestimate the importance of sensory handicaps and assume the existence of a major memory problem. Hearing losses, which are often subtle and difficult to detect, significantly reduce the ability to communicate effectively. Older persons with known hearing loss may not use their hearing aids or replace the batteries, circumstances family members and health care professionals should consider during the hearing examination.

Depression

It is well known that emotional disorders can impair thinking. Often it is a diagnostic challenge for the physician to determine whether severely depressed or anxious people have an irreversible brain disease or a severe but reversible emotional condition. Many depressed individuals are apathetic and often do not respond to what goes on around them. Others appear very restless and agitated. In most cases memory is affected, and most ADLs are performed with greater difficulty. The longer these con ditions persist, the harder they are to treat.

Depression is not the same as sadness. Depressed persons are usually sad, but their problem goes far beyond the sadness all of us experience in our lifetime. Clinical depression affects thinking, memory, sleep, and appetite and interferes with daily life. The term *depression* can be confusing because it is used to describe many different, albeit similar, conditions. The word can refer to a normal mood in the lives of healthy people. This mood is characterized by feelings of sadness, usually over a loss or in response to some memory. The clinical term *reactive depression* is used to describe a sudden shift in mood that is moderately incapacitating and lasts for a few weeks as a result of some crisis, usually a severe loss. The death of a close relative or friend, the loss of a job, the occurrence of a physical disorder, or any of a wide range of life changes can trigger a reactive depression. This is a normal response to such changes, but if the mood does not lift in a few weeks, then the onset of a more persistent depression should be of concern.

The word *depression* also applies to a major class of psychiatric disorders characterized mainly by sadness but also by many other symptoms. In some individuals with clinical depression, sadness is not even reported; the patient may just feel "empty." Appetite usually changes, resulting in significant weight loss or weight gain. Sleep is disrupted; affected persons may wake up early in the morning and sleep fewer hours, or alternatively, they may lie in bed and sleep too much. Loss of interest in pleasurable activities is another characteristic of clinical depression. Irritability and restlessness or the opposite—decreased energy and fatigue—

may be present. In addition, physical problems like pain, personal expressions of worthlessness or guilt, difficulty in thinking, a sense of hopelessness, helplessness, and worthlessness, and thoughts of death or of suicide are also frequently associated with clinical depression.

Depression is not always obvious to the observer. Among the aged it is perhaps the most unrecognized and underdiagnosed psychiatric disturbance. Older persons often complain about physical problems but say little about their feelings. Thus, when no medical reason can be found for a complaint and the person is not a hypochondriac, the possibility of depression should at least be considered. Physical diseases, personal losses, and the use of alcohol or a number of drugs can produce some depressive symptoms, making the diagnosis difficult even for the doctor.

Older depressed persons may not report feeling sadness but rather say that they feel empty and have the "blahs." Some older persons may deny being sad, but they cannot identify anything that gives them joy or pleasure. It is also common for depressed older persons to say that they just don't feel good, but they cannot be specific about where the pain or discomfort exists.

Isolation and Sensory Deprivation

Social isolation and sensory deprivation are also major causes of dementia-like behavior. Being with other people—talking, shopping, working, and otherwise interacting socially with them—creates a sense of well-being and fulfillment. A deprivation of human touch, activity, and excitement is experienced by many older persons who live alone or are homebound or institutionalized. The lack of meaningful human interactions and warmth has a potent effect. The human spirit withers. The mind may become dull or forgetful or confused.

This effect should not be surprising. Little has been written about the impact of the loneliness of old age, when family, friends, and companions are absent or the intimate circle is constricted. There are, however, situations to which all of us can relate. A long bout of illness that confines us to bed for days or perhaps weeks keeps us from our routine and severs most relationships with the outside world. When we recover and resume daily life, our body and mind may feel sluggish, awkward, and clumsy. Interactions with other people may seem strange and disconnected. Thoughts and words do not come easily. However, these experiences are transient; as we feel better and get back into the swing of things, our behavior becomes normal again.

Life apart from other people may create a major problem after enough time has passed. Just as a mirror shows us how we look, other people reflect whether our behavior is appropriate, acceptable, and desirable. Without rewarding relationships, our behavioral field is restricted and our behavior changes. The initial withdrawal may be subtle, but eventually it leads to confused and disoriented behavior. An extensive body of literature on sensory deprivation documents what isolation can do to human thought and behavior. Hearing problems, family moves or a recent move to another residence, loss of friends and not making new friends, all are factors that can contribute to social isolation.

Diagnosis Takes Time

As should be apparent, a good diagnostic evaluation for intellectual deterioration takes time. Indeed, several months may pass, and the doctor may repeat a number of tests before he or she is in a position to confirm a diagnosis. The symptoms may be baffling. If the doctor suspects medical disorders, drugs, or depression as the probable cause of the dementia, he or she will require some time to observe whether deficits improve with treatment. It is also possible that patients with Alzheimer's disease have coexisting reversible physical disorders that make the dementia much worse and prompt a trip to the doctor in the first place. In such instances, a partial reversal of dementia may occur as the secondary cause is eliminated, and there is unwarranted optimism that everything is under control.

Even though an individual and a family may be concerned enough to request professional help, the results of the examinations may be inconclusive. The mental-status testing may show only the mildest of deficits. Repeated examinations several months in the future may be necessary before the physician can ascertain whether the deficits are becoming worse. Remember, Alzheimer's disease is characterized by gradual, progressive, and hidden changes. A diagnosis of Alzheimer's disease should be rendered with the greatest of care. If the physician tells you he or she is unsure, wants the patient to return in the future, and provides assurance that he or she will be available if something happens before the next appointment, you are probably in good hands. A premature and incorrect diagnosis can have unfortunate and often irreversible psychological effects.

Mild Cognitive Impairment

Long-term studies of people with mild memory problems have identified what appears to be a prodromal stage of Alzheimer's disease. This new diagnostic group is called *mild cognitive impairment*, or MCI, where individuals have mild memory problems and word-naming difficulties. MCI is a borderland of mild but persistent memory losses that are greater than expected for a persons' age and education, but other clinical signs of dementia are not present. If an individual continues to forget important information that he or she wants and tries to remember, this may indicate a dementia process.

A diagnosis of MCI can be made if the individual meets the following criteria: the individual complains of memory problems; memory loss is abnormal for the person's age; ADLs are not affected; other cognitive abilities are intact; and there is no dementia.

About 40 percent of individuals given a diagnosis of MCI show progressive cognitive impairment and are diagnosed with Alzheimer's disease within three years. This is significantly higher than the 3 percent of healthy persons age sixty-five and older who develop Alzheimer's disease in a three-year period. As research continues, we should learn more about the predictors of MCI. This has important implications for drug treatment and hopefully prevention. Because people with MCI have a greater chance of developing Alzheimer's than do those without memory problems, they would be an ideal population to test the benefits of an Alzheimer's disease vaccine.

Nonreversible Causes of Dementia

When reversible causes of dementia have been ruled out, the differential diagnosis between Alzheimer's disease, cerebrovascular diseases, and other brain diseases with dementia may be easy or quite difficult. Although Alzheimer's disease is the most common irreversible dementia, cerebrovascular dementias rank as the second most common. Cerebrovascular diseases, conditions that result from problems involving the circulation of blood to the brain, are discussed in some detail in Chapter 14.

Small strokes may occur in as many as 15 to 20 percent of all persons with nonreversible dementias, and it is these strokes, and the resulting reduction in the flow of blood to parts of the brain, that lead to loss of memory. Since this condition involves many small strokes, it is sometimes called *multi-infarct dementia*. *Infarct* is the technical term for an area of cell death resulting from the blockage of circulation.

Although individuals with multi-infarct dementia, now termed *vascular dementia*, may seem very much like Alzheimer's patients to the family, there are subtle but important differences. The most conspicuous distinguishing features of vascular dementias, in contrast to Alzheimer's, are its relatively abrupt onset, the patchy quality of the cognitive deficits, and a stepwise progression, with losses often followed by partial recovery. Furthermore, since vascular dementia patients have circulatory problems rather than an unknown disease of the nervous system itself, there are medical approaches that may help to slow the progress of the condition.

Parkinson's disease, like Alzheimer's disease, is becoming more frequent as the population ages. Dementia and depression often accompany Parkinson's disease, and it is estimated that 30 to 60 percent of all Parkinson's patients have one or both of these associated conditions. The dementia is usually slow and progressive, with not only memory losses but also motor slowing and poor impulse control. The medications used to reduce the physical symptoms of Parkinson's can create severe psychiatric problems in some patients.

Frontal lobe dementias are now a subject of much interest as we learn more about Alzheimer's disease. Perhaps 5 to 25 percent of patients with irreversible dementias may have a frontal lobe dementia characterized by early severe language problems, spatial disorientation, and no insight into their behavior, as well as problems with self-control. Frontal lobe dementias have a genetic component. At least one study reported that 30 to 50 percent of patients have a close relative with the disease.

Pick's disease is one form of frontal lobe dementia, but it is very rare. The brains of people with Pick's disease have special lesions called *Pick's bodies*. The brain's cortex shrinks, especially in the frontal lobes, which is different from what happens with Alzheimer's disease. Pick's disease usually has an age of onset between forty and sixty years. The dementia progresses slowly, but the symptoms are different from those of Alzheimer's disease over the course of illness. Personality changes and inappropriate behaviors are more prominent in the early stages of Pick's than are memory losses, and the patient deteriorates into a profound dementia.

Another disorder is known as *diffuse Lewy body disease.* In Parkinson's disease these Lewy bodies develop in one part of the brain. In diffuse Lewy body disease, they appear throughout the brain, causing what is also known as the *Lewy body variant of Alzheimer's disease.* Lewy body dementia is characterized by great fluctuations in cognitive ability, bouts of parkinsonism, and visual hallucinations (i.e., seeing things that are not really there). Although relatively recently accepted as a separate entity, it is now believed to account for 7 to 28 percent of dementia cases.

Creutzfeldt-Jakob disease is another rare dementia with rapid onset and rapid progression. More than 50 percent of people with this disease die within six months, and very few live two years. Creutzfeldt-Jakob disease is associated with a virus-like agent called a *prion*—a protein with infection-like properties. The virus is harbored in the brain of affected animals such as sheep and cattle. It has become the subject of worldwide concern, with the occurrence of mad cow disease mostly in Great Britain. First reported in 1986, mad cow disease was traced to cattle feed that contained sheep meat infected with scrapie, a disease in sheep similar to Creutzfeldt-Jakob disease. To date, about sixty persons have died, most in Great Britain.

Creutzfeldt-Jakob disease progresses much more rapidly than most forms of Alzheimer's disease, with an average survival time of seven months from the onset of symptoms. Common features include myoclonus, which is muscular jerking and twitching of the arms, legs, and body; visual symptoms; ataxia or walking problems; dysarthria; and psychiatric symptoms. Until recently, the diagnosis was based on clinical symptoms and EEG findings as well as autopsy results. Attempts to treat Creutzfeldt-Jacob disease have been rare because the disease progresses so rapidly and it is so difficult to diagnose in the early stages. Recently, a protein in the cerebrospinal fluid called 14-3-3 has been identified as a diagnostic marker for the disease. Hopefully, this should help with early detection as well as research focused on treatment and prevention.

Other forms of dementia may be associated with brain tumors, lead poisoning, head trauma, nutritional deficiencies, HIV (acquired immunodeficiency syndrome, or AIDS) or other infectious agents, substance abuse including alcohol, postsurgical complications, indoor air pollutants, and a host of medically related problems.

How to Find a Good Doctor

Obtaining a careful diagnosis may not be easy in many places. More physicians are becoming informed about these diseases, and most major medical centers as well as hospitals have developed special programs for memory disorders. The appendices to this volume identify organizations and services throughout the United States that can help identify local clinical resources. For families fortunate enough to live near one of these sites, knowledgeable and caring professionals are usually available. The problem is what to do when these resources are not available.

There are several approaches to the search for caring medical professionals. Ask doctors and nurses in your community whom they would consult if someone in their family had a similar problem. Perhaps the best way to find professional help is through Alzheimer's disease organizations (see Appendix 1). These organizations are extremely valuable for many reasons. Their members may have information about good doctors and health resources as well as community services and agencies. Referral lists available from local medical societies or hospitals are often outdated and may or may not be useful. A telephone call to the physician will confirm whether he or she is interested and cares about older patients.

The Qualities of a Good Doctor

To identify competent, knowledgeable, and compassionate physicians, you can inquire about their training. Do they have special qualifications in geriatric medicine, geriatric psychiatry, or geriatric neurology? Have they had special training or experience in dealing with older patients or those with cognitive deficits? Ask what proportion of their practice involves people with dementia. Ask them questions, listen to their answers, and trust your own judgment. You might ask them such questions as "What causes memory loss in older people?" "What do you think causes Alzheimer's disease?" "What research is being done?" or "What can be done to treat the disease?" The answers to these questions, the willingness of the doctor to spend the time to talk about these problems, and the tone of voice reflect a great deal about the person. If the doctor seems uninterested or distant, or if you feel uncomfortable, you should find someone else. The objective is to find a doctor who is technically up-to-date and also cares about how the patient and family are coping.

The patient's internist or family-practice doctor will refer you to specialists in psychiatry and neurology. Find out whether the specialist is "board eligible" or "board certified." *Board eligible* means that the doctor has completed specialty training beyond medical school in an approved residency program. *Board certified* means the doctor also has passed a national examination and has been certified in that specialty. The examination is not mandatory and is not required for physicians to obtain a license to practice. Although passing the specialty board examination is not always the sign of a better physician, it does mean that the physician has had at least the minimum required training and experience in the specific area of medicine in which he or she is certified. You should try to make certain that the specialist you choose is at least board eligible.

It is important that you feel comfortable with your doctors and sense that they are willing to spend time with you and the patient. You will soon discover whether they are willing and able to provide you with the care and support you need. In our book *Caring for Your Aging Parents* (see Selected References and Internet Resources), we have written a special section to help you judge your doctor and other health professionals.

In this time of health maintenance organizations, or HMOs, special problems may arise in obtaining a careful evaluation. Your assigned or selected primary care physician may not be interested or knowledgeable about recent advances. Your primary care physician may not know about the range of treatment options, including behavioral and psychosocial interventions and family supports. He or she is likely to have less time with individual patients, and the HMO may not approve a referral to a specialist or the battery of diagnostic procedures recommended. Even Medicare itself has been limiting certain tests such as neuropsychological tests or MRIs unless specific reasons are given for the order.

Caregivers need to become advocates to get the quality of care the patient needs. See the reference list of books to help you challenge the HMO and managed care system. Recent history supports the value of challenging any organization that refuses to provide needed care in the interest of making a profit.

Do Patients Recognize They Need Help?

Long before professional help is sought and a diagnosis is established, individuals with cognitive problems and their families usually recognize that something is seriously wrong. Often, however, patients, as well as relatives and doctors, deny their problems and falsely attribute these changes to aging, problems at work, stress, or other life problems. The results of several studies suggest that family members are more accurate than patients in identifying a problem and that affected individuals are more likely to underestimate or deny their problems. Other studies show that families may overestimate or underestimate the ability of their patient-relatives.

Unfortunately, many individuals are so reluctant to recognize they have a problem that to even suggest something is wrong may provoke indignation and angry denial. Ann Sylvester and her husband had spent summers at their cabin on the lake over the past ten years. This summer Arthur noticed that Ann seemed more irritable and less interested in entertaining their friends. This withdrawal from social activities was disconcerting to Art because over the years they both had become very attached to the area and especially to their friends. Ann and Arthur had developed special friendships with four other couples, having become virtually inseparable.

When Ann first seemed detached and bored, everyone was supportive. Ann was a talented artist; Art and the others had grown accustomed to her periodic mood swings. However, this summer there was a raw edge to her personality. She argued over the simplest things—the amount of salt to put in the soup, the number of coals for the barbecue, the hour they had to leave to arrive at a concert on time, the type of mayonnaise to buy. Indeed, Ann became deeply insulted when Art bought a different brand of mayonnaise. Ann not only argued with her friends over trivial matters but even began to turn down opportunities to do things together.

Their friends shared their concerns with Arthur and each other. They even began to evolve a plan for confronting Ann with their belief that something was wrong and to ask her to see a doctor. However, it was Ann's sister Maria who finally questioned Ann about her behavior one evening as they sat together by the fire. Ann's response was as swift as a bolt of lightning. She asked Maria to mind her own business and even suggested that Maria could leave that weekend if she did not like her company.

More than two months passed before Ann saw a doctor. She fought with everyone and denied that anything was wrong. Finally, Maria called an old family friend who also was an internist and begged him to help get Ann in for an evaluation. Ann found many excuses and broke several appointments. The family decided to meet together for a Saturday evening meal and "gang up" on Ann. Arthur, their three children and their families, and Maria and her husband spent over four hours trying to persuade Ann to get a checkup. It was a stormy evening, but everyone was unrelenting. They gave Ann the room to be angry, continually reiterated how much they loved her, and insisted that there was no way they would let her go on like this. Everyone, including the grandchildren, emphasized how important she was to all of them.

It was the comments of her six-year-old granddaughter, Mary Jane, that brought the arguments to an end. "I'm afraid. Nana scares me sometimes," Mary Jane cried when Ann reached over to hug her. Ann finally gave in to her family's pleas to see a doctor.

The individual's inability to recognize that a serious problem exists delays the diagnosis of the problem. Furthermore, in such instances, the family members may fight among themselves as to whether to press the individual to see a doctor. This conflict is easily picked up by the patient, who justifies putting off professional help. As a result, families may continue to argue with their relative and escalate conflict rather than work with him or her more cooperatively and supportively.

Family members usually make the initial appointment for the diagnostic evaluation. Several factors appear to deter the "patient" from contacting the doctor personally, even when the individual is aware that something is wrong. However, in many situations one or more family members work together to pressure a loved one to see a doctor—then, once the individual has agreed, they set up the appointment without letting the patient take any initiative. Some family members become so overprotective that they not only arrange all the appointments but also talk with the doctors on their own and effectively exclude the patient from active participation in the entire diagnostic process. It is important to give patients opportunities to participate as much as possible. Let them help set up appointments if possible and talk with the doctors on their own if they wish.

The exclusion of the patient is sometimes reinforced by professionals who seem unaware of the insight the patient has into his or her own condition and who are more comfortable talking directly to family members. In meetings with professionals it is important to include the patient as well as available family members and to involve him or her in understanding the diagnostic process as early as possible. Exclusion of the patient may lead to suspicion that the purpose of the exam is to put them away, and the patient's paranoia may seem reasonable under the circumstances with unfortunate consequences.

Preparing to Hear the Diagnosis

Once the examination begins, ask the doctor to explain to everyone involved the steps in the diagnostic process as well as the signs or results that are being looked for. If the doctor does not do this, press for the information, but recognize that it may not be useful to demand the results of each individual test until the entire evaluation is over. Many individuals displaying symptoms of dementia can present puzzling diagnostic problems, and a careful health professional may need time to think and discuss his or her findings with knowledgeable colleagues.

There is something very specific family caregivers can do during this period. Bring the family members together and develop your own plan of action for the day you meet with the health professionals to hear their conclusions. Ask the doctor to give you an approximate date when the tests might be concluded, and tell him or her what the family is doing. Decide who wants to be present. Does the identified patient want to meet alone with the doctor first, before the spouse or other family members join the conference? As the agreed-upon date for the conference draws near, remind each other, especially the patient, several times. This tactic is a way of allowing the patient who wants little or no information to say so. This is extremely important when the patient lives alone and other family members are trying to help. Although most people want to hear the diagnosis, this is not always true. Well-meaning relatives should not impose their views on the patient.

When Marlene Van Dyk was told that she probably had Alzheimer's disease, she was alone with her doctors, at her request. Even though her husband and daughters had accompanied her to the various appointments and had met the doctors, Marlene was adamant about meeting with them first: "I knew something was terribly wrong. I wanted to hear the verdict without my family present. Yes, I even knew it was Alzheimer's before they told me. I was afraid when they said the words I would cry, and I needed to cry before I could face my family."

Not all people want to be alone when they hear the diagnosis. Craig McCarthy sat around a conference table with his wife and children when the doctors summarized the results of his examinations: "When I heard 'Alzheimer's disease,' the words struck me like a thunderclap. My heart began to ache, my knees trembled, and my body was numb. I felt like a gurgling whirlpool was sucking me down. I remember looking around the room at my family and the doctors. I needed them all to get my bearings again. Without them I would drown."

Receiving bad news is never easy. If you are fortunate, the doctor will spend the time you need, answer your questions, and listen carefully to what you say. The next chapter discusses common reactions to the diagnosis as well as what you can do to help the patient and yourself after the diagnosis has been made.

3

Reactions to the Diagnosis

*A sense of utter helplessness swept over me when the doctor said that I prob-
ably had Alzheimer's disease. The very words "Alzheimer's disease"
sounded harsh and unreal. I wanted to believe that he was talking about
someone else, not me.*

*I remember asking a few questions. Was he sure? Could it be some-
thing else? What could he do for me? I remember how he leaned forward
and stayed close to me when he answered, but I don't remember what he
said. I did not want to listen.*

*I wanted to talk; but I didn't want anyone to know how scared I was.
I had always imagined myself to be a strong person who could face anything. But now I was afraid of a disease I did not understand. How was I
going to live the rest of my life and take care of my family? All I could see
was darkness.*

When given the opportunity, many individuals will discuss their
thoughts and feelings after receiving the bad news—shock,
numbness, anger, disbelief, fear, despair. Jan Prescott, whose
words open this chapter, was aware of word-finding difficulties several years
before she finally submitted herself to a full battery of medical tests:

My memory lapses were humiliating. I couldn't depend upon myself anymore. Mysteriously I was changing. I knew about this
Alzheimer's disease, how it destroys intelligent behavior in bits and

pieces, but I was afraid to think that it was happening to me. When the doctor began to talk to me in the office, I began to get very nervous. I wanted to run away. It may sound absurd, but I thought if I didn't hear the words then I couldn't have the disease.

How do you tell someone he or she has Alzheimer's disease or a related dementia? There is very little research to guide the best practices for disclosing or witholding the diagnosis. The results of what has been done suggests that people who are told the diagnosis seem to be less troubled and cope better. Knowing the diagnosis provides a frame of reference to make sense of what happens to them on a daily basis.

People vary in their ability to accept the diagnosis, but telling an individual that they have Alzheimer's disease or a related dementia is the best course of action in most situations. Some individuals are relieved to know there is a cause for their problems and that they no longer have to cover up with family and friends. Others may deny they have Alzheimer's disease.

In a national survey of patients and caregivers, 65 percent of patients were told the diagnosis by a physician specializing in geriatrics; 11 percent were told by a spouse, adult child, or other relative; and 24 percent were not told what the diagnosis was. When caregivers were asked about the degree of insight the patient had about the diagnosis, they reported that 32 percent were partially aware of their problem, 19 percent were fully aware, 9 percent showed variable insight, 30 percent were unaware, and 10 percent denied the diagnosis. Furthermore, 50 percent of those not told had full or partial awareness of their illness.

In contrast to geriatric specialists, most primary care physicians do not tell the patient the diagnosis because they do not believe the person will understand it or they are concerned the patient will harm himself or herself. Some doctors deliver the diagnosis quickly and then offer a brief statement that little or nothing can be done. Many do not recommend currently available antidementia drugs (see Chapter 5). They tend to speak to the family members and leave them the job of informing the patient. Frequently, all those involved, professionals and family members, are uncomfortable and do not know how to talk or listen to the person who has been diagnosed. Listening carefully and actively to the person-turned-patient provides important clues about what the patient is prepared to hear.

In many instances once the individual and the family receive the diagnosis, all go home and are left to cope with the news with few resources. One woman told us:

> We lived in an atmosphere of silence. The doctor said that Jim had Alzheimer's disease. We didn't know whether to be thankful that the disease had a name or to be afraid. Jim would not talk about it. Sometimes at night, he would sit at the desk with his head in his hands, staring at a book. One evening I found him downstairs by the furnace, with a can of peas in his hand. He was crying, but turned quickly away when I entered. I pretended not to notice. He walked past me and pressed the can into my hand. "Choose a wine for dinner. I don't know whether to have red or white." And then I realized he had forgotten where the wine cellar was located. He had gone to the pantry instead.

Individuals do not have to suffer alone, but they often need help in voicing their emotions and coming to terms with them. By providing opportunities for people with dementia to talk and then listening supportively, one can help transform the initial grief and despair into acceptance. However, active listening is not always easy, because much of what patients say is painful for the listener. Jim Evans spoke the following words several months after the wine cellar episode:

> Alzheimer's disease is worse than death. It leaves bone and flesh intact while it erases judgment and memory. I could live with death. Death is a part of the cycle of life. It's like spring, the end of winter. But this disease—it's unnatural. It's the end of hope.

However, Jim and his wife Dee conquered his initial hopelessness and desperation. Dee learned to listen to Jim supportively when he felt sad, but then she always found ways to say how much they could still do together, which brought them both pleasure.

The attitude in general clinical practice of witholding the diagnosis of dementia is similar to the beliefs about telling patients about cancer thirty years ago. In the 1960s, 90 percent of doctors did not tell their patient the diagnosis, compared to 5 percent now. The change to disclosing rather than witholding the diagnosis came about for many reasons, including greater public awareness, the potential for effective treatments, and therapeutic optimism.

At the present there is significant public awareness about Alzheimer's disease, especially given the number of well-known and high-profile persons who have been affected such as President Ronald Reagan, Iris Murdoch, Willem DeKooning, and Lewis Mumford, to name only a few. With the explosion of research advances, there is also optimism about treatments and a cure. There are improved techniques for early detection and diagnosis, which make it possible to identify mildly impaired individuals at a time when they are able to deal with plans and adjustments for the future.

Disclosure is the beginning of a long process of change and adaptation to change over the course of the illness. After the diagnosis is made, there is a process of dealing with denial as well as sorting out emotions, feeling, and questions. Why me? What did I do to get this disease? As this chapter will show repeatedly, each patient and family deal with their reactions on an individual basis. The stories and guidelines of this chapter will provide a broad range of strategies for coping successfully.

If you pay close attention, patients will usually tell you how much they want to know. The rule of thumb is to *hear* what the patients wish to learn, and then to make responses tempered by their reactions and perhaps by what you are able to endure. Confirmation takes time, but it fosters the acceptance that lets people come to terms with themselves. One patient, a retired longshoreman, listened carefully to an explanation that he probably had Alzheimer's disease. His gaze shifted to the window for a brief moment. Then he looked back at his wife, the rest of his family, and the doctor and surprised them with his response, "More light." (These are the words Goethe said when he was dying.) "I want to know more. I need to prepare my family."

Although it may be emotionally difficult, it is valuable to share information with patients to the extent they are ready to receive it. Do not withhold information when asked a direct question, and above all do not lie. Listen carefully and gauge your response according to the question. When in doubt, say nothing! Sometimes you may not have to say very much at all. You may only need to show that you are ready to talk, and the patients will say a great deal. Confronting the disease gently and slowly is often the beginning of a successful treatment program that involves patients in discussions about their future. People with Alzheimer's disease have the right to determine how they will live their remaining years while they still have cognitive capacity in the early stages. Realistic discussions about the nature of their illness are the basis for plans for the future, before they become incapacitated.

One of the most difficult challenges after the diagnosis is to deal with patients who are upset and agitated but unable to express personal feelings. Patients are quite often afraid of upsetting other members of the family and wish to protect them. Some individuals, especially men, may never have spoken much about their feelings. The thought of becoming a burden on their wife or children may be too difficult for them to bear, and raising feelings about their loss of abilities is contrary to a lifelong pattern. In these circumstances the family must show its strength and gently create openings over time that may allow for the expression of unpleasant feelings. If this does not work, counseling by a minister, physician, or other professional may be the best approach.

Discussions also are likely to occur in the context of the need for legal and financial planning, which should be done soon after the diagnosis. A lawyer or accountant may be instrumental in helping patients begin to address the problem of planning for the future. Although the role of these professionals is not to focus on feelings, legal and financial issues often evoke emotions. The simple act of developing a financial legacy for members of the family may begin with financial and material matters, but it often evolves into the more significant emotional legacy that patients may need to express.

Marie Edwards told her lawyer that the disease had forced her to find a new meaning in life. Marie had been a successful businesswoman preoccupied with money, achievement, and constant activity. In order to face her dementia, she constructed a philosophy that measured her life in terms of values rather than time and money. She decided to concern herself with what gave her life meaning rather than with the number of years she had left. Her children were important to her, and she decided to visit them more often. She spoke with them about her desire to leave something for them to remember her by. One day she announced that she wanted to arrange the many hundreds of family photos into albums. With the help of her children, over a two-year period, she reviewed fifty years of photographs and seemed to become more contented emotionally. Mrs. Edwards felt that she had finished an important task with and for her family before the progressive dementia left her in oblivion.

Understanding the Patient's View

Understanding the individual-turned-patient's subjective experience during the early phases of the illness, beyond the results of medical tests, is essential to the integrity of the relationship. If you do not understand the person, clinical decisions will not represent the patient's needs in the caring transaction.

James John, a banker, described the impact of the diagnosis:

Having Alzheimer's disease made me face ultimate realities, not my bank account. My money, job, and other parts of my life were trivial issues that restricted my growth, my spiritual growth.

Alzheimer's disease transferred me from what I call the trivial plane to the spiritual plane. I have to face the absolute horror of the "A" word, and I began a dialogue with my existence, a dialogue with my life and my death.

The period following the diagnosis is the time when patients must deal with their feelings and begin to incorporate the disease into their lives. George Christos describes it to his doctor in the following dialogue:

DR.: How did you feel when you were told that you had Alzheimer's?
MR. C.: I was angry. I was confused. I was fighting against the diagnosis. I felt like it shouldn't happen to me.
DR.: Are you still fighting?
MR. C.: Yes, I'm still fighting, but not against the diagnosis. I am resigned to it. Now I am fighting to live each day. I'm fighting to live as it comes. I am fighting against my fears. Every morning when I wake up, I have to ask myself who I am. I am afraid of the day when I will not know who I am. But until that day the world will know that George Christos is alive!

Some patients do not seem to understand the diagnosis, whereas others admit to being at a loss as to how to deal with it. Many say that they feel as if they have been given a death sentence. Death and loss are frequent themes that surface early in discussions with certain patients and families. Often the issue of death begins as a reaction to the diagnosis. The labels "Alzheimer's disease" or even "dementia" convey the idea of profound loss as well as that of an incurable and life-shortening disease.

Such concerns reach deeply into an individual's emotions at a time when abilities are still largely intact, and many patients are capable not only of understanding what is at stake but also of feeling and reacting to their frustrations. Individuals with the disease are in the position of having to catch up psychologically with the consequences of the disease and what it means for their future life. In reaction to the diagnosis, one patient told us, "Death wasn't knocking on my door. Death kicked the door in to show his face."

Early in the disease many individuals are desperate to talk about what it means for their future and for their family. They will often confide in a compassionate friend or health professional. They have questions to be answered and need patience and support to overcome their anger, fears, and anxiety. Cognitive losses as well as speech and language problems often make this difficult. One woman spoke hesitantly about how difficult it was for her children and husband to talk with her. She knew how much love filled her family, but she lamented their fear of her disease and the breakdown in communication between them. One day, her eyes filled with tears, she quoted these lines from the poet Theodore Roethke: "Like the half-dead, I hug my last secrets. . . . I fall, more and more into my own silence. In the cold air, the spirit hardens."

Reactions of professionals and family members to patients are important. The task is to be honest with patients and inform them as much as possible about the nature of their disease, the prognosis, and the willingness of clinicians and family to help. Caregivers should work carefully with patients, giving them information as they are ready to accept it. This is made difficult by the patients' deficits and emotional responses as well as by the caregivers' own emotions. It also requires time and repetition. In the end, this sharing may foster the acceptance that allows patients to live with themselves.

In the following dialogue, Albert Johns, aged sixty-two, describes what he remembers feeling both at the time he was diagnosed and at the time of the interview:

DR.: When you were told that you had Alzheimer's disease, could you talk about the diagnosis easily with your wife?

MR. J.: No. I had trouble. It's an inevitable sort of thing, so you have to accept it. That's all. I didn't want to accept the truth then. Now I hope for the best and help other people who are going through the same thing—give them a little hand up.

DR.: Does that make you feel better?

MR. J.: Sure it does. You bet.

DR.: Do you think you and Dorothy have become closer?

MR. J.: Since working together on this? I think we have.

DR.: Do you ever feel very angry and frustrated?

MR. J.: Well, I suppose we all go through this. It's a continuing thing, but let's put it this way, I think I'm coping with it better now than I was a year ago.

DR.: What makes you say that? Why do you think you're coping better?

MR. J.: Well, maybe it's because I have more time to think about it and I realize what I'm doing wrong, where I'm making my mistakes. I won't say that I'm curing them, but I like to think that I'm on the right track.

DR.: Do you think very much about the future and what might happen as time goes by?

MR. J.: Yes.

DR.. Do you worry about the future?

MR. J.: Yes, but I am resigned. I know more about what's going to happen to me now than I did a year or two ago. A year or two ago I was shaken up quite a bit more. Now I can accept the situation. I might also say I am curious. I'm interested in what's on next.

DR.: What do you think is next?

MR. J.: Wish I had a clue.

Patients have a great deal to teach us about living with the anguish of what one man called "a living death." Jerome Lambert and his wife, Irene, invited us to their home to talk with them approximately two months after Mr. Lambert had been diagnosed with Alzheimer's disease. Mr. Lambert had some difficulty finding the right words, but he spoke slowly and effectively for several hours. He even gave us a small notebook to read. Together with his wife he had written a daily diary describing the changes in their lives as a result of his illness.

Mrs. Lambert cried several times and spoke of the anger she felt that her husband should be suffering such a cruel and senseless disease. He put his arm around her whenever she cried and said to us, "My brain is an attic, a place full of junk, but my shoulder is strong." Throughout the afternoon Mr. Lambert was enthusiastic about continuing to live. He was committed to telling his family what he wanted to do before he was incapacitated by the dementia.

Perhaps the most important concern many patients express after the diagnosis is the need to participate as actively as possible for as long as possible in family life. They want to have the information to make decisions relating to what is happening to them. Often individuals voice this concern because they feel excluded from the families' decision making too soon. They want to be involved in plans dealing with their future and the changes in their lives. A frequently expressed desire of many, though not all, patients is that heroic measures not be used when they are in the terminal phases of the illness. Firmly expressed too is the desire to avoid a nursing home, a wish that often comes back to haunt family members if institutionalization becomes necessary. Finally, most patients tell us that they want the primary goal of living to be "comfort" for themselves and for their family.

Many individuals share their fear and sadness that as the dementia progresses, their confused mental state will deprive them of the ability to relate to their family and themselves with dignity and self-respect. Although answers do not flow easily when these conversations occur, the act of letting persons express themselves is itself valuable. One way to respond may be to acknowledge that you understand their wishes and will help them with whatever happens in the future. It is important for family members to try to accept the reality of the future if the patients are to be able to do so. The emphasis should center on the present and what can be done to maximize comfort, pleasure, and meaningful activities. The focus should be on the patients' strengths. Challenge them to discuss with you how to use the time most valuably.

The courage of our patients and families is remarkable. Arthur Roberts, a successful writer, told us that he, his wife, and his family were living a life of "tranquil heroism." Mr. Roberts knew there was no cure, that the drugs available would only slow his deterioration, and that the disease would slowly leave him unable to function as a husband, father, writer, and man. But he was determined to fight to live. He regarded his wife as a heroine who had the courage to accept his limitations and continue to love him as a man who still gave her life a special quality. Mr. Roberts needed to feel that his wife, children, and friends would let him remain part of their lives. Although he was afraid of the future, he was helped by sharing that fear with them. For him it was the only way he could live, and die.

One man, a surgeon named Dr. Amos Baker, told us that he wanted to develop "the courage to make a series of silent retreats." He spoke of his need to gain power over his disease and to die a little each day without losing the desire to live. As a physician, and especially a surgeon, he had encountered life and death every day in the operating room. In that environment he was the man in control. Alzheimer's disease had leveled the playing field for him.

Arthur Kaiser was a deeply spiritual clergyman who shared his reflections with us several months following the diagnosis. He quoted freely from the scriptures in early discussions and continued to deliver Sunday sermons. Indeed, Rev. Kaiser wrote several sermons each week because he wanted to write while his mind still functioned. As the disease progressed over several years, he remembered less and less. However, Rev. Kaiser retained one important passage that he always quoted when asked how he was doing: "I am content. For all creatures, death has been prepared from the beginning."

Some individuals are reluctant or afraid to talk openly because they are embarrassed, ashamed, or frightened. Others will open up and overwhelm the receptive listener. The content is often surprising and unpredictable. The critical message for families and friends is to be ready to talk when patients want to do so.

With improved medical care, individuals with dementia are living longer. It is not easy to gauge the life expectancy of them at this time. Men and women can live with this disease for a long time. They have the same prevalence of physical health problems as persons without dementia, and the rate of change in memory may be very slow. Some professionals may not be well informed, but rather than confess their ignorance they may give patients and families incorrect information. Alex Georgio vividly recalled what he was told at the time of his wife's diagnosis: "She'll be in an institution within six months and dead in eighteen months." He repeated this often during the years following the event, and both he and his wife took particular pride in proving these words of doom wrong. He often emphasized that planning for his wife's demise as predicted by their neurologist was inappropriate. For years both he and his wife remained convinced that physicians knew little about the disease or its management: "What we learned about Alzheimer's we found out for ourselves."

Dealing with the Patient's Denial

What do you do when the patient flees from information? What tactics do you adopt when a close family member refuses to acknowledge what is occurring? The answers are complicated, and we can offer only guidelines. Most people need time to adjust to severe stress, and some simply require more time than others. The length of time needed to work through denial is a function of several factors, including the patient's personality, the rate of decline, the severity of cognitive impairment, lifestyle, the way the family system operates, and the availability of competent professional help. Dealing with the formidable diagnosis and prognosis of irreversible dementia brings up profound feelings. Some individuals may not make much progress accepting the reality of the disease after the diagnosis. And in these instances, family members should get professional help.

The family can take some very specific steps. First, family members should sit down and put their heads together to formulate a plan. If health professionals are available, they may be able to provide some valuable insights and assistance. If this form of help is not available, bring a clergyman, a trusted friend, or an outsider who may help you see the world a little more objectively.

Jesse Barker received a diagnosis of Alzheimer's disease at the age of forty-six. His wife Barbara and his two children described him as a gentle, quiet man. He had not only worked hard to provide for his own family but also supported his brother's wife and two small children. His younger brother, Bill, had been killed in a hunting accident.

Jesse refused to admit that he had Alzheimer's disease. He would sit through family meetings and listen attentively to others, but he would say very little. His sister described him as silently amused by the way everyone behaved. Jesse had always been a tolerant man, and nothing seemed to upset him. No one could remember him crying, even when his brother was killed. And whenever the family would reminisce about Bill, Jesse would seem not to listen. After Bill's death he took a second job and never complained about the long hours, even to his wife. But Jesse's wife wrote us several times about the family's frustration with his denial of his condition.

Dear Doctor,

Jesse goes about his days, business as usual. He quit one of his jobs last week. He just came home Friday and told me he would not drive a cab anymore. He said there were too many taxis for a town this size and business was slow for him. He had better things to do. There would be less money for a while, but he would find something else.

I called my daughter. I did not want him to take another job, and I also did not want him to continue in the second job. I am afraid he will be fired someday soon. He can still do his job as a salesman, at least with his old customers. But the new ones are a problem. We had dinner with his boss last week. Gerry told me that Jesse forgets appointments occasionally, and it had started to happen more frequently. Some of the customers have even started to complain. Although Jesse has been sick for almost a year now, we never told his boss or his friends at work. We wanted Jesse to be able to continue working as long as he could.

Doctor, I think the time has come for him to stop working altogether. I do not want him to be embarrassed by a pink slip. On the other hand, I am ashamed to tell his boss he has Alzheimer's disease. Each night I help him with the receipts because he cannot itemize the daily sales and deliveries. However, I cannot go out in the car with him. Someday he may forget to file an order for a big customer or he may have an accident. He hides it well, but I don't know how long he can go on like this. And I'm at the end of my rope.

Can you help us find a way out? When the kids and I talk to Jesse he listens but ignores us at the same time. He makes me so angry.

Several meetings were held with the members of the family to convince them they had done everything they could. Jesse's denial of his symptoms was consistent with his personality style. From all we could tell this was the only way he could deal with the illness, just as it had been his only way of dealing with his brother's death.

The employment issue was settled when Jesse was fired. However, his wife, Barbara, with the encouragement of her family, explained the situation to her husband's boss. The head of the company allowed Jesse to retire with disability compensation.

With time Barbara, the children, and the rest of the family became more comfortable with Jesse and his dementia. To fight him was ineffective and senseless. Jesse continued to live at home for five years before being institutionalized. The following excerpt is from a letter Barbara wrote after he died:

Dear Doctor,

I still think about Jesse every day. I did everything I could to care for him. He was my life, and now that he is gone I feel lost. Jesse was such a fighter. The entire time he was sick he stayed active. I always got the strangest feeling that he was determined to make it through every day, even towards the end. He never accepted the fact that he was sick, and he was determined to live. In his mind nothing had changed. In his own world he seemed so happy, so content, even though he appeared so confused to us.

I remember one time when he seemed to know what was going on. Last Christmas I visited him at the nursing home. In fact, it was Christmas Eve. We sat together in the day room for over an hour opening up his gifts. As the children and I prepared to leave, Jesse touched my cheek and he began to cry. He spoke slowly, "I guess I will never have a Christmas at home again."

Everyone was surprised. And everyone cried . . . me, the kids, and even the nurses. The children had to drag me out of the nursing home, and they brought me to their home for two weeks. I still think about that incident every day.

Jesse has been dead almost ten months now. We had so many wonderful years together. I am happy that he seemed not to know what was happening most of the time. I like to think that he died happy. Doctor, he lost his self with that disease, and I pray that he did not know what was happening.

How do you know when it is better to support rather than continue to confront the patient's denial? How do you deal with a patient with a strong denial system? The preceding example illustrates how important it is to analyze and understand the patient's reactions to severe stress in the past. If the patient's personality style has been to respond to stress and crises by avoidance and denial, it may be appropriate to quietly support the individual's denial.

There are strategies for working around the denial in certain crucial situations. Psychologically trained professionals may be successful in conjunction with appropriate attorneys to help families deal with specific problems involving financial assets and other legal issues.

Nancy Samuels turned to a psychiatrist and a lawyer to help her resolve an upsetting problem with her husband, who had recently been diagnosed as having Alzheimer's disease. Ronald Samuels had just been hospitalized because of internal bleeding. Mrs. Samuels was distressed by her husband's condition and by their financial straits. Mr. Samuels had a small business firm with several partners, and his wife thought the contract specified that all assets went to the firm when any of the partners died. Mr. Samuels completely denied that he had Alzheimer's disease and thus insisted that there was no need to deal with the matter. His wife was concerned about her ability to protect their assets.

The following conversation illustrates how the doctor was able to talk with Mr. Samuels and successfully work with him:

MR. S.: It is very nice of you to visit me, but I am doing quite well, thank you. I didn't ask to see a psychiatrist. Why are you here?

DR.: Your internist, Dr. Hanks, asked me to see you. He is a little worried about you and thought that I might help.

MR. S.: What do you mean? I am in perfect health except for this bleeding in my stomach. When they find out what's wrong, I will be out of here and back to work.

DR.: Mr. Samuels, I know you think everything is fine. However, both Dr. Hanks and I are worried about you. You have Alzheimer's disease. And there are several things we can do to help you.

MR. S.: Doctor, I do not have this Alzheimer's disease. My wife believes anything a doctor tells her. My memory is fine. I forget a few things now and then, but everyone does when they get older. It is nothing to get excited about. Everyone is making far too much fuss about this. Please leave me alone.

DR.: Mr. Samuels, I will leave you alone in a little while. May I ask you a few questions before I go? It would be very helpful to me.

MR. S.: Sure, go ahead.

DR.: How long have you and your wife, Nancy, been married?

MR. S.: She's my second wife. I think it has been twenty-six years now.

DR.: How would you describe your marriage to her?

MR. S.: (Silence) She is a wonderful woman. There is nothing I wouldn't do for her. Nancy *is part* of me, and I could not live without her devotion.

DR.: Has Nancy spoken to you about what the two of you should do to fight this Alzheimer's disease?

MR. S.: Doctor, nothing is wrong with me. Nancy wants me to talk with my partners. She says I have no life insurance and that I may lose my assets to the firm. I have plenty of money, and I intend to live a long and happy life with her. I will take good care of her. She deserves everything I can give her.

DR.: Ron, please, I must interrupt you. May I call you Ron and talk to you man to man?

MR. S.: Yes, you may call me Ron. What do you want?

DR.: If you love your wife as much as I suspect you do, why not talk to a lawyer with her? It will make her feel better and put her mind at rest.

A series of meetings took place between Mr. and Mrs. Samuels, the attorney, and the psychiatrist. Mr. Samuels never acknowledged that he had Alzheimer's disease. However, since he had such a strong relationship with his wife, this love became the key with which to open discussions about the business. In this instance, there was no need to confront him with the reality that he had Alzheimer's disease.

We have a great deal to learn about denial and how it helps or interferes with individuals' ability to cope with the dementia. For some patients denial may be an adaptive reaction to the need to survive; others are capable of mastering their painful emotions and of overcoming denial in dealing with their disease. However, the work must begin in the early phases of the illness, and the objective must be to do whatever brings the patients the greatest comfort, peace, and functional effectiveness.

Honest discussions after the diagnosis do not mean that the patient will not later deny the truth. Ivan Hackett asked his doctors endless questions about Alzheimer's disease during the diagnostic conference. The following day he told his wife that he didn't know what was wrong with him. The next week in the doctor's office he did not want to ask questions, and he told everyone that he was in good health. A week later he informed his doctor that even though he did not like it, he was going to die from this Alzheimer's disease. Ivan vacillated this way for several months. His family and doctors supported him by listening to him when he wanted to talk. Eventually, Ivan accepted the diagnosis.

Family Denial: A Common Reaction

In view of the many strange and disturbing incidents families experience before the diagnosis is finally made, it is startling to learn that the most common immediate response to the diagnosis itself is denial. Reactions vary, but expressions of surprise are typical. "No, it cannot be! It can't be happening to me, my husband, my mother." The same questions are put to the doctor, particularly when younger patients are involved. "Are you positive? Are you sure there's no mistake?" "Are you sure there's nothing we can do? Is there someone else who could help us?" These are all frequent queries, and for some families the doctor's answers are not satisfactory.

The denial can extend to some, if not all, people involved with the patient—spouse, children, in-laws, brothers, and sisters. Feuds may even develop if the reactions of different family members cannot be reconciled. Or the denial of family members, often living far away, will reinforce the reactions of the spouse or primary caregiver, sometimes resulting in a search for another diagnosis.

John Harriman first had difficulties at work. Although John could still sell a million dollars' worth of insurance a year, he could not fill out the forms correctly, if he remembered to do them at all. His wife, Bertha, would patiently organize the papers and calculate the premiums. His bridge game deteriorated to the point where he could not compete and members of the bridge club politely refused to be his partner. The final blow came when he received a new watch for his birthday. The wristwatch, a gift from his family, had small diamonds at four positions but no numbers. He could not tell the time. Finally, he and the family recognized that something was seriously wrong and that it could not be ignored any longer.

Almost on the heels of John's evaluation, the situation seemed to deteriorate rapidly. His wife, a strong and articulate person, began to take over. She arranged for a second diagnostic examination, then a third, a fourth, and even a fifth. By this time she was well known in the medical community, and everyone concurred about the nature of the problem and the completeness of the evaluation. Her relatives and friends urged her to put him in a good nursing home. He would receive expert care, and she could have a life of her own again.

Bertha shrugged off all advice concerning the diagnosis and about the need for institutional placement. She took her husband everywhere, involving him in many activities. John's brother, however, insisted from two thousand miles away that something more could be done. Out-of-town trips to more doctors and clinics were arranged. Finally, they found a physician who felt that a neurosurgical shunt should be tried as "a last resort."

John was operated on, placed on high doses of sedative medication, and then sent back home for care. This was more than seven years after the initial diagnosis. His condition had become aggravated by the post-operative complications of the neurosurgery. He was hospitalized and clearly could no longer be managed at home. Even then Bertha fought bitterly against his placement in an institution. She brought him home from the hospital, but three weeks later consented to let her doctor put him in a nursing home. At home he had struck her many times and yelled obscenities. It was only when he stabbed at her with a kitchen knife while she was preparing dinner that she let him go into a nursing home.

John Harriman's experience illustrates both the positive and the negative aspects of denial. The family's early refusal to follow medical opinions favoring institutionalization doubtless was appropriate for them. Keeping John a vital part of the family, challenging him to the extent possible, and relating to him in as normal a way as possible was helpful not only to John but also to his wife and children, all of whom remained close.

On the negative side were the emotional crises during the multiple diagnoses, the costs involved, the family feuding, and the anger at physicians, hospitals, and clinics for failing to deliver a more optimistic diagnosis and a cure. This in turn led to needless surgery and its complications, forcing the use of medication to control postsurgical agitation, and finally to an increasing complexity of care which required that he be hospitalized and then institutionalized. Furthermore, the reactions of geographically distant relatives strengthened Bertha's denial system. Her brother-in-law's insistence that something had been overlooked and that she seek further help from real specialists forced the diagnostic issue to be reopened. It was almost to prove a point to relatives not involved in his daily care that Bertha sought additional evaluations that eventually led to the neurosurgery. Dealing with the denial in the very beginning would have saved a lot of grief and resources and possibly would have improved the quality of life for the patient and the family. Sadly, the situation of John Harriman, his wife, children, and relatives is not rare.

The best way to begin to deal with your reactions to the diagnosis and to plan for the future is to understand exactly what examinations the doctors have conducted and to ask for a complete explanation of the results. If possible, the patient should participate in meetings with the doctors. The patient should not be excluded or made to feel that information is being discussed behind his or her back. Family members may also feel the need to have personal time with the doctor to ask for special help. If this is the case, let the patient know why you want to speak to the doctors privately. Explain briefly that you are worried about yourself. The patient may not understand your needs, but at least this gives him or her the courtesy of a brief simple explanation. Then too, the patient may understand.

Often the patient and family become engaged in a "silent battle" of which they are unaware. It is a battle over the control of information. Talking about Alzheimer's disease and what it does to the individual is painful. When something is unpleasant, people unconsciously respond by denying what is painful to them. The process of denial keeps information about Alzheimer's disease a "secret." More often than not, the patient and the family are trying to keep the "secret" from each other, in the hope they can spare each other the pain. Sadly, many families are out of sync, working against each other rather than with each other.

Difficulty in dealing with mental deterioration and death is a basic cause of communication problems with the patient. The attempt to control what is discussed undermines family members' efforts to communicate with each other. This is also an area where professionals are not always immune to blame. Too often they control the way information is exchanged about the disease because of either their own feelings or their fear of upsetting the patient and family. Their discomfort tends to become a barrier to a caring and effective relationship with the family. If you cannot talk openly with the patient's doctor or if you feel that he or she cannot speak easily with you, perhaps you should find another to help you.

In an effort to protect one another, family members sometimes consciously try to withhold information from the patient, or they communicate in a way that says very little. It is easy to spend time with a person during the day or night with little or no interaction, such as watching television, reading, writing, shopping, or listening to music. It is not unusual for family members to isolate themselves physically from the patient. People can control time by frequent business trips, shopping, meetings away from home—anything that precludes being with the patient.

Carroll Houck was unable to face his wife's illness, but he still managed to provide her with a high level of care. Kathleen Houck had begun to deteriorate in her late fifties. She was a beautiful, engaging woman who prior to the onset of Alzheimer's disease had enjoyed a successful business career. After its diagnosis Carroll began to live what his oldest daughter Karen called an "imitation of life." He could not face Kathleen's illness and spent long hours at the office, including business dinners each night of the week. Since it was well within his financial means, Carroll hired a suitable and attractive companion to live with Kathleen in their summer home. Since Kathleen loved to jog, swim, play tennis, work out in the gym, and lie in the sun, this life would be perfect for her. He would visit at least once a month. The other family members would visit less frequently but whenever they could.

The family carried out these plans, and Kathleen was happy to live in the villa. What Carroll and his family did not anticipate was her insistence on speaking with each member of the family on the telephone several times daily. Her question was always the same. When would they come to visit? This was a query she repeated with the regularity of a broken record. It was as if she had no recollection that she had ever asked the question. The usual family response was to answer her question the first time it was asked and to tell her they would see her next month. On subsequent questioning, they would simply ignore the query and tell her about whatever was going on at the moment, assure her of their love, and end the conversation . . . until the next phone call. Within a few months each of the family members had installed an answering machine.

On the surface it appeared that the family was in control of the situation, that Kathleen was secure and happy, and that the family members were organized and healthy. On one level, the family and the so-called patient were doing extremely well. The players, all family members, were engaged in their own lives. They spoke with one another and seemed to have a plan in which everyone was assuming a certain amount of responsibility.

Although the surface was calm, the deeper life of the family was in turmoil. The family members eventually sought professional assistance, and during several sessions they began to discuss the critical problem they had been successful in ignoring. They could not accept the fact that Kathleen had Alzheimer's disease. They wanted her to be comfortable. They wanted her to be happy and busy. Most important, they wanted her to be away from them, so that they did not have to see her and face the reality of her condition. Was the family doing the right thing? There is no right or wrong answer to this question.

Denial helps people deal with various aspects of their life in the face of potentially overwhelming emotions. There is, however, a paradox.

The process of denial that helps people deal with emotionally charged information by limiting the amount they handle may also blind them to information and feelings that can help. If you can recognize what is happening to you, the patient, and other relatives and if, even more important, you get help early, you will be in a better position to deal with your feelings as the disease progresses.

Genetic Vulnerability: Who's at Risk?

One of the most common reactions to the diagnosis of dementia is the fear on the part of other family members that they or perhaps their children are at risk. Some adult children even express concerns about having children of their own. Although it is common for family members to express anxiety when several family members have been diagnosed with Alzheimer's disease, many live with a sense of humor and perspective.

Richard Todd, a forty-two-year-old accountant, had a father as well as three uncles with Alzheimer's disease. All four had developed serious symptoms between the ages of sixty and sixty-five. Richard and his two brothers and two sisters lived close together and had shared the responsibility of caring for their father.

None of them seemed especially afraid of developing Alzheimer's even though their risk appeared to be reasonably high. Interviewed one evening on a local news channel as part of a fund-raising campaign, Richard described the burden of the family caring for relatives. After the broadcast, people in the studio stood around asking questions for several hours. Several individuals were in tears. Finally, someone asked Richard whether he worried about the prospect of getting Alzheimer's disease and whether he noticed any similarities between himself and his father and uncles. Richard appeared very serious as he answered, "Yes, I think my father, my uncles, and I are alike in one very important way. We are all oversexed!" The television crew began to laugh with him as Richard broke through their somber mood. Although Alzheimer's disease was possible, he could not afford to waste precious and happy years waiting for something that might or might not happen.

Chapter 14 provides an extensive discussion about the genetics of

Alzheimer's disease and how useful genetic testing may be in determining the risk of developing dementia. Alzheimer's disease is not caused by a single factor. In most cases, heredity alone is not sufficient to cause the disease. Other factors generally need to be present. Research studies of twins showed that even people with similar or identical genetic backgrounds do not experience the onset or progression of Alzheimer's disease in the same way. For example, in 10 percent of identical-twin pairs affected by the disease, only one of the two twins develops Alzheimer's.

Evidence for the role of heredity in Alzheimer's disease has been recognized for decades in a small number of families. The term *familial Alzheimer's disease* is used when Alzheimer's has been found in several family members, usually before age sixty-five, and generally in several generations of the family. It is estimated that only 10 percent of people with Alzheimer's disease have the familial type.

The most common type of Alzheimer's disease is called *sporadic Alzheimer's disease*, where there is no obvious pattern of inheritance. *Sporadic* means that the occurrence of Alzheimer's disease in families seems to be random. With continuing research breakthroughs we hope to learn more about the links among genetic predisposition, environmental factors, and other risk factors.

Guidelines for Developing Coping Strategies

What happens during the time immediately following the diagnosis affects the way the patient and the family deal with the disease and each other for years to come. Open, honest, and careful communication can minimize the difficulties ahead. A number of general guidelines may help the family deal with the situation right after the diagnosis.

1. *Go back to the patient's doctor or see another professional who is knowledgeable about dementias.* The meeting in which you learn about the diagnosis may be so emotional that much important information may be poorly heard, understood, or missing. A return visit is very valuable to the family. It should focus on informing you about what you can do. Find out whatever you can about the disease and ask for help to understand what the disease means. Ask about antidementia med-

ications that are available. Inquire about the location of Alzheimer's support groups in your area. If the doctor who makes the diagnosis is not the one to help you and the rest of the family understand the future, ask the doctor to recommend a knowledgeable professional with whom you are comfortable. Often a psychiatrist, psychologist, or social worker may be the person in the community most experienced with the disease and best informed about the resources available in your community.

2. *Ask, "What does the diagnosis mean to the patient (my husband, wife, father)?"* Hearing the diagnosis and understanding and accepting it are two different situations. It may be emotionally difficult to think clearly for a while. The diagnosis affects the entire family and everyone who cares about the relative or patient. One of the most important jobs facing everyone is to come to grips with what Alzheimer's disease really means in emotional terms for the patient and the family. What will the future be?

   Patients have the right to learn all the information they wish to handle. Ask for help if you need it to educate your relative about the nature of the diagnosis. Remember, it is usually easier for people to express anger than sadness, and anger once expressed is often misdirected. Like buckshot, it covers too much area and is very hard to control. Do not be hurt or frightened by the early outbursts of anger even if directed at you or someone else. Understand the cause of the patient's anger. It is important to allow people to blow off steam and then to deal with them rationally and constructively rather than to become guilty or to return the anger.

3. *Ask yourself, "What does the diagnosis mean to me?"* It is important to try to separate your own feelings about the diagnosis from what you think the patient may feel. This may sound simple but is usually extremely difficult. The bad news requires that all family members look inside themselves. Just as the patient has strong reactions, so will those close to the patient. However, caregivers usually have stronger reactions to the diagnosis than the identified patient.

4. *Do not say anything to the patient that is not true.* Although many patients will have difficulty accepting the diagnosis, methods usually can be found to educate them as they are ready. However, do not mislead them. Do not tell them that it is simply their age or that

they have nothing to worry about. Trust is essential in the management of the disease; once broken, it is hard to restore.

5. *Answer questions "in the here-and-now."* It is common for patients to worry about many issues: Do I really have Alzheimer's disease? How can the doctors be certain? Why me? Will I get worse? How long before I don't recognize my family? How long will it be before I no longer know myself?

When patients ask questions such as "Will I get worse?," respond with words that convey that, yes, someday in the future, but that for now, they are doing well. It is important to acknowledge that you take the questions seriously and that you are not going to run away from the answers and the patient. Answer the questions simply and honestly, but refocus the patient on the present and how well they are functioning. This reframing of issues to the present is part of living what so many people call "one day at a time."

6. *Talk with the patient but do not argue with denial.* Since it is characteristic for patients to deny the situation, do not argue or confront them too aggressively regardless of how illogical their denial appears. Patients will "hear" and believe the message when and if they are ready to deal with it. The denial is serving a short-term purpose by giving them more time to deal with the problem psychologically. It may be sufficient for a while just to inform them that Alzheimer's disease is the diagnosis and that things won't get much better.

A common sentiment expressed by patients is, "I'm going to beat this disease! I'm not going to let it destroy me!" Do not argue with these statements. Support the patient by saying you are going to help them beat it. This "fight" mentality is frequently expressed by people with other chronic illnesses as well as terminal diseases. It reflects the individual's ability to mobilize themselves to deal with the insurmountable odds, rather than give up.

7. *Do not lose hope.* Alzheimer's disease and related disorders do not cripple the individual overnight. Work with health professionals to understand your relative's strengths, needs, and desires. After the diagnosis there is often a great deal of time to fulfill a number of personal and family goals. Living one day at a time has become an important strategy for many families to cope with the disease successfully. Sharing becomes the key to dealing with the future.

8. *Keep a sense of humor.* Alzheimer's disease carries a black pall that is hurtful and frightening, but it is still acceptable to laugh and smile and feel joy in the ebb and flow of life with family and friends. Let yourself enjoy a television show, a movie comedy, or read a funny book. Laughing and smiling actually have a positive effect on the immune system, a natural way to keep you healthy.

9. *Find ways to vent your anger and sorrow.* Coping with the emotional reactions to the diagnosis is akin to riding an emotional roller coaster. Give yourself permission to cry and yell in your pillow. It is permissible to rail at God or the powers in which you believe. One patient's wife would yell out a phrase from Maria Rilke's poetry when she felt overwhelmed by her desperation: "Who when I cry out hears me from the order of angels?"

10. *Help yourself.* Recognize your own needs, fears, or anxiety and seek help. Living with a patient with the disease is a personally demanding burden. Finding a friend, clergyman, or professional to help you deal with your own feelings and reactions is a major step to helping the patient. Making a life for yourself in the midst of the tragic situation can also be crucial. Time out of the house—visits to friends, a movie, a restaurant, or a class—to take a break from the ceaseless problems at home not only are good for your physical and mental health but also are essential if you are to continue to provide care for the patient. Remember that if you break down, the patient suffers. Caregivers who do not take care of themselves are at high risk for physical and mental health problems as well as early mortality.

Putting life in order after a diagnosis is difficult. It is a time for everyone to come to grips with what one woman described as the "permanent uncertainty" of the diagnosis. Many changes and crises lie ahead. There will be days of fear, anxiety, and worry, and there will be times of tenderness, intimacy, and even humor. The next chapter offers some specific strategies for coping with the challenges of Alzheimer's disease.

4

Setting Goals after the Diagnosis

I am starting to lose control of myself. I feel robbed. I wish there were some way I could be repaired. Some of this brain must be good, or is it all rotting away? Must I disappear into oblivion? How much time will I have?

Last night my granddaughter Nydia sat on my lap watching television with me. My son walked into the room and reminded her that it was time for bed. Nydia began to cry and buried herself in the chair close to me.

Dear God, I can't get her words out of my mind. "Please don't take me away. I want to stay with Grandpa. You said that someday he will get so sick that he will not be able to take care of himself. You said that you don't know what to do. I know! I am going to stay and take care of him."

My son sat down next to me and began to cry. I cried too. We all held each other for a long time. I wish I could spare them my pain. —J.T.

We have offered some general suggestions about how to begin to deal effectively with the many psychological reactions of living with dementia, but understanding and doing are very different. Perhaps one of the most difficult challenges for everyone is to live daily with the frustration and suffering and to work to overcome it. James Thomas's diary entry not only exposes his inner turmoil but also gives us a sense of his personal courage. Nydia's behavior moved everyone and impelled the family to talk to a doctor about concrete strategies for dealing with the impact of dementia.

There are no life-saving machines for Alzheimer's disease or other progressive dementias. There are several antidementia drugs, and more that can improve functioning and skills in many persons for a period of time are sure to follow (see Chapter 5). However, the discovery of more effective therapeutic drugs will not negate the need for behavioral and psychological strategies to master the illness. There are many ways to maximize health and comfort and to help the patient adjust psychologically to the dementia. Alzheimer's disease challenges the patient and family to continually find new ways to cope with the progressive deterioration and incapacitations.

The challenge is to struggle to continue to care about living. Whoopie Adams described living with dementia as living in a dustbowl of hope and an oasis of despair. It was important to be a participant in her life as long as possible. She said success for her was playing the game, not necessarily winning it.

It is important to determine the preferences of the patient so that you can help him or her live as independently and comfortably as possible. As the disease progresses, consultations with professionals, exchanges of information about the patient's progress, regular checkups, and frequent discussions about family difficulties will help families and the patient exert control over their lives.

Dimensions of Caring: Setting Emotional Distance

Caregiving is not easy. The stages described in Chapter 1—handling denial and emotions, coping, maturation, and separation from self—challenge the caregiver to manage the patient as well as care for themselves and other members of the family. The challenge of caring is to be close to the patient and distant at the same time. You have to regard your relative as a loved one who is suffering and as a patient with a disease over which you have little control.

Developing at least a modest amount of emotional distance is helpful. It allows you to keep yourself psychologically more in control so that you can make decisions about the patient and about your personal and family life. If you are unable to separate yourself from your feelings about the tragedy of the situation, you will easily become overwhelmed with anger and with a sense of hopelessness or helplessness. As you learn to compartmentalize your feelings, you will be able to care for the patient more effectively and also protect yourself from total exhaustion.

Walter Eliot retired from his managerial job at the age of sixty-two. He looked forward to a life of travel and the "golden years" he had struggled to achieve. Within a year, though, he noticed his wife behaving very strangely. Evelyn would wear coats and sweaters inside out, use her bra to tie back her hair, and forget to put on earrings, belts, or stockings. Once she dressed casually in slacks for a black-tie affair and refused to change into an evening dress. On several occasions she served Walter sandwiches and beer for breakfast and fed the cat rice or cereal instead of Friskies. Within eighteen months he was stunned by the diagnosis of Alzheimer's disease and the neurologist's comment, "Sorry there's nothing we can do. She'll have to go to a nursing home."

Walter decided that this would not be. He tried to get help from an unresponsive community and was determined not to burden his children. Evelyn deteriorated quickly, and a succession of housekeepers were hired and fired. Evelyn did not sleep well at night, and Walter was up at all hours trying to keep control of the situation. Growing more and more upset, he began drinking heavily—a problem he had dealt with decades before—and became an alcoholic again, as he himself admitted. Only then did his children move in and force Walter to get help.

As he began to cope with his drinking problem, the overwhelming feelings about his life and Evelyn's condition emerged. Walter needed to find a way to care for Evelyn and also to have time for a life of his own. It took many months to control his drinking, and only when he became an active leader in a local Alzheimer's support group did he begin to deal more effectively with the situation at home. The support group had recommended a day-care center where Evelyn could spend five days a week, giving Walter the opportunity to be on his own. For Walter it was important in developing his emotional separation to keep Evelyn at home and also invest his energy in the local support group. Obviously, this is not everyone's solution.

Nancy Avery's friends made her "get out of the house." She did not want to join a support group or talk with anyone about the problems at home. She went to museums, where she could spend a few hours several days a week and focus on something else. For her it was "the pause that refreshed." Since she and her husband had always enjoyed collecting fine things, it gave her a feeling of wholeness in an otherwise difficult life of selfless and devoted care. Nancy felt guilty when she was away from her husband, but she achieved the recognition that the physical and emotional separation of a few hours each week improved her ability to care for him when they were together.

The enormous commitment involved in caring for an individual with progressive dementia requires that you develop a special relationship with the patient. You must understand and deal with his or her needs as well as yours in a way that does not emotionally, physically, and financially bankrupt you and the rest of the family. The process of evolving a special helping relationship has a technical name—approximation. *Approximation* is the process of forging a flexible or changeable relationship in which the caregiver must continually make decisions balancing the patient's needs with his or her own. There are numerous daily opportunities to make decisions—whether or not to be physically present, to do certain things, to react, to talk, to inquire, to inform, or to express feelings. The pattern of decisions and actions creates the unique relationship in the home and sets the tone for future decisions.

Approximation is not easy to achieve or to maintain, but you can learn to do it. Regardless of your personality, professional training, or background, it is hard to be close to the patient for long periods without feeling upset or uncomfortable. Learning how to distance yourself—not to avoid the patient or be insensitive, but to separate yourself on the basis of your knowledge of the patient's needs and your own—is helpful.

How do you learn the skills required for controlled distancing, which usually come with the professional training of clinicians? Here are eight guidelines we can offer.

1. Find Competent and Compassionate Mental Health Professionals.

Sometimes there is no substitute for individuals with special knowledge and skills to help you and your family share the burden of caring and keep from becoming overwhelmed. It can be very satisfying to be a caregiver, but the feelings engendered by caring for the Alzheimer's patient can affect your health (see Chapters 9 and 10). Like the patient, the caregiver may also feel abandoned and lonely and experience a profound loss of control. Many family members describe themselves as captives to the disease. These feelings may occur early on, or they may not surface for a while. Finding appropriate assistance after the diagnosis may prevent future problems.

Compassionate derives from the Latin word meaning "to suffer with," and there is a healing power in having someone to suffer with you. Having trained caregivers available will help you care for the patient and yourself by understanding the intensity of your emotions and their potential for disrupting or enhancing care. In years of training, mental health professionals have learned how to develop therapeutic relationships with patients, family members, and other caregivers.

Asking for assistance is often difficult. Moreover, many individuals are afraid of psychiatric help. The fear of the stigma of having mental illness prevents people from contacting precisely those professionals who are skilled in dealing with the difficult problems the patients and family encounter.

Unfortunately, many family members have serious misconceptions about mental health problems and the value of psychiatrists and mental health professionals. Psychiatric problems arc diseases of the brain and mind just as cardiovascular diseases are diseases of the heart and circulatory system. The couch and "talking therapies" are not the only tools of the psychiatrist. Psychiatrists are physicians with specialized training who are perhaps the best qualified to deal with human behavior and the many changes that affect the patient and the family living with Alzheimer's disease. They are also experienced in caring for people over long periods of time.

It is important to be forthright and ask the professionals you contact whether they can help you. Ask them to tell you about their interests, training, and experience with dementia. Their initial response will let you know immediately whether they will be helpful to you.

2. Find A Confidant.

Mental health professionals are not always available in your immediate community. Friends or confidants can be useful guides to help you measure off the distance between you and the patient. Friendships are stabilizing forces, and sharing feelings and experiences with someone you trust may simply make you feel better. Talking about your frustrations often helps you see the world a little more objectively. A trusted friend may also be a helpful critic who is able to compliment your stamina and courage and simultaneously urge you to be a little selfish and think of your own needs some of the time.

This seemingly simple advice may be difficult to follow. Many people are afraid and ashamed to let their friends know that a husband, wife, or family member has dementia. Some families have the financial resources to isolate the patient comfortably on an estate or in a luxury environment, hiding him or her away from the rest of the world. Although these arrangements may be done with the best of intentions, in the end the isolation may only create more problems.

Arnold Sands was stricken with Alzheimer's disease in his early fifties, ending a brilliant artistic career. His wife, Julia, and the children were devoted to him and financially able to construct a physical and social environment to simulate the activity of his previous existence. A chauffeur drove him to his studio. Young artists were employed to carry out the technical work associated with the production of his sculpture. Everything that money could buy was done to recreate his art world. Opening were even staged to show off new pieces at a local gallery.

As Arnold grew more impaired, he became unable to participate in any part of the artistic process. However, he was happy to watch the activity around him and continued to spend many hours each day in his studio. Julia Sands found it emotionally impossible to be with her husband as he deteriorated. Although she cared deeply for Arnold and took great pride in what the family did to keep him happy and comfortable, Julia had set up an emotional barricade between herself and Arnold after the diagnosis. She instructed her sons and daughters not to tell anyone what was wrong, and she withdrew from all of her friends, making excuses that the business was consuming her time and energy.

The entire family was concerned about her inability to accept the diagnosis and "go public" by letting her friends know about the Alzheimer's disease. Gradually, Julia became more irritable, drank heavily, and withdrew from many of her responsibilities in the family real estate business. Her children were able to take over at work, but they worried about her alcohol abuse. One evening Julia had a car accident while driving under the influence, injuring herself and a pedestrian. When she recovered, the family insisted she see a psychiatrist.

After several months of therapy Julia was able to deal honestly with the situation. Her fears of rejection were unrealistic, and her friends and family surrounded her with support that continued until her husband's death.

3. Hold Regular Family Meetings to Discuss How the Patient Is Functioning and Try to Anticipate Future Changes.

As long as the patient lives, the family will be caught emotionally between two different and changing worlds. One consists of memories of a time when the patient was an active, productive, and responsible member of the family or marriage partner. The second is the world of the present, in which the patient is changing and has diminished capacity to do many things. Families can help themselves by meeting to discuss the future needs and rights of various family members. Caring for someone with dementia changes the time family members have for other personal and social responsibilities. Meetings are the forum for relatives to begin negotiating their needs with one another and the patient.

Children should not be excluded from family discussions, but some may not wish to participate. The best way to proceed is to ask them and then accept their wishes. When they are included, they often show remarkable insights. Marion Talbot had been diagnosed with dementia for more than three years. Her husband and children were devoted to her, and together they did everything possible to keep Marion active and happy. Even Tim, her five-year-old grandson, showed a special involvement with his grandmother, visiting three or four days a week. On weekends, when Tim often spent the night, Marion would read him bedtime stories. As Marion's word-finding difficulties increased, Tim's father tried to prepare him for the changes in his grandmother by explaining that grandma could not read his books anymore because she had a disease that affected her ability to read and talk. Tim replied, "That's all right, you or Grandpa can join us. She can still hold me in her lap while you read the story to both of us! I like being with her."

Family cooperation in problem-solving activities around patient issues is not always easy. The larger the number of family members involved with the patient, the greater the room for family disagreements and arguments. These conflicts are not abnormal; indeed, they are necessary as different members voice divergent opinions and observations. The crucial variable is the family's ability finally to agree on solutions that represent the best interests of the patient as well as the family. By resolving problems together, families can achieve a sense of control over the situation. There are time-limited ways to control the dementia per se, but it is also possible to achieve an internal sense of limited mastery, which emerges from knowing that you have done everything in your power to deal with an impossible situation.

4. Do Not Blame the Patient or Yourself When Things Go Wrong and Your Frustration Level Is High.

Dementia changes the culture of family life. It is akin to living in a different country where you have to learn to find your way around strange places and learn a new layout. Everyone in the family needs to learn to change their roles and responsibilities as the dementia progresses. It is not the patient's fault or your fault when problems occur, emotions overwhelm you, or tempers flare.

George and Jennie Smith had just moved George's father with Alzheimer's disease into their home. A family ritual after dinner each night was to sit around the dining room table helping seven-year-old Janet and nine-year-old David with school homework. The older Mr. Smith would quickly become restless, pacing around the house in circles. George and Jennie would bring him back to the table, only to have him get more agitated.

After three nights George and Jennie were frustrated because it took so long to get the homework done. On the fourth night, Mr. Smith brought three bags of cookies to the table and emptied them out on David's book. George cursed his dad, told him to leave the table, and began sweeping the cookies off the book pages. David, however, took his grandfather by the hand and walked to the sofa in the living room, carrying his book. They sat down, and David opened the book to the middle where there was a map of the solar system. David took his grandfather's hand again and placed it on the page, asking "What world do you live in Pop-pop? I know part of you is here, but what part of you is somewhere else?"

5. Try to Sustain or Develop a Sense of Humor.

Humor is a healthy way to handle problems, and there are those who believe that it is better than any medication or elixir. Many daily circumstances and conversations elicit smiles and laughter. The ability to laugh at yourself and the world around you is therapeutic.

Larry Weiss had been diagnosed with Alzheimer's disease for about one year. He lived at home with his wife, Barbara. Both enjoyed living in their cottage on the lake. Larry could fish, work around the boat shed, and visit with friends at the marina. In the evenings when they did not entertain or visit friends, they would sit and read or watch television.

Each morning on rising, they would take a walk together around the lake. In the evenings when the weather was good, Larry would take Barbara out in the flatboat and row until he tired. Their time together had become even more precious since the doctor had told them that Larry probably had Alzheimer's disease. They were fearful of the uncertainty of the future, but they were both determined to enjoy their lives together as long as possible.

One evening in the fall, Larry and Barbara were getting dressed to go out on the lake. When Barbara entered the boat shed, she saw Larry standing with his hunter's vest on upside down and the life vest backward. He was struggling to put on a rain slicker, which would not fit over the life preserver. She burst out laughing, and within minutes both of them were laughing uncontrollably in each other's arms. Later, in the boat, Larry asked her what had been so funny. He had been unaware of what he was doing, and as Barbara described his actions, he became troubled. This was the part of the disease that scared him—that he could not do something as simple as dress himself.

Barbara admitted that she too was frightened but said that they could fight this disease together. For the moment and for the foreseeable future, they could still enjoy each other and find happiness and laughter.

Later, as they walked along the sandy beach near the dock, they watched a small puppy pull a large log along the beach. Larry walked over to the dog, dropped down on his hands and knees, eye to eye with the animal, and began to push the log with his head. Barbara froze in horror as she watched her husband. Within a few minutes Larry stood up and smiled broadly. She relaxed as she heard him say, "You're right, Barbara, it's good to play and be alive!"

6. When You Talk with Your Relative, It Is Sometimes More Important to Listen and Observe Than to Speak.

Part of the process of emotional distancing is to learn how to act like a paraprofessional. Since patients often have great difficulty with language or in remembering what happens around them, understanding of their needs and wants often requires you to become an "active listener." Observe and listen carefully. Sometimes it is helpful not to talk at all, but to give patients the time to speak or communicate in nonverbal ways what is on their mind.

Even the most devoted families may lose their ability to understand the patient and need help to rebalance their perspective of the patient's capabilities. Doris Watson had been caring for her husband, Alex, for more than ten years. Despite the dementia, she had kept him physically active. They walked six miles together each morning before breakfast. They played tennis and golf four or five times a week. They also went cycling and swimming every day at the health club. As Alex's dementia worsened, he could utter only a few words and required assistance with bathing and dressing. Doris began to leave him at home and did more activities on her own.

Alex became less active, gained weight, and began sleeping longer in the morning. Their friends continued to visit them at home, and several invited Alex to play tennis or golf. Doris discouraged their invitations, saying that Alex could no longer play well. However, Alex could still hit the ball and seemed thoroughly to enjoy the exercise. Doris refused to watch Alex play, insisting that her friends would grow tired of playing with him. They in turn were gently insistent that he was still a good partner. In the beginning Doris was insulted that her friends would challenge her ability to understand her husband. However, with time they were able to convince her that although Alex had changed, they still enjoyed his company and he theirs. Alex lost his excess weight, slept less, and regained his zest for doing things. Doris was grateful to her friends for helping her see Alex for the man he still was and for what he still had to give others.

7. *Honesty Is the Only Basis for a Relationship with Your Relative.*

Being honest is the first rule for treating a relative as a human being and a patient. Family members who learn to share the emotional burden of Alzheimer's disease with the patient can decrease the stresses and strains of daily life. Sharing the burden means working together and honestly accepting what the future brings, taking it one day at a time. Unfortunately, it is common for many family members to withhold the diagnosis or information from the patient, often for many years, or to refrain from answering a question many individuals ask—"Will I get worse?"

Being dishonest or avoiding answers creates psychological tension. Most, if not all, patients sense the discomfort or dishonesty on a nonverbal level. Some may respond by social withdrawal or retreating emotionally under the false assumption that this will make the family more comfortable. Patients' fears and anxieties then go unresolved and result in frustration, rage, and even violent acting out by the patients as well as their families.

Some patients place caregivers in a difficult position when they insist that no one outside the family be told about the dementia. This often forces the husband or wife into a stressful double existence—a social world where problems are denied and a personal and family world where problems are real. However, in both worlds tension increases because there is no basis for honest transactions in the family.

When the patient and family visit friends, shop, attend social events, or eat out, the family may be overprotective and make excuses for the patient rather than be honest with friends. However, as the dementia progresses, families may withdraw from social and leisure activities and become openly angry with the patient in public.

John Santini took his wife, Sonya, out to dinner four or five times a week because she enjoyed what had been a lifelong social pattern for them. Sonya had been diagnosed as having Alzheimer's disease but still enjoyed an active social life with her husband. And for many years after the diagnosis she had been a companion at business dinners. However, John was ashamed to tell anyone about the Alzheimer's disease. On those occasions when she had problems, he dismissed it with the excuse that she had had too much to drink.

As the disease progressed, John was becoming increasingly uncomfortable with his wife at business functions because of the way she dressed and acted. Sonya had begun to talk more at dinner and to giggle inappropriately, and sometimes she played with her food. One evening John exploded at his wife and stormed out of the restaurant when she insisted on pouring everyone's wine back into the bottle.

The Santinis' son, Frank, was successful in getting his father and mother to see someone. Frank was distressed that most of his father's friends thought his mother was an alcoholic. After several months the members of the Santini family were able to successfully confront the Alzheimer's disease and to do shuttle diplomacy with their friends and dispel the image of alcoholism.

8. Just as Parents Provide Consistency, Love, Security, and a Sense of Order for Children, So Do Family Members Provide a Stable Emotional Environment for the Patient.

Hundreds of books have been written about infant and child development and caring for children. Recently, more books have become available about aging and caring for older adults with health problems such as dementia. Many families are traveling in uncharted regions, trying to do the best they can, often walking a narrow trail between knowing and not knowing what to do. Sometimes they stumble onto answers by trial and error, sometimes knowledgeable experts or other families provide useful advice.

Patients with dementia often fear being isolated, rejected, and abandoned. This fear may be present even in the early phases of dementia and in the strongest of family relationships. Consequently, when caregivers have difficulty with their own emotional reactions and become so overwhelmed that they withdraw or avoid interactions with the patient, they cause significant reactions in the patient.

Jim Ricci and his wife, Gina, had been married for over forty years and raised ten children, all of whom were grown and married. After Jim was diagnosed as having Alzheimer's disease, Gina insisted that she was able to assume the additional responsibilities of the family business she and Jim had run together as partners. The children tried to persuade their parents to interview candidates to help them manage affairs, but neither would hear of it.

During the first year following the diagnosis, Gina and Jim quarreled more. Mario, the oldest son, and Anne Marie, the oldest daughter, who lived closest to their parents, had stopped by the store frequently throughout the years, and both became concerned about the increasing tension between their parents.

Mario and Anne Marie agreed that the first tactic was to talk with their parents separately—Mario to their mother and Anne Marie to their father. Afterward they would compare notes and plan accordingly. It was immediately obvious that Gina was frustrated and confused by her husband's behavior. She wanted to ask him to do things at the store, such as stock the shelves and inventory the items, and although Jim would agree to her request, he would then do something else. It was not his making mistakes in occasional confused periods that upset her; it was what she described as his deliberately doing something else to make her angry.

Jim was slow to confide in his daughter, and it was not until both Mario and Anne Marie cornered him at the store alone that the story began to emerge. Jim was deeply concerned about his memory losses and afraid that Gina would want to sell the store if she knew how much his difficulties troubled him. Jim was reluctant to do many tasks around the store because he was afraid of making errors, when in fact he was quite capable. The memory lapses were sporadic, and Gina was so sensitive to these periods that she would simply take over. Jim was embarrassed and ashamed that his wife would have to see him helpless and incompetent. He also secretly feared that she might begin to reject him.

Jim admitted that it was perhaps foolish for him to imagine that Gina would suddenly stop loving him after so many years. But he was beginning to dislike himself, and if he felt this way, she certainly could as well. Because Jim was so uncomfortable, rather than talk to his wife, he simply walked away from many tasks. This triggered arguments, which were becoming more frequent. Jim admitted to being ashamed, and since he was angry at the whole situation, he exploded at Gina. He felt trapped.

Mario and Anne Marie invited their parents to dinner and afterward spoke of what they had seen happening to their parents and expressed their desire to help. Both Gina and Jim were relieved by their children's intervention, although they admitted embarrassment that their own children could discern what they could not.

Gina and Jim continued to work in the store for several years. Jim became more comfortable asking for help, and they both agreed to hire someone to manage the store as well as a few salesmen, so that they could get away and travel as long as Jim was only mildly affected.

Alzheimer's disease can threaten even loving family ties that have existed for many years. Patients may consciously or unconsciously test the strength of their family bonds, somewhat in the way adolescents test parents. This analogy with children is used not to infantilize the patients but to emphasize the strong reactions and needs of individuals after the diagnosis. Some may repeatedly express a wish to die or a desire to kill themselves, a tactic reminiscent of many teenagers. Other patients may become angry and irritable and argue over trivial issues to get attention. If a relative is behaving in unusual ways, it may be difficult to determine whether there is a psychological or medical explanation for the behavior or whether it is a result of the dementia. Discussing a relative's behaviors with a professional may be helpful in seeking to understand disturbing threats and behaviors. A verbalized desire to die is deeply disturbing to the caregiver. However, it may be a way for the patient to communicate emotional pain, to get a loved one to say that he or she is needed and wanted.

Suicidal ideation is frequently observed in persons with dementia, but successful suicides are very rare. The existing literature suggests that 8 to 10 percent of depressed individuals living in the community may be at risk, and 5 to 10 percent attempt suicide. Expressions of the wish to die should not be ignored, and a mental health evaluation should be considered. Depression coexists in 30 to 60 percent of persons with dementia, and if undiagnosed and untreated leads to suicidal thoughts and behaviors. Suicide is discussed in greater detail in Chapter 13.

As the dementia progresses, many of the cognitive losses and behavioral changes cause extreme embarrassment for patients. Even persons with advanced dementia may be angry and ashamed. This anger may be expressed in strange ways because of the dementia and thus be misdirected at the caregiver.

It is hard to be supportive of someone who is difficult to live with. Sometimes the task may seem impossible. Remember, patients are adults who experience shame and hurt when they cannot finish a sentence, complete routine tasks, or do things that once came easily. Whereas babies must feel great relief when they wet their diaper, adults who have an accident and need help can only be deeply ashamed. Dealing with the humanity of shame and anger is one of the toughest challenges for families.

Although strong infant-parent bonds develop with the feeding, dressing, changing, holding, and playing as the child grows, different feelings and obligations may arise out of the daily activities of helping an impaired adult. The bond may be broken slowly by the demands of caring. Or a new intimacy may be achieved as the patient and caregivers adapt to different roles, which may be demanding but also fulfilling. Setting goals is an important step to maximize your well-being and that of your relative.

Setting Goals

The patient with Alzheimer's disease has many needs—physical, emotional, and social. The belief that patients cannot participate in their care and are untreatable often leads to an exclusive reliance on drugs and a failure to use other techniques that can be effective.

So where do you begin? Perhaps the first step is to define a clear set of plans. The process of establishing goals is helpful because it enables you to think of your relative both as a patient with specific disabilities and needs and as an individual who is a partner and who can make certain contributions to the family.

Goal 1: Evaluate the Patient's Ability to Work, as Well as Your Own.

In the beginning the individual-turned-patient can manage alone or with minimal help around the house or even at work. When Alzheimer's disease strikes a middle-aged or older adult who is still employed, the individual is usually not able to continue on the job. Indeed, the cognitive losses that ultimately bring about the diagnostic evaluation usually have disrupted the individual's ability to perform effectively, despite ingenious attempts to compensate for and hide these losses. Although the patient may be able to continue part-time work, this often requires an extremely supportive network of friends. Some individuals have worked as salesmen in stores or as volunteers in hospitals, social agencies, or libraries, and some have even continued to tutor children in art, music, and other school subjects.

The patient's continued ability to work needs to be evaluated carefully in terms of safety and competence. What is the nature of the individual's work history, accomplishments, and motivations to continue any type of work? What resources or opportunities are available for the creation of a viable structured work situation for the patient? How acceptable are any arrangements with current or prospective employers?

In certain instances it is imperative to discourage the patients from working, whereas in others there may be merit in supporting continued employment. In many jobs impaired individuals cannot perform the work safely or the level of impairment is so high that adequate performance is not possible. However, in some situations individuals can go to their place of work and feel that they still have a place to go with people they know and enjoy, when in reality they can no longer work. Many businesses, schools, law firms, and even factories have supported the presence of impaired partners or former employees.

Patients and families may find it very difficult to deal with the dilemmas of retirement from work. Virginia Rich and her husband, Dale, both aged fifty-five, lived together in a small town. Dale recently was diagnosed as having Alzheimer's disease, after the completion of the full series of diagnostic evaluations in another state. He and his wife deliberately flew out of town to hide the situation from their friends and from Dale's employer. Dale was determined to continue to work as long as he was able to drive safely and handle his accounts. Virginia helped her husband with the paperwork in the evenings, but she was concerned about his ability to continue to drive safely as the dementia progressed. Fortunately, Dale was senior enough that he did not have to take on any new accounts, and at least for a while he was able to handle all of his old clients successfully.

Dale and Virginia decided that they would take each day as it came. Dale agreed to see a psychologist and have his ability to drive evaluated by a series of tests. As long as he passed these examinations, he would continue to drive. And as long as he felt comfortable talking with his old clients and with Virginia's help on the books, he could keep going.

Although Dale continued to work for more than a year after the diagnosis, Virginia began to feel more and more frustrated. She worried about the future and became increasingly distressed from the isolation, having no one with whom to share her concerns. She could not speak with her friends or even join the local Alzheimer's self-help group because Dale's diagnosis was a secret.

How could they balance Dale's need to continue working and to feel worthwhile with Virginia's need to support her husband and also be supported in her caregiving role? Two years after receiving the diagnosis, Dale finally retired voluntarily. He had to do so because his speech and memory problems had worsened and it was dangerous for him to drive. When he failed his last driving test with the psychologist, Virginia urged him to retire. She wanted him alive, and the risk of a car accident was too great.

A number of serious work dilemmas emerge for working caregivers. A husband or wife may continue to work until the needs of the patient force him or her to stop. If the caregiver is fortunate enough to be financially capable of paying for home help, he or she may continue to work. However, even in these situations the emotional toll affects the productivity and efficiency of the healthy spouse in the work role.

Children involved in the care of their parents or relatives may lose time from work and feel torn between loyalty to their parents and the need to support themselves and their family. The oldest daughter or daughter-in-law seems to inherit or assume the role of primary caregiver when a parent is affected. The combined pressures of parent caring, family, and job can be intense. About one-quarter of working women shorten their work hours and another quarter quit work to care for an impaired parent.

Jean and Armand Ansel had been struggling to build their own lives and to care for their parents over the past nine years. Armand's eighty-five-year-old mother had a history of strokes over the years, and Jean's seventy-year-old father had Alzheimer's disease. They had placed Armand's mother, a widow of fifteen years, in a nursing home six months earlier because she could no longer live at home. The cost of a twenty-four-hour home attendant had depleted their resources, and another stroke had further debilitated her. Jean's father, Pierre, continued to live alone in his cooperative apartment several miles away from his children. Since he was one of the few men in the apartment complex where he had lived as a widower for more than ten years, several ladies and a few men formed a tight group of friends who helped him get along each day.

However, as Pierre's condition began to deteriorate, Jean and Armand found themselves making daily visits in the evening to check on Pierre. Furthermore, without Armand's knowledge Jean began to visit Pierre's apartment over the lunch hour and also called him several times daily. Jean's distress began to interfere with her performance at work.

Jean was an administrative assistant to the president of a large corporation. She was brilliant in her job and was able to keep up with her work and with Pierre, at least for a while. After several months Jean's boss invited her to lunch to find out why she had begun to have so much trouble on the job. Jean had made significant errors in his calendar and in travel arrangements. Business files were incomplete for administrative meetings, and she was neglecting several important projects. Jean's boss suggested she take several weeks off to deal with her family problem and find another living situation for her father-in-law.

To avoid problems at the office or job, it is often helpful to sit down with your boss or supervisor, apprise him or her of the situation, and if necessary, ask for some time off to get family affairs organized. Time invested in planning after the diagnosis will pay off later. The amount of time off from work is necessarily limited, and you will have to juggle work deadlines with the immediacy of family demands. Work-life issues during the course of caregiving are discussed in Chapter 15.

Goal 2: Choose the Primary Caregiver.

Although this may sound simple, it is important to decide who the primary caregiver or caregivers will be. Even in situations in which the patient has a living husband or wife at home, the spouse's physical and mental health may limit his or her capacity to be responsible for the patient on a daily basis. Family discussions should focus on this topic. The primary caregiver lives with demanding daily responsibilities, and even a healthy, dedicated spouse will need help. It is not unusual for small groups of people in the family, such as a daughter and son-in-law or several children, to function as primary caregivers. Primary caregivers may also change with time. In some families in which the patient is alone, children and other relatives may decide to rotate caring responsibilities in order to give each person time off on a regular basis.

Goal 3: Take a Good Look at Family Relationships and How Your Family Operates.

Care planning and caregiving occur in the context of the family system. Take a close look at your family. Every family is different, and not all family members are able or willing to work together caring for a relative with dementia. However, to be effective you need to understand the talents, liabilities, and availability of who is or who ought to be involved. The size, composition, structure, and resources of your family affect your ability to mobilize individuals to be involved in the plan of care. These factors include divorce and remarriage, geographical distance, economics, previous conflicts, solidarity, and differences in values and beliefs. The complexities of family caregiving, including marital strain, sibling rivalry, intergenerational commitments, and ethnic and cultural issues are reviewed in Chapter 9.

Goal 4: Assess Whether Disturbed Family Relationships May Disrupt the Routine.

A number of family problems may surface if the Alzheimer's patient has had a strained, disturbed, or severed relationship with a spouse, son, daughter, brother, sister, or any other significant relative or friend. Conflicts, arguments, and disagreements occur in every relationship. However, marital problems, separation, divorce, intense sibling rivalry, angry relationships between parents and children, or any combination of emotionally discordant relationships among family members can stand in the way of helping the patient.

Caring for an Alzheimer's patient can be complicated by any number of disruptive situations. When a husband or wife separates or divorces a patient, conflict with children and other family members may result. Children and spouses from previous marriages of the patient may be excluded from contact with the patient by the present family. An estranged adult child of the patient may refuse to visit the patient and cause additional emotional distress for the patient as well as the entire family.

A trained professional or clergyman is a valuable source of help for the entire family in dealing with these situations. When relationships have been estranged or significant legal, financial, or personal catastrophes have occurred in the family, attempts at reconciliation are not usually successful. It is important to focus on mobilizing family members and others who can work together.

Goal 5: Establish a Structured Daily Routine.

The development of a structured daily routine is perhaps one of the most important tasks to be accomplished. Since dementia gradually impairs patients' abilities to plan activities and do things for themselves and others, an organized schedule keeps them active and involved to the limits of their abilities. Furthermore, a structured routine helps maintain the patients' abilities and develops a sense of security and accomplishment.

Setting up a routine requires an accurate analysis of the patients' capabilities as well as of the families' resources. Unfortunately, many families and their physicians encourage a premature dependency and reinforce a helplessness that often leads to the "one-person nursing home." It is natural to worry about relatives' safety and their reliability in carrying out various tasks. The mistake is to allow these feelings to interfere unnecessarily with the individuals' freedom to function and express themselves. These are tough decisions. The patient has the right to continue to live as independently as possible. Likewise, the patient is only one member of a family system in which other individuals also have legitimate rights and needs.

Negotiations regarding the patient's limitations arouse feelings of discomfort in caregivers and feelings of anger and sadness in the patient. The patient has losses that require alterations in lifestyle. Just as an individual with a broken neck or back is restricted in many activities, the individual with dementia must deal with the reality of undeniable limitations. Facing these life changes is painful, but one can deal with these feelings by implementing a plan of action and by living one day at a time.

Since the patient will change over time, the daily routine inevitably will need to be altered. If changes are anticipated in advance and alternative solutions are prepared, the patient and family members will feel more in control of changes as they occur.

A psychological evaluation by a professional will determine the patient's strengths and weaknesses and assets and liabilities. This information is the basis on which to recommend life and work roles for the patient. Although memory and attention losses often make the successful completion of such household tasks as cooking, cleaning, and shopping impossible, individuals nonetheless may be able to perform some portion of these tasks. An impaired adult may be incapable of doing the weekly shopping but may derive enormous satisfaction from running a simple errand, such as buying a loaf of bread or a quart of milk. Cognitive testing highlights the skills an individual retains during the progression of the illness. It also gives the family or caregivers a realistic baseline for what to expect from the patient, whether at home or in an institutional environment.

Remember that dementia is often a slowly progressing disease. In most patients not only are the losses gradual, but also a number of intellectual skills are preserved for years. Individuals are not immediately and totally incapacitated. Furthermore, many everyday activities require little in the way of higher-order reasoning and thinking. Some of the most important and rewarding experiences in our lives are the special times we share with those we love by simply being together.

Amy and Archie Thompson had lived together for more than thirty-five years. At the age of sixty Archie began to complain of memory problems. He also had trouble finding words and finishing his sentences. This went on for six years before he and the entire family decided that a complete speech and hearing evaluation was in order.

The results documented what Archie and his family already knew. Now there was a technical report that described his language disturbance as an aphasia. Archie's internist, who gave him a clean bill of physical health, insisted on a neurological examination. The neurologist informed them that Archie probably had Alzheimer's disease. The entire family was deeply concerned, except for Archie.

In a subsequent family meeting Archie tried to tell everyone that he was coming to grips with the dementia. Yes, the day he heard the diagnosis he felt numb. However, as he walked to the car after leaving the neurologist's office, a trivial event occurred that had a special personal significance. A bright red leaf fell in his hand. Its simple beauty was overwhelming. Archie stumbled over his words as he tried to tell his family how he identified with that leaf. He and the leaf were both old. It was autumn and the leaf had aged, turned color, and was dying in resplendent color. He, too, was growing older, and now he had a disease that would someday affect him greatly. But for now he simply felt rich and proud to be surrounded by his family. "If only I could turn a bright color and you could look at me and say, 'How beautiful!'"

Archie was able to live with his speech problems. There was much he could still do. He and Amy lived in a small country town. He enjoyed working in the yard and also derived special pleasure doing carpentry in the basement workroom. His great love, however, was his personal computer, and he would spend hours in the den. Although Archie had difficulty with some of the computer programs, he still enjoyed many of the computer games, especially the airplane cockpit simulations. He had been a pilot in World War II and the Korean War, and his hours at the computer brought back memories of times past.

Goal 6: Establish and Maintain a Program of Physical Exercise for the Patient.

Physical activity is important. A simple daily program including walks, jogging, gardening, exercise regimens, or even dancing can maintain the patient's physical condition and contribute to a restful night's sleep. Exercise may reduce the need for sedative medication and will also help the patient maintain a healthy appetite. Sports like golf, tennis, and swimming can be especially therapeutic for the individual who enjoyed such physical activities before the onset of the illness.

Some patients and families have arranged the entire day's schedule around exercise. Although Karen Hart, aged fifty-eight, had been diagnosed six years earlier, she and her husband, Calvin, continued to play golf and tennis together daily throughout the year. What changed after the diagnosis was the amount of time devoted to physical activity. Each morning they did thirty minutes of calisthenics before breakfast, and after eating they jogged and walked two miles around the neighborhood. This was followed by a tennis game or golf. In the afternoon they went to the health club to work out on the equipment and swim. This was also an opportunity for Calvin to leave his wife for a few hours and have some time alone. He had met with the health spa staff after the diagnosis and informed them of his wife's problem. From the beginning everyone was supportive, and indeed amazed at her physical endurance and stamina.

Not everyone can afford a health spa or tennis club, but there are many other ways to get exercise, such as following along with exercise shows on television, gardening, riding a stationary bicycle, and taking long walks. Even when the patient has had dementia for years and is severely impaired, physical exercise and walking should be programmed several times a day, ideally after each meal. This not only is conducive to good physical health but also gives the individual a sense of personal achievement. As cognitive powers diminish, many patients report taking great pride in physical accomplishments. Feeling good about oneself is a cognitive act.

Goal 7: Monitor the Patient's General Health.

Keeping physically healthy is an important aspect of care. Patients who are as comfortable as possible will be much more able to function at their best. Since many patients cannot explain aches and pains and other phys ical problems, the caregiver must be attentive to their physical well-being.

Francis Coco had been hospitalized for over a year. None of the local nursing homes would admit him because he screamed much of the day and was a difficult patient to manage. Mr. Coco had a vascular dementia but had originally been admitted to the hospital a year earlier when he fell and broke his hip. Multiple medical complications had developed in the intervening months.

In the tenth month of hospitalization, Mr. Coco became a "screamer," raving whenever someone entered his room. In the course of each day, the screaming decreased in the afternoon and evening as he became hoarse. The yelling was especially intense when his wife visited. The only way to quiet Mr. Coco was to give him his Bible or prayer book. However, there were days when this did not console him either.

Mrs. Coco insisted that something was wrong with her husband, but everyone—the doctors, nurses, and social workers—insisted that his screaming was part of the disease and that they hoped to get him into a good nursing home. Finally, Mrs. Coco was successful in locating a geriatric specialist for a consultation.

On the day of the visit, Mr. Coco had just finished lunch before the doctor entered the room with his wife. The doctor sat down and introduced himself, whereupon Mr. Coco began to scream, showering the doctor with food and saliva. Mr. Coco continued to yell, but the doctor said nothing and wiped the food from his face. After a few minutes the screaming stopped, and Mr. Coco only stared hard at the doctor. The doctor began his examination with Mr. Coco's quiet consent. It was not until he moved Mr. Coco's leg that the patient screamed in pain. A review of the chart revealed that he had a history of phlebitis, and further tests revealed that it was clearly a current problem. Psychological studies also revealed that Mr. Coco was capable of reading and writing and that he retained skills which nobody had imagined because of his difficult behavior.

Mr. Coco's phlebitis was controlled successfully, and the staff members were able to maintain some limited conversation with him. The screaming stopped, and for the first time Mr. Coco seemed happy. However, placement in a nursing home was still necessary because of the heavy nursing care he required. Within a short time, an appropriate institution was found, and Mr. Coco lived out the next two years comfortably.

Patients with Alzheimer's disease become more susceptible to infections and other illnesses because of a weakened immune system. Regular checkups with the family doctor will avert many types of health hazards. The patient's health program should also include good hygiene, a suitable exercise program, dental care, and a balanced diet. A carefully managed health program may avoid an unnecessary drop in functioning as a result of problems with vision, diet, or teeth or of any other problems otherwise unrecognized.

In the early stages of Alzheimer's disease, patients do not appear to be physically less healthy than the rest of the older population. In its later stages, though, especially when patients are long-term residents in nursing homes, multiple physical illnesses incapacitate them and often severely limit their activities. However, certain exercises to maintain body tone and circulation can be done in bed or a wheelchair. Ask your doctor to recommend a physical therapist and also consult some of the caregiver books in the reading list. When patients do become ill, they should be treated with at least as much care as other members of the family. Caregivers should never feel shy about using the medical profession when needed. It is important to remember that a commonplace illness can be more dangerous for persons with dementia than for a healthy person.

Goal 8: Monitor the Patient's Vision and Hearing.

Sight and hearing should be tested at least once a year. As the dementia progresses, it will become more and more difficult for an ophthalmologist and audiologist to evaluate vision and hearing because of poor cognition and unreliable responses. Patients are not always capable of answering the questions posed by the examiner, for example, "Is this sound higher or lower than the last sound?" or "Can you hear this sound?" or "Which letters are clearer—the letters on the right or the letters on the left?" Alert the doctor to the problem. Ask him or her to make the procedure and the questions as simple as possible. Inquire about the availability of special tests designed for young children. Consult with specialists in your area who work with autistic children or developmentally disabled children, since special procedures developed to test sensory acuity in learning-disabled children may be modified for adults with dementia.

Goal 9: Monitor the Patient's Emotional Health.

Many people lead relatively functional lives for years after the diagnosis. They find their own ways of coping with the dementia and with the major changes that occur in their personal and family lives. Others, however, develop emotional disorders. Depression and anxiety, which lower the ability to think clearly, are the most common ones and are usually treatable. Successful treatment of emotional problems does not correct the intellectual losses caused by Alzheimer's disease, but it often helps the patients function at the highest possible level.

Rebecca Hunt became extremely agitated when she was unable to dress herself or when she forgot her thoughts in the middle of a sentence. Her husband and children tried hard to help and comfort her, but

Rebecca usually burst into tears and ran from the room. "I just seem to go to pieces . . . I feel so awful," she said in a family interview. "Sometimes I feel good, and then, when it gets to be too much, I go all to pieces, and I want to die."

Mrs. Hunt was successfully treated by her physician for her anxiety. In addition, she and her family identified a number of tasks that were not too difficult for her to perform. As time went by, Mrs. Hunt became more comfortable asking for help. She and her husband even rehearsed together what they would do if she forgot her thoughts or said inappropriate things when they were out in public. Mr. Hunt would put his arm around her and pat her shoulder. This anticipatory coping gave them both a sense that they were at least prepared to deal with the future.

When symptoms of anxiety and depression occur, they should be treated as soon as possible. They may include loss of appetite, irritability or apathy, hyperactivity or a marked slowing in behavior, changes in sleep pattern, and often a noticeable drop in cognitive status (see Chapter 10). If you think the patient might be suffering from serious depression or anxiety, seek help from a psychiatric clinic, community mental health center, or mental health practitioner. If there are no professionals knowledgeable about geriatrics in your community, contact a self-help group near you or the Alzheimer's Association office for information (see Appendix 1).

Goal 10: Make Living Areas More Accessible in Your Home.

The home environment may have to be rearranged, or in some cases even remodeled, to make the living space more usable by the patient. Many activities—dressing, eating, bathing, resting, doing housework, and playing—can be hampered without these alterations. Changing the environment also allows the patient to exert more direct control over his or her world and be as independent as possible. Take time to examine the physical environment of your home, room by room. If available, an architect or home designer may be useful (although perhaps costly) to help you identify ways to make the physical environment more accessible. Chapter 8 provides some guidelines for evaluating ways to change your home to make it barrier-free and more comfortable and safe for the patient.

The following case illustrates the dramatic impact of certain simple environmental changes even in later stages of dementia. Harold Jacobs had been diagnosed as having Alzheimer's nine years earlier and lived with his wife, Angela, in a small house along a ship canal. Angela left him at home while she went to work each day, and neighbors would check on Harold during lunch and in the late afternoon. He enjoyed sitting in the backyard watching the boats or gardening.

They had managed well together until he began to deteriorate significantly in the ninth year. Angela came home one day to find some neighborhood children in front of their house making fun of her husband, who was shrieking at them and striking the fence with a small garden tool. She chased them away angrily. Angela was deeply shaken to see her husband act like a wild man. She was afraid to unlock the gate.

A neighbor and close friend heard the disturbance and brought Angela to her home, where together they watched Harold from the window. After he calmed down, they went outside. Harold waved to them and seemed not to remember anything that happened. He lay down to sleep for several hours while Angela talked with her neighbor.

It was time to get help. Angela did not want to place Harold in a nursing home, but there seemed to be no choice. She had to continue working to pay the bills. The neighbors were willing to watch over Harold, but his violent behavior was frightening. Angela was also scared, angry, and embarrassed. She was troubled by the change in Harold's behavior. Angela did not understand his rage until her neighbors told her about some experiences their children had had while checking on him. Three teenagers had taken turns looking in on him over the years. Recently, on several occasions they found Harold clinging to the front gate, shaking it violently. They were afraid to enter the yard because he acted so crazy. The day Angela discovered them, several strange teenagers had begun to tease him.

A plan emerged one weekend when several neighbors were visiting. Harold's closest friend and neighbor, George, noticed that over the last few months he had become more restless. Harold paced around the yard and appeared lost and scared. George suggested that he would build a porch on the back of their house and enclose it with glass. The sunporch would give Harold a comfortable place to sit and watch the boats, and perhaps he would feel more secure in a more structured environment.

The solution worked. For the next year Harold seemed happy to sit on the porch, which gave him a magnificent view of the water. Angela was able to continue working with the close support of her neighbors and friends. A year later Harold died peacefully in his sleep at home.

Goal 11: Examine Your Financial Situation and Get Help to Plan for the Future.

Financial planning is often the last issue with which family members want to be bothered after the diagnosis. The newly diagnosed person will usually still be competent to handle money matters and may remain so for some time. In these cases family members may feel uncomfortable talking about money matters. However, as difficult as this may be, financial concerns should be taken up as soon as possible, while the individual is still capable of participating in the decision making. If financial planning is delayed, the family could find itself in economic trouble when it is too late to do anything.

Since caring for the patient usually becomes more of a burden than caregivers can handle alone, home attendants, assisted living, or a nursing home usually become necessary at some stage. These options are expensive and inevitably drain the family's resources. Chapter 15 includes a discussion of what Medicare and Medicaid will and will not cover; it also reviews the usefulness of Medigap insurance, long-term-care insurance, and other health insurance alternatives. With early financial planning, the family may be able to arrange its finances so that it can feel confident in paying for a relative's care and having a more secure future.

Because the legal and financial problems are complex, families should get legal advice to make the best decisions for their particular situation. Patients also have a right to make decisions about their assets, and this can be done only while they have the capacity to sign legally binding documents. Planning ahead and taking action before the dementia incapacitates patients and before crises occur will prevent unnecessary emotional distress, protect assets, and avert needless legal proceedings.

You can gather some basic information even when it may be difficult to talk about money matters. At the very minimum you should know the things listed below. Set up a worksheet of what you have and what you need to know.

1. Where the patient keeps his or her will, bankbooks, insurance policies, stock certificates and bonds, treasury bills, real estate documents, and other important papers
2. Social Security and Medicare numbers
3. Name, address, and phone numbers of his or her lawyer, insurance agents, financial advisor, and accountant
4. Names and addresses of banks, numbers of checking and savings accounts, and location of safe-deposit box
5. Names of life, health, homeowners, and other insurance companies as well as numbers of the policies
6. With whom he or she has a pension plan, IRAs, Keogh, profit sharing, deferred compensation, or other retirement plans

You may be able to work out an arrangement whereby you help your relative organize his or her financial matters and pay bills. Consider the following:

1. Arrange to have access to the safe-deposit box so that you can get important papers in the event your relative is hospitalized.
2. Consider a joint bank account so that you can get cash for your relative's emerging needs.
3. Arrange to pay insurance premiums so that policies will not lapse, and make sure you know what terms are in effect when your relative dies.
4. Find out when bills are due—rent or mortgage, taxes, utilities, credit card and charge accounts—and offer to sit down once a month to help write out the checks.
5. Make sure Social Security checks, interest checks, and other sources of income are deposited in your relative's account. The easiest way to ensure that Social Security checks are not lost is to have the patient sign Form SF-1199, authorizing the Social Security Administration to send the check directly to the bank.

It is frightening when you first realize that your relative is making financial errors—losing or not depositing checks, writing large checks that bounce, forgetting to pay bills. It can also be upsetting to try to work with your relative to handle financial matters as he or she becomes more impaired. However, it is vital to monitor the income and outflow of money and to manage assets to protect the patient and yourself.

How do you judge when it is time to intervene with your relative? This is a difficult philosophical and legal issue, as well as a personal one. However, it is better to discuss this question within the family, including the patient when possible, rather than to let the courts decide it after the patient has significantly deteriorated. At some point your relative may become unwilling and unable to manage money or to do what is necessary to protect assets. Lack of proper maintenance of his or her life may harm your relative or others. Remember, help in these instances provides crucial protection.

There are several ways of dealing with financial problems. Each involves giving to someone else a degree of control over the patient's assets. This may be a member of the family, a close friend, or an institution. The crucial variable is that this be someone who is trusted. Furthermore, expert advice is necessary because the alternatives available vary from state to state. Chapter 15 describes some of the alternatives available in different parts of the country. Regardless of which option you choose to pursue, it is important that you recognize the need for examining the choices open to you.

Goal 12: In Addition to Publications on Alzheimer's Disease and Related Disorders, Read Other Literature.

Edith Shelley, who at the age of seventy-five had been diagnosed for sixteen months, spoke about the impact of reading Eudora Welty's "A Worn Path" and *One Writer's Beginnings*. "A Worn Path," the story of a grandmother's love in spite of poverty and frailty, helped Mrs. Shelley talk to her grandchildren about her fears of rejection.

However, the book *One Writer's Beginnings* troubled her because it evoked sad longing for the life that was being taken away from her. But after laboring to read the book several times, Mrs. Shelley spoke insistently about an important message for Alzheimer's patients in Welty's work:

The book has helped me to review my own childhood, my relationship with my parents and to think about those moments in life that are precious to me. It also allowed me to gently face my eventual loss of memory and still dare to live. My memory is the treasure most dearly regarded by me. Eudora Welty helped me put my losses in perspective: "Memory is a living thing, and it too is in transit. But during its movement, all that is remembered joins and lives, the old and the young, the past and the present, the living and the dead." As you know, I am a woman who, like Ms. Welty, came of a sheltered life. "A sheltered life can be a daring life as well. For all serious daring starts from within."

Several books, monographs, and articles have been written about dementia and its impact on the patient, the family, and society. The reference section at the end of this book offers a selected reading list. In the early phases of dementia the patient may want to read what has been published. When small print, poor vision, or limited reading skills make this difficult, read to the patient or summarize some of the material for him or her.

Although handbooks on Alzheimer's disease contain information about practical problems and solutions, it is important to read other material—adventures and mysteries, romance, science fiction, short stories, commentary, drama, and poetry. Literature provides a resource for reflecting on the personal challenge of growing older and living with Alzheimer's disease. Reading is also an escape, a hobby, and a source of great pleasure to many. It may remain an important part of the patient's life. For those with visual problems, there are talking books, and many books are available on cassettes or records.

Alzheimer's disease changes everything in the patients' life, forcing them and their family to live what one patient called a "speeded-up version of life." Max DuBois responded to the diagnosis of dementia by making a list of everything he wanted to accomplish before the dementia made these goals impossible. Max wanted to live the good times left to him by keeping busy and conducting his affairs as usual: "I do not want to live an imitation of life just because I have this disease. There are books to be read, plays and movies to be seen, and time to be spent with my wife, children, and grandchildren. I also want to go to London one more time . . . to say good-bye."

Max traveled to London with his wife, Jean, and on his return began to collect every book he could about the city—travel guides, photography books, even novels about London. His library expenditures became part of the family's weekly budget, and even when Max could no longer read his books, he seemed to enjoy collecting them. Jean reported that in the later stages of the illness, when he became agitated, she would sit with him in the library and read excerpts from a "London book." This calmed him, and often he fell asleep next to her. Jean seemed to derive great comfort from feeling that Max had lovely dreams about the city, where they had first met and married.

Many books are not only entertaining and inspiring but also tools for understanding and coping with the future (See "Bibliotherapy" in the reference list). Patients and families who seem to adapt best are those who anticipate many of their future problems and conceive alternative solutions. Many also attribute their successful coping style to the growth and self-awareness that come from reading. Books help them focus on the challenge of finding joy and pleasure and meaning in their daily lives. Reading becomes an outlet for private emotions and fantasies, a way to reassess their own nurturing needs.

The choice of reading material depends on many factors—health, educational interests and preferences, as well as special needs for tapes and recorders. A number of resources are available in many community libraries, community centers, and hospitals, and senior citizen organizations may offer special guided-reading programs. Many hospitals and long-term-care facilities have programs in bibliotherapy for patients who are hospitalized or institutionalized. *Bibliotherapy* is the use of selected reading materials and specific techniques to help individuals deal with personal problems. Here a trained librarian, teacher, or counselor evaluates the individuals' literary needs and involves them in private or group reading sessions. Even illiterate patients can be brought into group reading sessions.

Bibliotherapy proved to be a valuable addition to family therapy sessions with the relatives of Harry James, who had been institutionalized for six years with dementia. Harry and several members of his family were Holocaust survivors. Everyone in the family had strong feelings of isolation and great difficulty in accepting Harry's extended deterioration.

The institution's librarian suggested that Harry's grandson Hy read *Mr. Sammler's Planet* by Saul Bellow. The novel shows how Mr. Sammler, a seventy-two-year-old Holocaust survivor, successfully adapts to the alien environment of Manhattan in the 1960s. After Hy read the book, he suggested that the entire family do so, and that became the focus of discussions about Harry and their own feelings of disassociation. Even though Harry was bedridden with advanced dementia and unable to participate in family sessions, members of his family found that their reactions to the Bellow novel allowed them to sort through their feelings as individuals and as a family and to deal emotionally with Harry's psychological death and the pending physical death.

Goal 13: Locate a Family Support Group in Your Area.

Alzheimer's disease family support groups exist all over the United States and much of the world. Most of them are chapters of the national Alzheimer's Association. Information about national and international organizations can be found in Appendix 1. The Alzheimer's Association can put you in touch with a local group or even help you organize a group if one is not conveniently located near you.

The experience of participating in or organizing a family support group is a valuable one. Groups provide the opportunity for families to discover others with common problems. Members provide essential support and help each other cope with the many changes in their personal and family life. The following excerpt from a letter describes one wife's experience with a group of caregivers:

> I am thankful for the family group. When I first joined I felt hope for the first time. It may sound strange, but seeing others with the same problem gave me hope for the future. Their strength gave me the confidence to face my own problems. I knew that I was no longer alone.
>
> Some people were worse off than I was. I realized that I could reach out and help them, and I felt better. It was as if I could make part of me whole again by helping others.
>
> With time I came to appreciate the group more and more. I was able to talk freely. I did not have to hold anything inside.

They understood my anger and my sadness. I could cry and not feel ashamed. And whenever I felt down I could call someone.

The group has given Jim and me a sense of being connected again. I used to feel alone and abandoned like a sailor who had fallen overboard during the night.

Groups are a safe place to talk. Family members can express many complicated feelings and not be afraid that others will misunderstand or think unkindly of them. For example, it is common to feel anger toward the patient or even wish that he or she were dead. This is the kind of feeling that should be shared with others because such feelings are normal. Hearing this same message firsthand from others in similar situations is even more powerful. Learning that others whom you respect as good and caring people, like yourself, have experienced such feelings has a remarkable effect. Sharing normalizes the experience of wishing you or the patient to be dead.

Groups help families retain a sense of hope for the future. "Hope" may sound like a strange word in this setting, but it often emerges from a sense that others are in this with you and are prepared to be of help. Groups can help family members understand that life is not hopeless and that others are there to help. It is especially important for caregivers, especially men, to know that their wish that the patient were dead is normal. Unfortunately, about 20 percent of homicide-suicides, where an older husband kills his wife and then commits suicide, involve a wife with dementia. Hopelessness and helplessness as well as depression in the husband caregiver motivate the tragic, lethal act. These are discussed further in Chapter 13.

Groups provide practical information about Alzheimer's disease and related disorders. Most groups establish good relationships with local health professionals who offer lectures and seminars about the latest research in the field. Larger groups publish newsletters with updated information about current issues on the national and local scene as well as about clinical progress.

In support group meetings family members are encouraged to ask questions freely. Factual information can remove misconceptions about dementia and often relieves anxiety. Relatives who have lived with an impaired family member can teach each other many things by drawing on their own experiences—for example, what personality and mental changes may occur, how to evaluate the needs of the patient and the rest of the family, how to minimize or alter distressing behavior, how to adjust expectations, and how to maximize the quality of life for the patient and each other. There is the added value of knowing that families will hear about scientific advances as soon as they are made.

Groups also develop a sense of cohesiveness and social belonging. *Cohesiveness* refers to feelings of belonging that are so important to our mental health. Group membership often decreases the social isolation experienced by dementia patients and their families. Many families are surprised and pleased to find that their group becomes an extended family.

Groups give family members opportunities to help society as well as themselves through research and consumer advocacy activities. The support of research into the causes, prevention, and cure of the disease becomes a significant goal for many families. There is also much value in acting together to deal with problems of government health policy, long-term care, and reimbursement and organization of services (see Chapter 15). These are important issues for the relief of those suffering with dementia. Through group efforts individuals may derive a genuine sense of accomplishment, of moving a step closer to controlling or eradicating dementia and thus benefiting future generations as well as their own.

Not everyone finds support group meetings to be helpful. Some family members do not see themselves as "caregivers" when the diagnosis has been made early and the patient is only mildly impaired. In the early stages some individuals shy away from support groups and prefer the intimacy of friends. It is also common for spouses to find support groups more helpful than the patients find them. Newly diagnosed individuals often find it upsetting to see others who have deteriorated because they see a real portrayal of what they will be like in the future.

Many family members find that the meeting times do not mesh with their schedule, transportation may be lacking, or there may not be any groups in their local area. There are a number of sites on the Internet with electronic support groups and chat rooms (see Selected Readings and Internet Resources).

Goal 14: Identify Resources in the Community.

A number of programs and services available in many communities are focused on the aged and may be useful to families caring for relatives with dementia. An important organization is the Area Agency on Aging (consult the local government or agency listings of your telephone directory). If it is not located in your immediate community, you can find out where it is in your region. Area Agencies on Aging also may have different names such as Council on Aging and Area Planning Councils. Refer to Appendix 3 for the addresses and phone numbers of your state Agency on Aging.

The Agency on Aging should help you identify several programs and areas of assistance:

Your eligibility for income maintenance programs
Health and mental health services
Transportation services
Legal assistance
Nutrition programs
Employment and volunteer programs
Multipurpose service centers
Housing
Adult day-care programs
In-home services
Long-term-care institutions

Sometimes resources are difficult to find, especially when you do not live in a large city or if your relatives live far away from you. Chapter 7 includes a detailed discussion of various programs and various ways to go about finding them.

Goal 15: Become an Advocate for Reforming Policy on Alzheimer's Disease.

Learn what is happening at the national, state, and local levels. Get the names and addresses of your U.S. senators and congressperson, of your state assemblyman or woman, as well as of appropriate state, county, and city officials, including your governor and mayor. Write and tell them about the needs of patients with dementia and their families. Educate them about your needs and problems and seek their help. Inquire about the existence of any pending bills to support research, about tax exemptions for families caring for a relative at home, and about community-based home-care and day-care programs.

Work with the Alzheimer's Association, which has an active public advocacy program. Since its birth in 1979, the Alzheimer's Association has been effectively lobbying Congress.

Goal 16: "Go with the Flow."

Obviously, the way patients and families cope with the impact of dementia is influenced by many factors—early diagnosis, the course of the dementia and the severity of the losses, the effectiveness of antidementia drugs, the availability of family members and friends, the technical competence of professionals, as well as family lifestyle, values, and philosophy of life. One daughter of a patient, Iona Fleming, admitted that her job became easier and the household calmer when she was able to adopt a strategy "to go with the flow." It took time to accept the complexity of dealing with her father's needs and safety as well as those of her family and herself. Although there were times when she imposed certain limits, such as not allowing her father to drive the family car, do the weekly shopping, or baby-sit with the children alone, she found ways to involve him, respecting his need to contribute something to daily family life. There were days her father could barely cope with the world around him and required constant help. There were others when it was hard to believe anything was wrong. Mrs. Fleming said she had to get over asking herself why and to live day by day with the changes.

The Future: Living and Caring

Living with Alzheimer's disease or related dementias is a herculean task for everyone—patients, family members, and other caregivers. However, the odyssey of care can be made less stressful if one identifies goals and implements plans. There are no specific rules for providing the best care as the disease progresses, but families can do a great deal to break through what one patient's wife called a "cycle of despair." Norma Hull told us, "For months after George was diagnosed, I felt beaten. I wanted to re-treat from everybody and everything. However, one day I watched George in the garage carefully organizing his tools, and the truth became clear to me. With some help I could do a lot for us. We had each other, our home, and our future."

Medications to Cure Alzheimer's Disease

Where Are We?

When the night has come, and the land is dark
And the moon is the only light we will see.
No, I won't be afraid, oh, I won't be afraid.
Just as long as you stand, stand by me.
So darlin', darlin' stand by me.
Oh stand by me.
Oh stand, stand by me, stand by me.

If the sky that we look upon should tumble and fall
Or the mountains should crumble to the sea
I won't cry, I won't cry, no, I won't shed a tear
Just as long as you stand, stand by me
And darlin', darlin' stand by me
Oh stand by me
Whoa stand now, stand by me, stand by me

"Stand By Me"—Jerry Lieber, Mike Stoller, and Ben E. King

"Stand By Me" has become the motto of the Alzheimer's Association, and the song sung by Ben E. King has been adopted as a theme or fight song by patients and families. The power of the song symbolizes the power of patients and families who stand together as "warriors and heroes and martyrs," in the words of Oliver Sacks, in the fight against the unrelenting losses of dementia illnesses.

Since the first edition of *The Loss of Self*, several antidementia drugs have been approved by the Food and Drug Administration (FDA), many more are in development, and several substances are promising for prevention. However, as of this writing, there are no cures for the disease, a reality that breaks the hearts of those afflicted and those who love them. Nonetheless, the race is on to clarify the causes of Alzheimer's disease and other dementias, and as researchers learn more about the causes, they are searching for new medications to halt, treat, reverse, and prevent dementia.

"Stand By Me" carries a special poignancy during the search for the magic bullets in this brave new world of scientific discoveries. When someone you care for has Alzheimer's disease or a related disorder, it is almost impossible to accept the idea that there is no cure. We live in an era when newspapers report medical miracles every day, including the transplantation of vital parts of the body, new cures for other diseases, and important scientific discoveries about the body and the world we live in. Each news story evokes the hope that a cure for Alzheimer's disease will soon be forthcoming.

Because Alzheimer's disease affects so many persons and has received so much national media attention, any new lead, no matter how unsupported, is widely publicized, giving grounds for optimism to families and clinicians alike. Misleading or exaggerated information in the newspapers is explained later in the scientific literature with a full and accurate story that is usually more conservative in its implications, but this does not make the headlines. Meanwhile, the family rides an emotional roller coaster from excitement and hope to despair, and this may aggravate the problems of caring for the patient. Therefore, it is valuable to have access to informed physicians and other professionals. Information from the Alzheimer's Association is also important to translate the meaning of new findings and place them in perspective.

To state it simply, no drug is known at this time to prevent, stop, or reverse the destruction of brain cells and cognitive losses that occur in Alzheimer's disease. There have been some successes in slowing the course of cognitive and functional losses as well as treating behavioral changes with drugs, and pharmaceutical research throughout the world has intensified to find a cure. A major breakthrough is probably years away, yet advancements are being made, fueling optimism and hope for the future, which are effective albeit partial antidotes for despair.

In the mid–1970s researchers discovered that the levels of one of the brain's neurotransmitters, chemicals that help transmit information from brain cell to brain cell, was very low in persons with Alzheimer's disease. Almost 90 percent of the neurotransmitter called acetylcholine was depleted in the brains of patients with advanced Alzheimer's disease compared to the brains of older people without the dementia. This was an important discovery because acetylcholine in animals plays an important role in memory, and it is found in many neurons in the hippocampus and cerebral cortex of persons who had Alzheimer's disease. (Neurotransmitter changes are described in detail in Chapter 14.)

For several years research efforts focused on the study of medications to increase the amount of acetylcholine. Although replacement of acetylcholine should have theoretically helped patients with Alzheimer's disease, studies showed that administration of pure acetylcholine did not get into the brain. However, acetylcholine brain levels could be enhanced by giving the patient lecithin and choline orally. These substances are metabolized in the body to form acetylcholine, which is then more available in the brain. Early clinical trials attempted to measure whether taking choline and lecithin could improve memory in patients, but unfortunately these compounds have not been beneficial in patient care.

The rationale for the use of choline and lecithin was to repeat the success achieved with replacement therapy in the treatment of Parkinson's disease. Patients with Parkinson's disease have uncontrolled tremors, body stiffness, problems in walking, changes in facial expression, and a number of other neurological problems. No cure is known, but drugs have provided a modest degree of relief for some patients with the disease. In Parkinson's disease the neurotransmitter dopamine is diminished in specific areas of the brain. Dopamine given directly cannot enter the brain, but the compound L–dopa (levodihydroxyphenylalanine) taken by mouth does get there, and it sets off a chemical reaction increasing the production of the needed dopamine. L-dopa has been used successfully to manage the tremors and rigidity of Parkinson's disease in about 75 percent of the patients treated, changing their lives dramatically. However, other disabling symptoms, which may also include dementia in

40 percent of patients, are not relieved, and the course of the disease is only modestly changed.

Cholinesterase Inhibitors

The marked declines in acetylcholine levels stimulated researchers to learn more about the cholinergic system—the brain cells that use acetylcholine and the enzymes that manufacture it or influence its activity. The goals were to find substances that would increase the amount of acetylcholine, replace it, or slow its breakdown.

All of the antidementia drugs approved for use in the United States belong to a class of drugs known as *acetylcholinesterase inhibitors*. These therapies are targeted on increasing the amount of acetylcholine and prolonging its activity in brain cells. When acetylcholine is released by nerve cells communicating with other nerve cells, it must pass through a space called the *synapse*. Specific chemicals known as *enzymes* are found in the synapse, and they facilitate the breakdown and recovery of neurotransmitters by the neurons that make and release them. The enzyme that breaks down the neurotransmitter acetylcholine in the synapse is called *acetylcholinesterase*. By blocking or inhibiting the activity of acetylcholinesterase in the brain, the supply of acetylcholine in the synapse is increased.

As of this writing the FDA has approved the use of three drugs in the United States. The drugs are marketed under the trade names Cognex (tacrine), Aricept (donepezil), and Exelon (rivastigmine). All are acetylcholinesterase inhibitors with different formulas and differing side effects. What is noteworthy about these medications is that they do not claim to reverse the symptoms of Alzheimer's disease. They are neuroprotective and slow the progress of the dementia, giving more months of quality life to the patient and family. Thus, the earlier the drug is used, the better the effect on the patient because a higher level of functioning will be maintained for a longer period. The value of using these medications over long periods of time has not been reported.

Cognex, which was first on the market, was reportedly effective in about 30 percent of patients by slowing the rate of change of cognitive losses, but about half of patients also showed elevated values for certain liver enzymes. This was not usually serious, but patients had to have regular blood tests to make sure that elevations did not become so high that it would necessitate stopping the drug. Because of the risk for liver toxicity, the complex management schedule, and the limited positive effect, Cognex is no longer a treatment of choice and its use has dropped considerably.

Aricept and Exelon are the current drugs of choice for treating people with dementia in most countries around the world. About one million people in over thirty countries have been prescribed these drugs. Aricept is given once a day and requires no liver function testing. The results of drug studies using 5-mg and 10-mg daily doses for three to six months indicate improvement in functioning in mild to moderately impaired patients. The drug keeps some patients from deteriorating for about nine months, and it is becoming a popular medication, largely replacing Cognex.

Exelon was released in the United States in April 2000, although it had been tested widely and used in Europe and Latin America. Patients seem to tolerate Exelon well, since it is eliminated by the kidney not the liver, and they show significant improvement in their cognitive abilities compared with patients taking a placebo. Exelon is given twice a day, starting at 1.5 mg daily and moving up to a maximum dose of 6 mg daily. Improvement is usually seen in about thirteen weeks. The side effects include nausea, vomiting, and other gastrointestinal symptoms in some patients, but these are potentially reduced by taking the medication with meals and increasing the dose slowly.

Exelon appears to enhance overall cerebral metabolism, and therefore it improves the functioning of not only patients with Alzheimer's disease but also those with vascular and Lewy body dementias. It reportedly enhances behavioral functioning in more severely impaired patients as well as those with other physical illnesses. Exelon may be more effective in certain patients because it affects another enzyme in the synapse in addition to acetylcholinesterase. Both Exelon and Aricept are acetylcholinesterase inhibitors. However, Exelon also inhibits butylcholinesterase, a related substance that normally exists in much smaller amounts than acetylcholinesterase. Thus, the drug has a two-track effect. Furthermore, in

Alzheimer's disease levels of acetylcholinesterase and acetylcholine decrease whereas levels of butylcholinesterase increase with advancing disease. As a result Exelon is effective in later stages of the illness as well as early stages.

Other acetylcholinesterase inhibitors are being developed and tested in clinical trials. Metrifonate is an acetylcholinesterase inhibitor that is chemically different from the others. It is reported to significantly improve everyday abilities, such as doing chores around the home, participating in leisure activities, using money and the telephone, and performing other activities of daily living. Metrifonate also is reported to improve behavior significantly by reducing agitation, depression, and aggression, and it may have a role in the inhibition of butylcholinesterase. While metrifonate seems to be a helpful medication, the FDA is scrutinizing it closely for its safety profile. In the doses studied, a small proportion of the patients had adverse reactions to the drug involving severe respiratory muscle weakness, and a few required assistance in breathing. The prospects for the expected approval of this medication await addressing the concerns of the FDA and the likely need for further testing.

Galantamine is in a different class of acetylcholinesterase inhibitors under review by the FDA. This experimental drug is believed to increase the amount of acetylcholine in the brain in two ways. It inhibits the cholinesterase that breaks down acetylcholine, and it also stimulates other receptors in the nerve cells to release more acetylcholine. A limited amount of information is currently available, but research on this compound is ongoing in preparation for application to the FDA for approval.

Another acetylcholinesterase inhibitor is heptylphysostigmine (Eptastigmine), which has a longer-term effect in the body than Aricept. The cognitive and behavioral data have been promising, and most patients have tolerated the drug reasonably well, although a few have shown serious adverse effects. The drug has not been studied in the United States at this time. The results of European tests show that Eptastigmine is a helpful treatment for cognitive losses as well as behavioral disturbances, and adverse effects have not been reported.

All acetylcholinesterase inhibitor drugs act to slow down the metabolic breakdown of acetylcholine, protect the nerve, slow the patient's cognitive decline, as well as have a positive effect on overall behavioral functioning. However, none of these compounds change the long-term course of Alzheimer's disease. Clinical trials are currently being conducted to study the effectiveness of these drugs on delaying the onset of Alzheimer's disease, especially in persons diagnosed with mild cognitive impairment (see Chapter 2). In addition to acetylcholinesterase inhibitors, totally different approaches to Alzheimer's disease are being developed and tested.

Antioxidants

Antioxidant therapies, which include vitamin E, vitamin C, and selenium, have been used in older people with memory complaints. Antioxidant compounds are believed to protect nerve cells from what is known as *oxidative damage.* Oxygen is essential to life, but during normal metabolism oxygen also breaks down into free oxygen radicals that damage proteins and cell membranes. Researchers have hypothesized that free radicals play a role in aging as well as brain degeneration in Alzheimer's disease, and the search is on for agents that stop or protect against oxidative damage. Vitamin E (alpha-tocopherol), one of the most important antioxidants, has been described to slow progressive decline in severe dementia for about seven months.

The basal ganglia in the brain, which has large amounts of the neurotransmitter dopamine, are particularly vulnerable to oxidative damage. The antioxidant medication selegiline (Eldepryl), used for Parkinson's disease as a substitute for L-dopa or as an antidepressant medication, has shown positive results in people with Alzheimer's disease. Selegiline enhances dopamine activity. Whether its role as an antidepressant or its antioxidant properties are responsible for the positive effects seen in patients is not yet clear, but the drug is a good candidate for protecting nerves. The negative sides of using this drug are the dietary restrictions that must be followed by persons taking monoamine oxidase (MAO) inhibitors as an antidepressant and the potential for interactions with other medications (see Chapter 6).

Ginkgo

Derived from one of the oldest trees on earth, *Ginkgo biloba*, gingko is widely used in Europe for its effects on circulation and metabolism. Ginkgo, in the form of concentrated extracts from the leaves, has been shown to have a variety of positive effects, including recovery from strokes, macular degeneration, ringing in the ears, chronic dizziness, and vascular impotence (caused by reduced blood supply to the penis). Studies in the United States and abroad on the effects of ginkgo for Alzheimer's patients have yielded promising results. It seems particularly effective when the dementia is caused or complicated by vascular insufficiency. Since changes in the aging brain may be related to reduced circulation, ginkgo may be effective even though Alzheimer's disease is not primarily vascular in origin. The federal government is now initiating larger-scale studies of ginkgo. Since it is a naturally occurring substance, the FDA has not reviewed it for effectiveness or safety.

Estrogen

It has been reported that women receiving estrogen replacement therapy have a reduced risk for developing Alzheimer's disease. A medication designed to treat breast cancer, tamoxifen, which is similar to estrogen, also has been reported to reduce the risk for Alzheimer's disease. While the role of estrogen is not entirely clear, it does enhance acetylcholine production in certain neurons, and it has both antioxidant and anti-inflammatory properties. Estrogen appears to improve blood flow in the brain and reduce the body's production of beta-amyloid, which is the basis for the amyloid plaques. As described in Chapter 14 on the causes of Alzheimer's disease, a high concentration of amyloid plaques in the brain is destructive to nerve cells. At this time, however, the case for the value of estrogen is still somewhat controversial. Not all studies have yielded positive results.

Several studies are targeting the value of estrogen in the prevention of Alzheimer's disease. What is the effect of estrogen replacement therapy on cognitive decline in postmenopausal women who have had a hysterectomy? Will estrogen replacement therapy decrease the incidence of dementia? Will the use of estrogen in women who do not have Alzheimer's disease but who have a family history prevent Alzheimer's disease?

Nonsteroidal Anti-inflammatory Drugs

An entirely different approach to drug treatment comes from observations that patients with rheumatoid arthritis treated with anti-inflammatory medications are less likely to show symptoms of Alzheimer's disease. Trials of these nonsteroidal anti-inflammatory drugs (NSAIDs) have been underway to test the value of medications such as ibuprofen and indomethacin. Low doses of steroids such as prednisone also have been tested. Why steroids or other anti-inflammatory medications might be effective is not entirely clear. It may be that in the process of neuronal loss, local inflammatory responses in the brain may emerge and this in turn could worsen the condition of the brain. Despite the lack of a strong body of data, many experts are recommending NSAIDs to their patients, since the side-effect profile is minimal in most instances.

Neural Growth Factor

In recent years scientists have become interested in the value of neural growth factor (NGF) in degenerative neuron diseases. This factor has been shown to stimulate the regrowth of dendrites and nerve cells in the laboratory. To date the NGF medication has had to be delivered to the exact site by neurosurgical approaches. Now, genetically modified cells able to produce NGF can be injected into the brain without implantation of fetal tissue or other cells. The potential of this approach is quite exciting, although, once again, caution is advised in becoming overly optimistic about its immediate value.

Larnitin

Larnitin, a marketing name for acetyl-L-carnitine, has been shown to offer some protection from cognitive decline in Alzheimer's disease. In several studies, those who were given carnitine showed less decline over six months to a year. Carnitine itself is a combination of two amino acids, lysine and methionine. Why it seems effective is not clear, but it does give support to those scientists who think that acetylcholine deficiency is not the exclusive problem in Alzheimer's disease.

Future Developments

Although other classes of drugs are not currently available, several new strategies are being considered. One is the search for an analogue of acetylcholine, a drug that mimics acetylcholine at the synapse. More basic approaches are also being examined. Since we know that a pathway to Alzheimer's disease is the overproduction of amyloid in the brain (discussed in Chapter 14), drugs that will inhibit the production of brain amyloid should slow or prevent the disease. As we learn more about how amyloid precursor genes as well as other factors produce amyloid, we can develop improved strategies. While these are years away, they represent an important approach to the problem.

Living with the Search for the Cure

Individuals living with incurable illnesses face the personal challenge of living with optimism and hope as scientists search for the cure. Progress is being made, but useful knowledge develops slowly. Rational thinking is often compromised when someone has a devastating, incurable illness. It is natural for patients and families to hope for a miracle, and for some the pressure to search for one is intense. Families desperate for a cure are easy prey for individuals who promote new but unproved treatments. The vulnerability of Alzheimer's families to quacks and charlatans is extraordinarily high. The family may go on a frantic search for a miracle, often losing out emotionally as well as financially.

Experimental drug trials are critical for determining the safety and efficacy of new prospective drugs, and we learn from the courage and determination of patients who lend themselves as research subjects. Participating in clinical drug trials can be a fulfilling and hopeful experience for patients and family members. Many patients express a burning desire to someday be freed of the yoke, to be able to think and function again, and to beat the oblivion. Chapter 6 gives a fuller account of issues to be considered in drug trials.

Not all individuals are needed or accepted into drug trials. Some are too far along in the disease or too mildly affected to meet the criteria of the research protocol, while others are dropped for medical and other reasons. When persons are unable to participate or are excluded from clinical trials, health professionals have a responsibility to refer the families for appropriate general care and follow-up. Although the following story is a rare circumstance it does emphasize the risks.

Anita Fitzgerald, a sixty-three-year-old woman diagnosed with Alzheimer's disease and vascular dementia shot and killed her ninety-three-year-old mother, Erica Good. She then shot herself in the chest. Although Mrs. Fitzgerald was not expected to live, she did recover. She was charged with second-degree murder and spent two weeks in jail. A judge then released her to the home of her own daughter on $50,000 bail. Because of declining health, including multiple small strokes, the judge sentenced Mrs. Fitzgerald to probation so that her family could continue to care for her at home.

Before this happened, Mrs. Fitzgerald had been dropped from an antidementia drug trial because of side effects, and there had been no follow-up or referral by the investigative team. For three weeks after the drug trial was discontinued, she became increasingly depressed and agitated. She expressed anger to her family that her brain was not good enough for the doctors, and she would get even. One afternoon awakening from a nap, Mrs. Fitzgerald was agitated and angry that her family would not take her to get the drugs. That day she went into her son-in-law's study to get the gun. Mrs. Fitzgerald walked out into the kitchen and shot her mother who was sitting at the counter eating her lunch.

Caring Is Tougher Than Curing

As researchers search for the cure, there are still many medical treatments that can be helpful in dealing with many aspects of Alzheimer's disease, and these interventions can make the burden of caring a little easier for the family. Close contact with informed and caring physicians who take a real interest in the patient and family is essential to everyone's physical and mental health. Doctors with good clinical judgment appreciate three elements: the patient, the disease, and the illness. Families should feel that the doctors understand the lifestyle, personal goals, and special needs of everyone—the patient as well as individual family members. Doctors obviously need to be knowledgeable about the disease and to be aware of the latest scientific developments. Finally, physicians must recognize that the illness, which refers to the way the disease affects the patient, may not be the same in any two individuals with an identical diagnosis. It is particularly important in Alzheimer's disease to recognize how the illness will vary from one patient to another.

As we point out in other sections of this book, not all dementias are Alzheimer's disease, and what appears to be Alzheimer's disease may turn out, on closer inspection, to be another condition. Years ago studies of what was called *senile dementia* confused the vascular dementias with Alzheimer's disease, and investigators tested the same drug for both. Recent research showed that Lewy body dementia, frontotemporal dementias, and HIV-related dementias exist, and that early-onset dementias ultimately may appear to be distinguishable from later-onset illness. Since there are at least five genes involved in Alzheimer's disease as well as a range of risk factors, researchers will likely discover that one treatment does not fit all apparent forms of Alzheimer's disease.

With the expected scientific advances, we hope to learn more about different forms of Alzheimer's disease as well as improved diagnosis and treatment. The next chapter reviews what drugs are helpful to manage or treat coexisting psychiatric problems such as depression, anxiety, and paranoia, which are seen frequently in patients.

tissues also means that it may take the older person longer to eliminate drugs after they stop taking them.

The bodies of older people, especially those with medical illnesses, are less efficient at metabolizing drugs. The body breaks down most medications into less active or inactive compounds, and this is usually done by enzymes produced in the liver. After this process occurs, drug by-products or the parent drug itself pass from the body through the kidneys, the gastrointestinal system, or the lungs. Dementia patients with diseases involving the liver, kidneys, or lungs will have trouble deactivating or eliminating drugs from the body. In such cases, very low dosages must be used to prevent undesirable side effects. However, these low doses in turn may have a less intensive effect. The patient's weight, activity level, nutritional status, and genetic makeup may play a role as well.

The sensitivity of various parts of the body to a given drug also increases with age. The older brain, and especially the Alzheimer's brain, appears to be more sensitive to medication. As a consequence, relatively low doses of a drug can have powerful effects not only in the brain but also in the rest of the body. Considering the possible effects of alcohol, nutritional status, health status, and other factors, it is difficult to predict the frequency and severity of side effects. All of these changes make the management of medications complicated, but a working partnership between the patient, family, other caregivers, and the physician can go a long way to resolve the complexity.

Guidelines for Caregivers

Drugs must be used appropriately in order to have the desired effect. For example, they should be taken at the times listed on the label of the bottle. However, the high cost of drugs may lead to an attempt to be thrifty by cutting down on medications, or in the hustle and bustle of the daily routine, drugs may be forgotten. Furthermore, when individuals take several different medications at various times of the day or night, it is common to forget a pill or to take one at the wrong time. Special pill boxes for storing pills by the day and the time can be purchased at the pharmacy. Remember, a change in the use of a drug without the doctor's knowledge may create a serious set of problems.

Alcohol is a drug worth particular attention because it has significant effects, including the way it changes the body's ability to handle other drugs. The use of beer, wine, and whiskeys should be discussed openly with the doctor. In almost no instance can patients handle large amounts of alcohol without complications. Small amounts of alcohol—a beer, cocktail, or glass of wine at lunch or dinner—may be quite enjoyable and even desirable if there are no medical contraindications. When alcohol use has been a regular part of the patient's social activity, social drinking is often pleasurable, but sensible judgment is important. For some households it is better to restrict the amount of beer, wine, or liquor kept in the home or perhaps to eliminate it altogether. Sometimes patients will drink themselves into a stupor, not because they are alcoholic but because they forget how much they have consumed.

Frequently, the patient is using several different drugs, which can become a serious problem for several reasons. Drugs affect each other, and the breakdown and elimination of drugs by the liver or kidneys may set up a set of competitive chemical reactions. The number and dosage of medications challenge the body's ability to handle them. Family members should question their family physician about possible interactions different drugs have with one another. Drugs prescribed by different physicians, the use of old drugs that are not discarded, drugs "borrowed" from other people, or mixtures of drugs, alcohol, and over-the-counter preparations used together can lead to these competitive reactions known as "drug-drug interactions."

The manner in which drugs are taken also can be important. Injections are generally the fastest way of getting drugs to act in the body, but most medications are taken orally. The absorption of drugs from the stomach and the rest of the gastrointestinal system can be affected by the contents of the stomach, such as the presence of food recently eaten (especially fatty food), the availability or the lack of certain enzymes in the digestive system, the size of the meal, and the person's emotional state. Inadequate fluid intake, the use of laxatives, and irregular eating habits also have an impact on how drugs are absorbed from the stomach and intestines.

Giving drugs in later stages of the disease can be a problem. Some patients will spit out pills and capsules or simply not swallow them. Some may have trouble swallowing and gag, and others may resist going to the doctor if a shot is involved. If this is a problem, check with the doctor prescribing the medication. Is it available in liquid form? Can the number of times it is given per day be minimized? Can the number of pills or capsules be reduced? Can the patient tolerate a drug-free day or weekend? The physician is usually happy to work with you to create an optimal program to ensure that medications are more likely to be used correctly.

The following checklist may be helpful:

1. Keep a written list of the names and doses of all drugs the patient is using.
2. Make a daily chart of times for which drugs are prescribed. Check off drugs as they are given.
3. Check with the patient's doctor or pharmacist to clarify whether a specific drug should be taken before, during, or after meals.
4. Make sure every doctor prescribing medications knows all the drugs being taken, including prescribed as well as over-the-counter medications.
5. Keep a record of any drugs that have caused a problem in the past. Allergic reactions can be serious or even fatal. Be prepared to report this to doctors, nurses, hospitals, and other medical professionals.
6. If the patient has had a history of taking a particular drug that has been helpful for the same condition, tell the doctor. It can save time finding the effective treatment.
7. If the patient is taken off of a drug, throw out the pills, capsules, or liquids remaining in the medicine cabinet. The temptation to use them again may be too difficult to resist.
8. If you feel that the drug is too expensive, tell the doctor. If you cannot afford the cost of the medication, there may be ways of reducing the expense. The physician often can save you money by prescribing an alternative form of the same medication. In some states this is automatic, while in others you may need to discuss it with the physician or a pharmacist. Be honest with the doctor. No competent physician will be offended if you explain your problem. If the doctor is irritated by this discussion, you may wish to consider changing doctors.
9. Many drugs sold without a prescription can affect the patient. Among the most dangerous of these over-the-counter drugs are alcohol and

sedatives (sleeping pills). It is generally a good idea not to give the patient over-the-counter drugs without consulting the physician. These drugs often alter the action of prescription drugs. This warning even applies to aspirin or similar drugs, as well as "herbal" medications.

It is a mistake to think of the many psychotropic drugs as only tranquilizers or medications that do pretty much the same thing. There are several major classes of psychotropics, each of which has a specific purpose. They include antipsychotics, antidepressants, mood-stabilizing drugs, antianxiety drugs, sedative-hypnotics, and cognitive-acting medications. Each of these affects the body differently, and subclasses within each group have differing patterns of action.

The remainder of this chapter reviews basic information on psychiatric symptoms and behavioral problems and the major classes of psychotropic drugs used to treat them. Cognitive-acting drugs were discussed in Chapter 5. Our objective is to help you judge when drugs may be needed and used effectively to help the patient function at the highest level possible. The information is also intended to help you understand the different types of drugs and ask questions of the doctors. It cannot be a substitute for the care of a trained physician, nor should it be seen as the final word about the safety or effectiveness of the drugs mentioned.

Agitation, Irritability, and Assaultiveness

Agitation is among the most distressing features accompanying dementia, and it is perhaps the most disturbing one reported by caregivers. Agitation occurs frequently and is reported in almost 85 percent of patients who have had the disease for more than five years. Sometimes it is verbal, but many patients exhibit physical violence, such as hitting, kicking, and biting, several times a week. Understanding the cause of agitation is the basis for successful treatment. The decision to use drugs requires careful consideration. Psychotropic medications are usually effective and helpful when used properly, but they should be considered only after several other steps have been taken.

Patients become agitated for many reasons: medical conditions, drugs, dehydration, hunger, fatigue, boredom, changes in the environment, personal needs and habits, as well as pain and injury. Therefore, before any drug treatment is initiated, the cause of the agitation must be evaluated. Such questions as the following should be answered:

1. Is there a medical condition superimposed on the dementia?
2. Is the patient receiving a new or different dose of a medication, prescribed or not?
3. Is the patient allergic to the drug or are there side effects that may cause agitation?
4. Does the patient have pain or discomfort from an injury, cut, fall, corns, hemorrhoids, or heartburn?
5. Are shoes or clothes making the patient uncomfortable because they are the wrong size?
6. Is the patient bored or overstimulated?
7. Have there been changes in the physical or social environment of the patient?
8. Is there a temporal pattern? Does the patient get agitated before meals or when dressing, eating, bathing, toileting, or watching television?
9. Do certain people create distress in the patient?
10. How do attending caregivers deal with the patient's agitation?
11. If the patient is of an ethnic minority, do cultural, ethnic, or racial issues need to be considered in the care of the patient? These may range from language to food.

Watching the patient carefully, doing a behavioral analysis of when and where he or she becomes agitated, as well as noting associated events and circumstances are essential before drugs are prescribed. If the patient is violent and uncontrollable, drugs can be used. However, a behavioral analysis and plan of care should be implemented immediately thereafter with a staff trained to implement a consistent plan in response to the agitation. The first objective is to attempt to treat, ameliorate, modify, or change the conditions precipitating the agitation. It may involve changing medications, treating underlying infection, or in rare cases, checking for possible broken bones from falls, or even severe constipation and impaction, which can cause behavioral disturbances in patients who cannot otherwise communicate. The patient's hearing and sight must be checked periodically since sensory impairment leads to impaired communication. For example, a patient who has good hearing but impaired eyesight may be frightened by shadows and cry out, and if the patient is not attended to, cries may escalate into screaming.

Antipsychotic Medications

Antipsychotic medications affect the activity of several neurotransmitters in the brain—notably dopamine, norepinephrine, and serotonin. They are widely used to control the paranoia and irrational behavior of patients who are a threat to themselves or others. There are six major chemical classifications of antipsychotic drugs: (1) atypical psychotics such as risperidone (Risperdal) and olanzapine (Zyprexa); (2) phenothiazines such as chlorpromazine (Thorazine), fluphenazine (Prolixin), trifluoperazine (Stelazine), and thioridazine (Mellaril); (3) butyrophenones such as haloperidol (Haldol); (4) thiothixene (Navane); (5) molindones (Lidone, Moban); and (6) dibenzoxazepines, such as loxapine (Loxitane). All of these drugs are powerful and, consequently, also can have powerful side effects.

Antipsychotic medications are helpful, but they should be used in small doses. However, even smaller doses of medications such as chloropromazine, haloperidol, thioridazine, or thiothixene can and do have significant side effects. In recent years a new class of medication has emerged, and the older traditional antipsychotic medications have largely been supplanted by what are referred to as *atypical antipsychotics* because of their different modes of actions and reduced side effects. The older medications may still be used, partially because they are more economical and may be effective for patients who have used them successfully in the past. However, they must be used carefully and sparingly. Recent consensus guidelines on the use of medication for agitation, established by polling a large number of geriatric psychiatrists, emphasize the use of atypical antipsychotics as a first-line medication. The atypical antipsychotics have a more focused effect on specific brain pathways.

For protracted periods of severe agitation, the atypical drugs play a prominent role. The consensus guidelines specifically identify the drugs risperidone, olanzapine, divalproex (Depakote), and trazodone (Desyrel) as effective for long-term management of severe agitation. These atypical antipsychotic medications also may have a positive effect on cognitive performance, mood, and ability to perform activities of daily living and may be beneficial when given together with some of the newer antidementia drugs.

For milder agitation, the antianxiety medications and a drug known as buspirone (Buspar), which is a nonbenzodiazepine drug, may be effective. Trazodone and benzodiazepines may be appropriate for short acute-care management of agitation. When agitation is associated with depression as well as anxiety, there is a role for the antidepressant medications known as *selective serotonin reuptake inhibitors* (SSRIs), discussed later in the chapter.

In addition to agitation and assaultiveness, antipsychotic and atypical antipsychotic medications can be used for the treatment of other disturbing behaviors such as yelling and screaming, irrational violence, and bizarre thoughts, including hallucination and paranoid states. They can be particularly valuable for the patient whose paranoia becomes the basis for aggressive behavior that the patient adopts for protection. Antipsychotics also can be used for restlessness and irritability. In small doses they may be used quite effectively to eliminate the confusion noticed in some patients in the early evening, frequently called the *sundown syndrome.*

The agitation, irritability, and hostility frequently seen in dementia can be controlled by medication prescribed by a knowledgeable and careful physician. However, it is important that lowered frustration, appropriate levels of stimulation, regular exercise, and meaningful activities be part of the plan of care. They are extremely effective in managing restlessness and irritability. Drugs are a poor substitute for regular physical activity.

Antipsychotic drugs will not improve or reverse memory loss or other intellectual problems that characterize Alzheimer's disease or vascular dementia. However, as stated before, the atypical antipsychotics may enhance cognition and overall behavioral functions in some patients. The antipsychotics often help with the management of behavioral problems associated with dementia, but they are not always successful in treating them. One reason for this is the difficulty in regulating the dosage in older persons with dementia to maximize the desired effect while minimizing side ef-

fects. Adjusting the amount of medication may be a delicate matter, requiring patience from everyone—patient, family, and doctor.

Once a drug is selected, the doctor will want to use the lowest effective dose. The usual procedure is to start with a low dose, look for
side effects, gradually increase the dose to an effective level, and then adjust the daily amount slightly until the best balance is reached. When the
individual does not show the expected response to a drug, the doctor
may wish to test the level of the drug in the blood. For some drugs, laboratory techniques can determine whether a therapeutic dose of a certain drug is present in the body. After an antipsychotic drug has been
used for a while with stable effects, ask the physician whether it is advisable to stop the use of the drug for a short period, perhaps over a
weekend, to determine whether it is necessary to continue treatment, or
at least reduce the amount of the drug.

All the typical antipsychotic medications seem to be equally effective,
but they differ in their potency and the specific side effects they produce.
Some antipsychotic drugs have a greater sedative effect than others. However, because sedation causes clouded consciousness, the more sedating
antipsychotic drugs also may cause slightly more daytime confusion and
disorientation. Thus, observing and understanding the patient and knowing about drug actions are essential to help the patient and minimize the
number of medications.

Side Effects of Traditional Antipsychotics

Side effects to drugs are by no means universal, but they are not rare.
When administering any drugs, certainly for antipsychotic medications,
it is as important to watch for the appearance of side effects as it is to
monitor the beneficial effect on the behavioral problem. When side effects are harmful or make the patient extremely uncomfortable, even
after an appropriate period of drug administration, the drug should be
withdrawn. In some patients a surprising effect may occur with antipsychotic medications: a patient who is agitated and given antipsychotic
medication may become more agitated. If this happens, the dosage should
be decreased, the medication changed, or the drug should be stopped
altogether.

Among the most common side effects of the traditional antipsychotics are sleepiness, dry mouth, constipation, blurred vision, and bladder problems. Patients taking them also may have problems like stiffness of the joints and occasional drooling. In extreme cases, regular use will produce parkinsonian symptoms such as rigidities and tremors. When such problems occur, as they may in 20 to 30 percent of patients, antiparkinsonian drugs often are used to reverse these symptoms. However, as mentioned earlier, this causes the patient to use two drugs in combination and therefore increases the possibility of other side effects.

Other side effects include low blood pressure and a sensation of being dizzy or light-headed, particularly when the patient moves from a seated or lying-down position to standing upright. This condition is known as *postural hypotension*, a drop in blood pressure as a result of sudden changes in posture. It can be managed by making sure that the patient gets up from the bed slowly, first to a sitting position, and then standing up at the side of the bed, or holding on to the arms of a chair for the time it takes the head to clear, before starting to walk.

Tardive dyskinesia, a disorder associated with long-term use (usually years) of psychotropic drugs, occurs in as many as 15 percent of individuals. Patients develop uncontrolled and exaggerated movements of the mouth, tongue, and jaw area. At the moment the best approach is to recognize these signs early and stop use of the drug. Regular examination of the mouth and tongue will detect the presence of unusual movements before it becomes a manifest problem. Poorly fitting dentures also can cause the individual with dementia to make strange mouth movements, which should not be confused with tardive dyskinesia. However, the best way to prevent this serious condition is to minimize and regulate the dosage given. Whatever the drug, it should be used sparingly. Drug-free periods or total cessation of the drugs should also be considered. Medications vary in their likelihood of causing tardive dyskinesia, and you should talk with the doctor.

While we have focused on the negative side effects as precautions, we come back to the problem of the severely agitated, often abusive, and impossible-to-manage patient. Psychotropic medications can and do help, but a cost-benefit approach is needed. The benefits are clear, and the cost in this case is more than money. It is the possibility of negative side effects. Medication management is a combination of science, the healing art, and careful monitoring of the patient.

Atypical Antipsychotics

As described earlier, the more traditional antipsychotic medications are being supplanted and largely replaced by newer medications, referred to as *atypical antipsychotics* in view of their different spectrum of activity and side effect pattern. These newer drugs have a wide range of activity that goes beyond calming the patient. They seem to have a beneficial effect on depression and cognition, while causing fewer parkinsonian features often seen with the older antipsychotics. Since these newer medications have been shown to be effective in the management of agitated patients, many experts have supported the use of low-dosage atypical antipsychotics as a first approach to the patient. At this time however, price is an issue. The atypical antipsychotics, still under patent, tend to be far more expensive than the traditional antipsychotics, some of which are being sold in generic forms. This trade-off between economic cost and value is an important debate in health care. Drugs such as olanzapine and risperidone have been studied in older patients, and recent reviews of the treatment of agitation in older patients indicate that geriatric psychiatrists who specialize in such care recommend these medications, in low doses, to their colleagues. These consensus guidelines are complex but are published and available to the treating physician through various sources (also see recommended readings).

The field of psychopharmacology is expanding rapidly, and newer medications are being produced regularly. The growth of the aging population and the increase in the number of older patients makes this an attractive market for major pharmaceutical firms, most of whom see this as a priority for research and product development. The physician should stay abreast of the latest information through scientific journals, continuing education, conferences, and computer searches. Caregivers also can access this information. The Web site of the national Alzheimer's Association can be helpful, particularly where new drugs are concerned. Drug companies themselves also are advertising directly to the public on television and in the print media, which can be informative if it is discussed with the physician.

Cautions and Warnings

It should be clear that doctors make complex decisions when they prescribe drugs. Which drug will cause the least harm and provide the best treatment for the right patient? What side effects are most likely to occur? How can they be managed? What are the alternatives to medications—exercise, nutrition, changes in the physical or social environment, or supportive discussions and behavioral management?

Although any physician can prescribe drugs, it is important for you to ask several questions. Is the physician knowledgeable about the psychopharmacology of aging and associated psychiatric problems? Will the physician consult with a colleague who specializes in geriatrics? Has the doctor done a careful analysis of what happens when the patient shows behavioral problems? Does the doctor listen to you when you describe the patient and the patient's reaction to the drug(s)?

Depression and Dementia

Clinical depression can affect thinking, memory, sleep, and appetite and interfere with daily life. Therefore, the existence of depression in patients with dementia clearly complicates and worsens their ability to function. Depression has been observed in 20 to 30 percent of patients with early-stage dementia. However, recognizing depression is often a challenge. Memory-impaired individuals are less able to act and communicate effectively. Even early in the disease individuals may not report they are sad or depressed but rather that they feel empty or apathetic. Nothing gives them pleasure, and they simply "don't care" about things. Sometimes apathy and withdrawal or conversely, agitation, are symptoms of depression rather than of worsening dementia.

Severe depressive symptoms may appear as the result of diseases unrelated to dementia or the psychological state of the individual, such as thyroid conditions or other metabolic disorders. Depression also can occur as a side effect of drugs used to treat physical disorders, such as certain antihypertensive or high blood pressure medications.

Since the major objective of patient care is to maintain the highest possible level of functioning, treating depression successfully can reduce apathy, inattention, and irritability. One problem, apart from possible side effects of the medication, may be the family's initial enthusiasm that the patient is being "cured." Although this can happen in patients in whom depression alone causes the dementia, it is not to be confused with a "cure" for Alzheimer's disease or related disorders. Family members still denying the presence of Alzheimer's disease or vascular dementia often grasp at straws and once again go on the emotional roller coaster of optimism and disappointment, and then develop their own reactive depression.

Antidepressant Medications

Several types of drugs are used to treat major depression in patients with dementia. These include tricyclic antidepressants, monoamine oxidase (MAO) inhibitors, selective serotonin reuptake inhibitors (SSRIs), and other unique drugs. Each class has several specific medications, and each drug has a slightly different profile of main effects and side effects. Depression appears to be associated primarily with a diminished supply or balance of at least two neurotransmitters, serotonin and norepinephrine, and antidepressant drugs act by altering the level of these neurotransmitters in those areas of the brain.

Until recently the most commonly prescribed medications for depression have been a group of chemical compounds known as *tricyclic antidepressants*. Effective in most instances, tricyclic antidepressants also often have caused adverse side effects. Even newer medications, such as maprotiline (Ludiomil) or mirtazapine (Remeron), which have selective effects on serotonin and norepinephrine, may cause fewer of the side effects associated with tricyclics such as dry mouth, but they may enhance intraocular pressure, urinary retention, and response to alcohol.

Tricyclic antidepressants are still valuable medications, and many physicians know these drugs and have good results. They generally cost less, and side-effect patterns may be benign for a particular patient, so they may still be the drug of choice. One side effect, alteration of the electrocardiographic (EKG) pattern with an effect on heart rate, is a signal to change antidepressants. The newer SSRIs do not influence EKG patterns and have become the treatment of first choice. These drugs seem to act more effectively, require smaller dosages, and cause fewer side effects than do either the tricyclics or the MAO inhibitors.

The first of the SSRIs to be released was fluoxetine, under the brand name Prozac, which slows the reuptake of serotonin, norepinephrine, and sometimes even dopamine into the neurons, with the resultant antidepressant effect. The SSRIs have become popular and are supplanting the older tricyclics as the drug of choice for many patients. In addition to fluoxetine, other drugs in this category include such brand names as Zoloft, Paxil, Efexxor, Serzone, and Celexa, to name a few. Each of these has a similar mechanism of action but a somewhat different side effect profile, and therefore individual patients may tolerate them differently. The SSRIs take time to have an effect. Patience is essential because weeks (four to six weeks is not unusual) may elapse before the full value of these medications can be realized. In the case of lower dosages used for older persons, it may take longer.

Another class of drugs used to treat severe depression are the MAO inhibitors. They block the action of a chemical called *monoamine oxidase* (MAO), which is normally found in the nervous system. MAO acts to maintain the chemical balance in certain parts of the brain by breaking down excess amounts of the neurotransmitter norepinephrine (noradrenaline). One of the major theories of depression proposes that it is caused by the shortage of norepinephrine or serotonin, or both, in key areas of the brain. Whether this shortage is caused by the presence of too much MAO, inadequate production of norepinephrine, or other factors is not clear. However, since MAO reduces the level of norepinephrine in the brain, a drug blocking the action of MAO will increase the availability of norepinephrine, and the therapeutic result is relief for the depressed patient.

When MAO inhibitors are used to treat depression in dementia patients, caregivers must be careful to follow strict dietary and medical guidelines. These drugs can produce undesirable interactions with certain foods, drugs, and other medications. Mixing MAO inhibitors with any of the substances listed below can cause severe headaches, neck stiffness, increased heart rate, and increased blood pressure. These restrictions apply while the drug is being taken as well as for a period of ten days to two weeks after its discontinuation.

Avoid These Foods:
1. All cheese (except cottage cheese, cream cheese, and ricotta cheese), including cheese crackers, cheese sauces, and pizzas
2. Liver

3. Smoked or pickled fish
4. Foods containing brewer's yeast
5. Fava beans, broad bean pods
6. Fermented sausages

Avoid or Limit These Drinks:
1. Red wine
2. Beer
3. Other alcoholic drinks
4. Drinks containing caffeine or chocolate

Avoid or Limit These Medications:
1. Over-the-counter cold, cough, decongestant, and allergy items
2. Hay fever and sinus medications
3. Appetite suppressants
4. Pain relievers
5. Other psychotropic drugs
6. Any prescription medications not first discussed with the doctor

An overdosage of MAO inhibitors can be dangerous. Symptoms may include confusion, agitation or drowsiness, hallucination, changes in heart rate or heart failure, enlarged pupils of the eyes, convulsions, vomiting, high fever, muscle stiffness, or coma. The individual should always be taken to a hospital emergency room along with the medicine bottle, and the patient's doctor should be contacted immediately.

Other antidepressants such as bupropion (Wellbutrin) are effective for some patients. While the exact mode of operation is not clear, bupropion also blocks the uptake of serotonin, norepinephrine, and dopamine. Once again, this is an alternative option depending on the physician's assessment of the individual patient, other drugs being taken, medical conditions, and the efficacy of drugs used earlier.

Buspirone (Buspar) is another compound that may be helpful in depression. It is more frequently prescribed primarily for its antianxiety effects and is favored by many clinicians for older patients. In addition to treating anxiety with less sedation, buspirone seems to have serotonin-like properties, which may make it useful for minor depression and even agitation.

When to Use Antidepressant Drugs

It is important to emphasize that drugs are not necessary or even appropriate in treating all forms of depression. Patients may have reactive depressions, characterized by grief or sadness in reaction to some loss. Supportive counseling and social interventions are the treatments of choice in such instances. Particularly for minor depression, drugs may not necessarily be a good choice. In early phases of the disorder, individuals may be acutely aware of their losses. They may remember and grieve over the death of a relative when they attend a funeral or feel the loss of friends or pets. Sadness about losses is normal and is best dealt with by quiet, frequent discussions, learning how to cope and put things in perspective. Drugs should be reserved for the more serious conditions.

Antidepressant medications may be effective for the treatment of depressive disorders characterized by a change in mood and the following symptoms:

1. Sleep disturbances (either a noticeable increase or decrease in sleep)
2. Appetite changes and weight changes (either a significant gain or a loss over a four- to six-week period)
3. Loss of energy and complaints of being tired
4. Agitated behavior or a marked slowing of behavior
5. Loss of interest in pleasurable activities
6. Difficulty with concentration and thinking
7. Impaired ability to carry out activities of daily living
8. Low self-esteem, guilt, and negative feelings about self
9. Thoughts of death or suicide
10. Persistence of depressive symptoms for several weeks, including crying, sadness, and social isolation

These signs or symptoms should be a trigger for referring the patient for a full evaluation. Depression is eminently treatable and with treatment has a good prognosis. The major barrier to the treatment of depression is the failure to evaluate and diagnose it. Since busy physicians often overlook these indicators when treating the patient's physical problems, sharing information about the patient's behavior and emotions at home presents valuable data to the caring physician.

Choice of an Antidepressant

The choice of a particular antidepressant drug is determined by many factors. The patient may not be able to tolerate a certain medication because of side effects. Some antidepressant drugs will aggravate other physical illnesses or interfere with the action of other medications. As discussed in the section on antipsychotic medications, the characteristics of the specific drug need to be considered thoughtfully in relation to the patient's problem. For example, some medications have a sedative effect, which may be useful for a patient with dementia who is very agitated and has sleep disturbances. Conversely, for depressed patients who lack energy and are inactive, a medication with activating effects may be useful.

Some medications should be given in divided doses or in one dose at bedtime. This reduces the possibility of the patient's developing postural hypotension, the drop in blood pressure when the patient stands up from a lying or seated position. Postural hypotension can cause falls and injuries, which in turn may require major nursing care. As a general rule, individuals who show clear differences in blood pressure when they change from a sitting to a standing position, even before medications are given, should not be treated with tricyclics. As described earlier in the discussion on antipsychotic medications, patients should be encouraged to get up from bed slowly.

Determining the appropriate dose of medication for the older patient is often a challenge. Drugs are metabolized differently in older persons because of biological changes with aging, as discussed earlier in this chapter. The activity level of the person and other medications being taken also affect dosages. It is easy to understand that some trial and error may be involved in getting the correct balance of medication. The task is to get the lowest effective dose to the patient. If the dose is too low, it will be useless; if too high, the resulting side effects will be possibly harmful.

Once a positive effect is achieved, the antidepressant medication should be maintained for at least six months or longer. The dose can be decreased, and maintenance levels determined if depressive symptoms do not recur. The physician's clinical judgment is the key to successful drug management, and the family caregiver is an important partner to provide information on the patient's behalf. Once again patience is important. Often, experience with a new medication will be less than satisfactory for the first day or two, but if the side effects are not too severe, it is important to continue the drug. The physician will alert you to the severe side effects that should be a signal to stop the medication immediately and to call the doctor.

Side Effects

The different antidepressants have several types of side effects. Some cause sedation, dry mouth, and blurred vision. The tricyclics also can cause tremors and sweating. These occur more often with tricyclics like desipramine, imipramine, and protriptyline. Therefore, these medications may not be the drug of choice for some older patients. Tricyclic antidepressants also can affect heart rate and present a problem for certain patients who also have heart disease. Although no persistent damaging effects of tricyclics on the heart have been reported, a conservative assumption is that the tricyclic antidepressants should not be used within two months after a heart attack or other major disturbance in the heart's functioning. Patients with certain uncontrolled and irregular heart rhythms and those with uncontrolled angina or poorly controlled congestive heart failure should probably not be on tricyclics.

SSRIs can cause nausea, a bad taste in the mouth, reduced appetite, or other gastrointestinal symptoms. These should be monitored carefully, particularly if weight gain or loss occurs. Similarly some SSRIs lead to feelings of tension often confused with anxiety, and some patients do not tolerate these feelings very well. They may pass or be ameliorated by an antianxiety medication taken during the first few weeks of SSRI administration. If the drug cannot be tolerated, substituting another medication may help. Some patients experience insomnia when they begin an SSRI. They may have a hard time falling asleep, which is different from the "terminal" insomnia of depression in which the patient wakes up very early in the morning and is not able to get back to sleep. The insomnia and gastrointestinal problems are usually manageable by taking the drugs in the morning after a meal and adjusting the dose. While the

SSRIs are usually effective, good care management requires patience, communication with the doctor, and compliance with the way the drug is prescribed.

Mood Swings

A different class of drugs is used for patients with a history of significant mood swings. These medications act to smooth out and prevent exaggerated ups and downs of the depression–mania cycle that affects some individuals. For patients with a history of manic–depressive disorder, also known as *bipolar disorder*, antidepressants should be administered in conjunction with one of the following medications. Lithium is the most commonly used drug, but recent drugs such as divalproex (Depakote) and lamotrigine (Lamictal) are effective in protecting against exaggerated mood swings that can result in severe behavioral problems. The important consideration is to make sure that the patient's emotional history is given to anyone prescribing an antidepressant. For vulnerable individuals, a new cycle of ups and downs can be precipitated by the sole use of an antidepressant. Ongoing psychiatric consultation is advisable for persons with a history of bipolar illness.

Anxiety

Anxiety is a normal reaction to certain stressful situations but can become severe enough to be crippling in its own right. The severity of symptoms and the extent to which they disrupt a person's effectiveness are considerations when one is deciding whether the anxiety is a minor psychological upset to be treated by psychological and social support alone, or a more serious and disabling psychiatric disturbance for which medication is also advised. It is sometimes difficult to diagnose anxiety in the patient with dementia, but the symptoms of irritability, emotional upset, increased activity and wandering, agitation, and fear that characterize anxiety are easy to recognize. Careful observation of the patient over the day to note periods of upset and a review of the patient's history prior to the diagnosis are useful to detect anxiety. People who were anxious prior to being diagnosed with dementia are likely to show anxiety with the disease, fearing the loss of mental powers and isolation from the family.

Nondrug as well as drug interventions may be useful to reduce the anxiety of patients with dementia. A supportive social and physical environment is essential, and the search for activities appropriate to the level of the patients is a constant challenge as the dementia progresses. A regular routine can reduce anxiety by preventing overstimulation. Caregivers must recognize patients' fears and anxieties and encourage them to talk about it if they want to and are ready to handle it. Giving patients positive messages that there is support for them, that they are still part of the family, and that they can make a positive contribution is a helpful strategy.

Antianxiety Medications

Antianxiety medications, most of which are benzodiazepines, may help. However, they should not be used routinely or for prolonged periods without careful monitoring. Long-term use is not recommended because they may have the paradoxical effect of making the patient more anxious. Meprobamate and other drugs containing barbiturates frequently used for anxiety and sedation in the past are not safe medications for older patients. Barbiturates such as meprobamate can lead to physical and psychological dependence. Furthermore, confused patients may kill themselves with an accidental overdose if they have easy access to the medication.

The most common side effect of all antianxiety drugs is drowsiness, which leaves many patients less able to enjoy daily activities. The benzodiazepines, however, may have additional and serious adverse drug effects: apathy, dry mouth, confusion, depression, slurred speech, nausea, headaches, dizziness, constipation, urinary incontinence, change in heart rhythm, lowered blood pressure, blurred vision, rash and itching, nervousness, water retention, liver dysfunction, and inability to fall asleep. If the patient develops any of these symptoms, stop use of the medication and call the doctor.

Patients taking antianxiety and sedative medications should avoid smoking, alcohol, barbiturates, narcotics, antihistamines, and antidepressants for the most part. Benzodiazepines should not be used if the patient has used one of these compounds in the past and developed an allergic reaction. They should also be avoided if the patient has narrow-angle glaucoma, but they may be taken by a patient with open-angle glaucoma. While antianxiety drugs are not addictive in the technical sense, for most individuals they do create psychological dependence, and thus, their long-term use is to be avoided.

Patients can accidentally overdose on any of these drugs. Symptoms of overdose include disorientation, sleepiness, shallow breathing, low blood pressure, lack of response to pain such as that caused by a pinprick or a pinch, and coma. Take the patient to a hospital emergency room and bring the bottle. It is a good idea to keep only a modest number of pills around the house. In instances where prescribing services provide large quantities, hide the majority of the pills and only provide a few days' supply in the medicine cabinet. In some instances, after long-term use, abruptly stopping barbiturates can be associated with a withdrawal reaction including convulsions. Care must be taken to taper off these drugs, and a physician's help is a must.

Sleep Problems

Sleep problems are common in the patient with dementia, and they often become more upsetting as the dementia progresses. The wakefulness and nighttime wandering of a patient often wear family members out. Indeed, sleep disturbances are among the problems that most frequently cause families to place the patient in a nursing home.

A routine, organized approach to sleeping is helpful. Behavioral approaches are the treatment of choice to prevent sleep problems, particularly in the early stages of dementia. Simple strategies such as rising at the same time each morning, elimination or minimization of afternoon naps, daily physical exercise, proper nutrition, and a carefully planned active day can go a long way toward improving the patient's sleep pattern. Patients who live through a meaningful and reasonably stimulating day will tire and sleep at night. It is unreasonable to expect that people who are passive all day and encouraged to nap after lunch will use their nighttime for sleep in the same way as others do.

Avoiding liquids for two to three hours before bedtime will reduce the likelihood of awakening to go to the bathroom, with its consequent destruction of the sleep cycle and difficulty returning to sleep. Finally, the bed should be used for sleeping—get the patient out of bed in the morning and use the bed for sleep rather than lounging. The patient who spends hours dozing throughout the day will not have a full night's sleep, and this will add to the burden of the caregiver who needs the sleep after a busy, stressful day.

Sedative-Hypnotic Medications

Two major classes of drugs are commonly used to treat sleep problems— barbiturates and benzodiazepines. As indicated earlier, the latter are also employed to deal with anxiety, but barbiturates are not appropriate for use by older persons. They are addictive and render sleep problems worse, not better. In some instances, barbiturates can make patients more upset and irritable.

A group of short-acting benzodiazepines may have some value if used for relatively brief periods, but they should not be relied on for the long-term management of sleep problems in dementia patients. The drugs currently available can help improve sleep initially, but their long-term use interferes with sleep. In addition, sleep medications can create dependency in the patient and problems for family members who may feel emotional conflict about whether or not to provide such medication. The sedating benzodiazepines initially can help the patient sleep, thereby giving the tired spouse the opportunity to sleep. However, they also can cause residual drowsiness and cognitive impairment the next day, thus increasing the burden of care. It is not uncommon to observe family members caught in a vicious cycle of giving the patient sleeping pills in large doses, "hoping" that the pills will work, and then developing anger and frustration over the patient's increasing disorientation during the following days. Here the family must carefully make a risk-benefit analysis and advise the doctor about its wishes. Most physicians will be glad to work with the family in this complex management task.

For sleep a short-acting medication is preferred. Some benzodiazepines have the advantage of clearing from the bloodstream and brain in a few hours, minimizing drowsiness and confusion the next day. However, older persons, particularly those on other medications, may not clear out the medication as rapidly as hoped, for all the reasons discussed earlier in the chapter.

As with all classes of drugs, the individual compounds vary in effectiveness, and their effects also can vary greatly in different patients. Some drugs used for a long time cause problems when they are stopped, including sleeplessness, agitation, anxiety, and the need for even higher doses to achieve normal sleep for a few days. Although rare, some reactions to stopping the drug, such as convulsions, may be serious. In general, we suggest that any medication used for sleep should be given only for relatively brief periods, that is, for a few nights or weeks and for problems due to a short-term stressful situation. This will prevent the physical or psychological dependence that leads to increased drug use and a vicious spiral.

If not monitored carefully, sedative-hypnotics can be dangerous in the patient with dementia. An accidental overdose can occur if the patient takes one dose but then forgets about it in the mild confusion that can occur as the drug begins to take effect. The result may be that the patient takes too many pills. In the event this occurs, the patient and the medicine bottle should be taken to a hospital emergency room. Caregivers should be very vigilant in controlling access to such medication.

General Rules for Psychotropic Drug Use in Dementia

Families and caregivers should become knowledgeable enough to judge when drugs are being used appropriately and effectively for the well-being of their loved one. The following principles are important to keep in mind:

1. The doctor should start with a low dose and increase it gradually, if necessary, particularly if the drug is new to the patient.
2. A drug should be given only for the patient's benefit, not primarily for the benefit of the family or professional staff.
3. Some drugs have side effects that can make the patient uncomfortable and aggravate the dementia. Be alert to changes in behavior, as the patient is often not able to tell you how he or she feels.
4. Side effects themselves are not necessarily adequate reasons to stop drug treatment. Such side effects may be appropriately managed or

be less serious than the initial problem being treated. Some are transient and will disappear after a few days or weeks.

5. When the doctor starts the patient on a drug, plans also should be made for withdrawing the drug in the future. Do not be afraid to ask the doctor about future plans for the drug.
6. A patient's physical condition affects the way a drug acts.
7. The use of over-the-counter medications or alcohol should be avoided, unless discussed otherwise with the physician.
8. Outdated medicines in the medicine cabinet should be thrown out.
9. Every physician prescribing medication should know about all other medications being taken by the patient.
10. Drugs interact with each other and can cause serious problems. Be alert every time medications are changed.
11. Drugs should be used in conjunction with psychological, social, and environmental therapies as appropriate.
12. Drugs may be harmful to the patient if not used appropriately.
13. Drugs may not work at all.

It is almost never advisable to give the patient more than one drug in a major psychotropic drug class at the same time. This means a person should not receive two or more antidepressant or two or more antipsychotic drugs at once. However, under certain circumstances, it may be appropriate to administer an antipsychotic drug with an antidepressant, such as when the individual with depression also has severe delusions or hallucinations, or to administer an antianxiety drug with an SSRI when the patient is severely agitated. The advice of a psychiatrist or other physician experienced with such medications is essential. If a patient is seeing several physicians, it is possible that each will prescribe different psychotropic drugs. Therefore, it is critical to alert the lead doctor and have him or her review the need for multiple medications and work with the others. In general, less is better and certainly safer.

Herbal Medication

St. Johns Wort has been promoted widely as a mild antidepressant. Since it is an herbal medication, its efficacy is not well known. It may be helpful, but it does interact with a range of other medications, and the physician should be aware that the patient is taking this medication. Melatonin, used by some for sleep, is again untested, though widely advertised. Here again, it is wrong to assume that because a drug is not prescribed, it is not powerful or does not have an untoward effect, particularly if the patient is on other medications.

Clinical Drug Trials

The doctor may offer or even recommend that you consider enrolling your relative in a clinical drug trial to test the usefulness of an experimental drug to treat the symptoms of dementia or some other condition in the patient. This may be a valuable opportunity, and it may be of help to the patient. Clinical trials are essential for the development of new, safe, and effective treatments. However, there are some important considerations when enrolling in a drug trial.

Participating in a drug trial is a personal decision, for you and the patient. If you agree, some precautions are in order. Ask questions about the safety of the new compound and about previous research results. Find out whether the study has been approved for scientific merit and ethical use of human subjects by an accredited medical institution. Before signing any consent forms, make sure you understand the risks of harm to the patient as well as the potential benefits. Also consider the patient's wishes when possible. Issues of informed consent by the patient require that there be an evaluation of competence or that you have legal authority to give such consent.

In general, the medication being tested should have direct relevance for the patient or the patient's condition. In the latter instance, the research will help others, not the patient. Having said this, altruism can play a role if there is informed consent and full disclosure. Everyone in the family needs to understand the consequences so there are no false beliefs or expectations.

Make sure that you have a clear understanding of what your responsibilities are throughout the study. Do you have to travel to the clinic or physician's office on a regular basis? Are you expected to fill out forms based on your observations of the patient's behavior? Do you have to keep close track of diets, other medications taken by the patient, and side effects? If you have to visit the clinic frequently, will there be compensation for expenses?

Some studies may involve use of a placebo, that is, an inactive ingredient looking like the "real thing." In such studies the doctor usually does not know which patients are given the trial drug and which are given the placebo. In some studies the treatment will be switched in the middle of the study so that patients first taking the placebo will then take the trial drug and vice versa. This is to test whether the active drug under study really works better than the alternative. Ask if there are provisions for continuing to receive the drug for a period after the study, if the drug turns out to be effective.

In short, find out everything you can. Be clear about any side effects or possible dangerous consequences and assess the risks and benefits carefully. Find out whether the study will pay for treatment of side effects. Remember the first overriding rule is to protect the patient. One final issue—make sure that there are backup plans if something unanticipated happens. You should have a card with a phone number that you can call in case of emergency.

7

Ways of Caring

"Herman, you really need to start playing tennis again. Look at your stomach. You need it." Sue Ellen, a victim of Alzheimer's disease, spoke these words to her husband as she lay in her hospital bed. As she talked, Herman simply stared at her, then caught himself and replied, "Yes, you're right." And she was. After a few more exchanges Sue Ellen changed the subject. "When do you fly to Rome? Will you take Jamie with you? He so enjoys working with you in the business, and he wants you to be proud of him." Herman gently protested that he, Jamie, and the rest of the family would stay near her until she left the hospital. Sue Ellen sat up in her bed and summoned Herman to move closer. "Please go away. You need a break. I won't die before you return. This disease won't let me die. It's just changing me, but I'll be okay.

Families and other caregivers are often surprised to hear patients voice relevant thoughts and concerns or see them behave appropriately. Sue Ellen Williams had been hospitalized following a fall in which she fractured her hip. The pain and the general stress of being in a hospital had caused her to be even more confused and disoriented much of the time. Sue Ellen's physicians had given her the best medical care, and everyone was optimistic that she would heal and walk again. Even though the doctors were pleasant with Sue Ellen, they said little except hello, how are you feeling, and good-bye. Sue Ellen would often try to ask them questions, but they seemed unable to understand what she said. Indeed, they hardly seemed to listen. However, as the opening interchange shows, her family had just begun to listen.

It is important that Alzheimer's disease not become a stigma. It is a label as well as a disease. When the diagnosis is mentioned, we immediately change the way we perceive and act toward the person with the disorder. Perhaps one of the most significant barriers to providing good care is our difficulty in recognizing the human qualities of those who have been diagnosed. There is a tendency for everyone, from physicians and other professionals to friends and family members, to act differently around the patients or to avoid dealing with them in a natural way once they are diagnosed. Cognitive deficits, communication difficulties, and strange behaviors make most of us uncomfortable, and we may become angry, sad, and even frightened. These feelings color our abilities to see and react to the "humanity" of the patient. Many patients sense this and withdraw as a result.

It is important to identify and overcome false beliefs and fears about dementia in order to be able to meet the daily challenge of living with a person with the disease. While Alzheimer's disease involves the slow, irrevocable loss of ability and ultimately even the sense of self, the stereotypical notion that victims of dementia lose the ability to think, write, read, talk, work, or love overnight is a tragic error. Changes do occur, but skills and abilities decline at different rates. In fact, some skills and feelings remain relatively preserved for many years. When changes do occur, they may require that we modify our behavior, but how we change and what we say and do can make the patient function better or worse.

The following letter illustrates how even the most loving caregivers may lose their perspective in relation to the person with dementia.

Dear Sis,

Mom has changed so much in the past several months. She sits in the house most of the day and cries a lot. She talks, or at least strings words together, but they seldom make sense. However, Dad seems to know what she is saying most of the time. I guess it comes from their fifty years together.

Dad would not say "Alzheimer's disease" in front of her. He also would not allow me to talk about Alzheimer's while I was visiting. However, she knows she has a problem. Several times during the day, usually at meals, she asks him, "What's wrong with me?" His reply is always the same: "Your memory is not what it used to be, dear. Don't worry." It took all my strength not to get angry with him. After all he is the one living with her and taking care of her all of the time.

Something happened, however, that convinced me that she understands more than he gives her credit for. Mom and I took a walk together around the orchard while Dad ran some errands. She seemed happy just to be with me. We walked for several hours. Once she stopped to look at a bed of wildflowers that grew by the old woodshed. I bent to pick a small bouquet for her, but she stopped me. I tried to explain that they would look lovely on the kitchen table. She became terribly upset: "Please, no . . . let them live. Don't . . . Cut flowers die slowly—like me."

Sis, I froze when she spoke those words. I looked into her eyes, and she—we—began to cry. We walked back to the house slowly, arm in arm. We knew we—Mom and I—had to have a long talk with Dad.

And talk we did. And for the first time I think they both were honest with each other about Mom's disease. Even though Mom said very little, I think she understood. She and Dad sat together on the couch after I went to bed.

In this letter Alan Hodges shares a story containing one of the most important lessons families must learn in order to cope successfully with the changes dementia imposes on them.

When loved ones have Alzheimer's disease, they are still members of the family, and despite their dementia, they communicate a great deal about their personal needs and feelings. They do this by the way they act as well as by what they say. However, for them to be understood, those close to the patients need to be open to such communication and relate to the individuals both as patients with deficits and as persons with many human strengths. And who should be more capable of compassion, patience, and understanding than the family? However, the situation is complicated.

Caregivers are often unaware of the patient's feelings. This is not because they do not care. Indeed, quite the opposite is true. Family members care so much that they develop psychological ways to cope with the intensity of their emotional pain. When they protect themselves from their own feelings, they often block their ability to accurately recognize the feelings of others.

What can the family do to cope successfully with the patient's emotional needs as well as their own? Fortunately, there are well-tested ways of dealing with such needs, and they are a key to living life to the fullest. The first of these techniques involves a reorganizing of family life in ways that make room for the patient. As discussed in Chapter 4, one of the first goals after the diagnosis is not only to identify appropriate activities and design a structured program for the patient, but also to determine what changes need to be made in the family lifestyle to accommodate the patient's needs. This type of planning is a simple and powerful way to reduce stress on the family.

Adjustments in response to the patient's losses do not come easily, even in the healthiest families, and a great deal of emotional energy is expended in dealing with the many changes. Different feelings surface—sadness, anger, guilt, death wishes—and people need to find ways to control them.

Barney Tate lived in a small rural town with his wife of twenty-three years, an Alzheimer's victim. Selma had fractured her hip in a car accident and was confined to a wheelchair. Barney took care of her with the help of their two sons, both of whom lived nearby with their families.

One winter night their younger son, Doug, sat with them by the fire. It was snowing too hard for them to drive home. Doug was a Vietnam War veteran, and he had just finished writing a novel about the war years. He decided to read several chapters to his mother and father. That night Selma sat quietly on the couch, content to be with her family. She insisted, though, that Doug sit by her side on the couch. She even held his arm while he read. It was unusual for Selma to be so attentive. She watched Doug carefully while he read about the night his best friend was killed and about his desire to die and end it all. When Doug finished reading, Selma took the book from his hand. She held it to her forehead and said, "Me too. I want to die."

After Selma fell asleep, Barney and Doug stayed up talking for several hours. For the first time they spoke openly about the awful feelings each had kept private. Both had secretly wished Selma were dead rather than live a meaningless existence. Hearing her death wish had stunned them. That night Selma had taught them a valuable lesson. Part of her was still very much alive, and she was still at the emotional center of the family. And they needed her to be part of the family. Before the Alzheimer's disease had been diagnosed, she had always been the person in the family who settled arguments and helped everyone get what he or she wanted. Strangely enough, through the expression of her own wish to die in spite of her dementia, Selma had forced her family to deal with their conflicts.

This chapter reviews the more common problems that families face and some useful techniques in solving them. The problems fall into four major categories: (1) cognitive deficits, (2) communication impairments, (3) behavioral problems, and (4) maintaining marital and other relationships. The list is not all-inclusive but covers some of the troublesome issues that have to be overcome.

Cognitive Deficits

Cognition means more than the ability to learn and remember. Broadly defined, *cognition* refers to perceiving, understanding, imagining, willing, thinking, and moving around intelligently in the environment. The mind of the patient can be thought of as a cognitive sieve, in that the individual loses various types of information and then has less and less capacity to act as an intelligent and accepted participant in the world. Following the diagnosis, families and professionals too often assume that the losses occur immediately and affect all aspects of behavior. Thus, they condemn the patient to a more helpless position than he or she deserves. It is important, therefore, to see that the individual's cognitive strengths and weaknesses are carefully evaluated and that a plan of action to complement them is formulated. Otherwise, chances are high that patients and families will be deprived of important opportunities to enjoy each other and find pleasure in life. One patient told his wife, "The question is not can I talk or think or reason. The question is whether I can suffer. And without you close to me, helping me, I would suffer."

It is important to understand patients' individuality, even in the later stages of dementia. Their feelings, beliefs, desires, hopes, and plans are unique and need to be respected. It follows then that it is necessary to provide opportunities for patients to express themselves. Their expressions may not be readily interpretable, but the simple act of setting aside a regular, quiet time for them to talk, however incomprehensible their remarks may seem, can fulfill a human need to be close to and communicate with a loved one. By listening carefully, you can sometimes piece together broken patterns of thoughts or themes to be communicated from pain or discomfort from heat or cold, anger, and hunger. If these feelings and thoughts are not communicated quietly in such a setting, they may be reflected in behavior that will certainly get the attention of the caregivers. Agitation, aggressiveness, and many troublesome behaviors seen in Alzheimer's victims are not always the result of brain destruction. They may be the result of frustrated attempts to communicate, evolving over time in persons whose needs are not understood by those around them.

Alison Barnes had been living in a nursing home for more than a year. She was a forty-nine-year-old, legally blind widow with Alzheimer's disease. The nursing staff had labeled her as a belligerent, unpleasant woman who was difficult to dress and get out of bed in the morning. Mrs. Barnes yelled at the aides and often struck them. She was frail and therefore unable to hurt people, unless she bit them, which had happened on several occasions.

A newly hired nurse's aide assigned to Mrs. Barnes was responsible for making an important discovery that changed the staff's attitudes toward Mrs. Barnes. During her first week on the job, the aide would introduce herself by name and chat about the daily news or weather as she raised the blinds, arranged the breakfast tray, and straightened up magazines on the bedside table. Then she would sit down close to Mrs. Barnes and ask her how she was feeling, whether she was ready to eat, or whether she wanted to freshen up before breakfast.

For the first two days Mrs. Barnes complained and yelled. However, on the third day she told the aide that she wanted to wash up before eating. After this was done, the aide and Mrs. Barnes talked while she ate her breakfast. Then Mrs. Barnes dressed herself with little assistance and asked to watch the morning news. As the aide prepared to leave, Mrs. Barnes took her hand and spoke slowly, "Thank you for making me feel real again."

The rest of the staff took their cues from the aide's talking with Mrs. Barnes and learning about her as the woman she once was. They learned to be gentle with her in the morning and listen to what she needed to say. The angry behavior toward the staff had developed out of her frustration and feelings of being ignored when she wanted to wash herself before eating her breakfast.

Although patients often lose their train of thought and are not able to carry out even simple tasks, they are conscious of many things about themselves and their world throughout much of the illness, and they react to changes in their environment. Unfortunately, their difficulty in expressing themselves, and particularly in modulating their feelings, too often isolates them from family and friends.

It is common for many patients in the early or middle phases of dementia to be angry and privately yearn for a return to their former competence. Frustration mounts when individuals cannot find a way to overcome their losses. One man cried, "I can't live and I can't die. And no one understands how lonely my life is." Even in later stages patients can express a silent anger by the way they act. Another man, who had dementia for eight years, would walk to the window and raise his fist, almost in defiance, whenever he could not express himself.

Cognitive-training strategies may help improve communication between patients and family members. In order to develop any sort of cognitive-training program, a complete evaluation of cognitive skills is necessary, if available. The results of cognitive testing should provide a basis for family members to develop realistic expectations for a patient's performance and to find meaningful tasks, however simple, in the family. The evaluation may be expensive, but it is worth spending the money for a complete interview and battery of tests if the psychologist has the training and experience to use the examination and test results to identify the practical implications of the patient's deficits and strengths. The psychologist should be able to help you understand the patient's awareness of others; ability to find his or her way in the home environment; and capacity to plan realistically for the future, to deal with financial matters, and to communicate effectively. Knowledge about these and several other areas of abilities and weaknesses will help you to adjust your expectations for what the patient can or cannot do. The patient is able to fill many roles in the family if the activities are within his or her cognitive limits.

Many of the activities family members report as happy, intimate moments are those when they are doing something together—playing with a child or a pet, sharing a meal, taking a walk, or sitting together reading, listening to music, watching television, or talking. Families successful in keeping the patient at the emotional center of the family are able to find a place or meaningful role for the patient. Jerome Gardner had cared for his wife, Sarah, for more than seven years after the diagnosis. Even as Sarah declined, Jerome continued to take her camping and fishing in the summer, and during the winter he kept her active in community and church activities:

> Sarah is not the woman I married, but she needs me . . . and I still love her. There are times when we are together, and for a second I forget that she has Alzheimer's disease. Several times a week she washes my hair in the kitchen . . . the warm water, the massage, and the intimacy relax me. These are special times when I forget that she is sick.

Finding appropriate activities beyond quiet, intimate involvement is often a challenge, and this is where the results of cognitive testing can be valuable. Accurate evaluations provide the framework for recommendations about life and work roles for the patient. As the son of an Alzheimer's patient told us,

> Mom has lived with us fifteen years since Dad died, and she had run the house, since my wife and I both work. Things have been rough since this Alzheimer's started. However, she is still able to do some of the weekly shopping. We try not to stress her. She gets enormous satisfaction if we let her walk to the 7-Eleven to buy a single item once or twice a day. She still feels that we need her.

Dementia can affect concentration such that individuals stop in the middle of a task or lose track of their thoughts in midsentence. Because of these lapses in attention, you cannot depend on the patient to complete an assignment. When attentional and memory lapses occur together, it is difficult to trust the patient to do anything without supervision. But although deficits may make the successful completion of household chores like cooking, cleaning, and shopping impossible, patients often succeed in performing aspects of these tasks. And when they are so impaired that they cannot help, keeping them close by often gives them the security of being part of the hustle and bustle of family life. It is important not to block patients from emotional involvement, even when they are at a loss cognitively.

Social behaviors—the way we act around other people—usually remain fairly well preserved in most patients for long periods. Indeed, it is remarkable that when losses in memory and attention disrupt many routine behaviors, individuals are still capable of behaving in a socially intelligent way. Many activities with other people remain pleasurable—going to concerts or art museums; playing sports like tennis, golf, bowling, and cycling; boating, camping, dancing, gardening, and walking. Many patients are so aware of their limitations that they monitor their behavior closely in public surroundings for fear of "giving themselves away." One woman remarked, "I enjoy going on television. My husband and I just tell the interviewers not to ask me hard questions, especially anything to do with numbers. If you ask me things I know—about the disease or my family—I can answer you."

Many steps can be taken to develop a cognitively stimulating and constructive situation at home. The following checklist should help guide family discussions:

1. If you live in a city with a major university or medical center with geriatric specialists, inquire about the existence of a memory clinic.
2. Make a list of all the hobbies and leisure activities that gave your relative pleasure before the diagnosis of Alzheimer's disease. Which ones can he or she still do alone and which of them require assistance? Which ones are dangerous? Is your relative still able to do things with his or her hands, and can someone help while the patient does the actual building, modeling, or planting?
3. List the household chores your relative did and reconsider the division of responsibilities. Investigate the availability of a homemaker or someone to help with chores when your relative lives alone or when you need assistance. Assign some simple tasks to the patient, such as folding laundry, cutting vegetables, filling pots with dirt, or any repetitive task that is useful.
4. For as long as possible, continue social activities that involve you

and the patient with other people—lunch or dinner with friends, picnics, clubs, bowling, golf, tennis, exercise classes, movies, theater, or anything you all enjoy.

5. Find acceptable ways to involve the patient in a routine of new physical activities—jogging, swimming, cycling, walking, or gardening.

6. As the dementia progresses, find new ways for the patient to contribute to the household or family activities, no matter how simple. Talk to the person and ask about his or her day. Make everyday conversation. Feeling needed is a powerful emotional force.

7. Anticipate changes and discuss ways to deal with them in the future. What will happen when the patient cannot drive safely? What if some household help is necessary? If the patient loses his or her bearings in the home or elsewhere, what should the patient do? When the patient has trouble finishing a sentence or forgets a word, how might he or she ask for help?

8. Keep the patient active and mentally stimulated. Many patients still enjoy reading or being read to even though they may forget much of what they read. If the patient cannot read, records, tapes, and talking books are available. In many cases you may need to sit with the patient during these activities, but this creates the connectedness that so many patients crave, even into the late stages of the disease.

9. Take daily walks with the patient and when possible, visit different places several times a week—a zoo, a museum, a park, a botanical garden, or a shopping center or mall—any place full of sights and sounds. Even when the patient is institutionalized or confined to a wheelchair, try to schedule trips or visits out of the residence. Decorate the room with pictures or memorabilia to fit the individual's tastes.

10. When friends or relatives visit, introduce them by name and give a clue to their identity. Alert the patient to visitors before they arrive; then, when they arrive, say, "Oh, here's your cousin Peter." This may make you uncomfortable at first, particularly when close friends or relatives are involved, but they usually understand. And while the patient may seem irritated and say, "Of course, I know," the tactic can be helpful. Frequently, relatives report that after a pleasant evening visit, the patient will say something like "Who was that nice young man?" At this point a simple statement will suffice: "Oh, Mother, that was Joe, your favorite grandson."

No amount of cognitive retraining will replace the skills and abilities affected by a "failing" brain. However, often unrecognized are the human attributes that make the individual very much a participant, albeit sometimes a passive one, in the family. The challenge is to interact as a family, looking for opportunities to enhance the quality of life, rather than deal with the patient as someone simply destined to suffer progressive loss and nonexistence. Patience and an awareness of what is lost and what may be corrected are called for.

Communication Impairments

Patients are capable of higher-order thinking and reasoning to varying degrees, depending on the individual's education and experience as well as the progression of his or her illness. Whatever these abilities are, they are often eclipsed by clear and growing limitations as the dementia progresses. What becomes destructive to the patient's relationships with other people is the inability to articulate thoughts and feelings and to be understood by others. One of the important reasons to have complete psychological studies done early in the illness is to understand the patient's cognitive strengths as well as weaknesses and to develop ways to communicate effectively. These evaluations also should be done at regular intervals throughout the course of the dementia, to track changes in cognition and adjust communication strategies appropriately. A certain amount of trial and error will probably occur throughout the illness as people try to communicate with each other.

Alzheimer's disease and other dementias often impair language and speech, but so do other disorders that can be treated. More than half of adults over the age of sixty-five without dementia have communication impairments. Such disorders, if left untreated, will significantly decrease the quality of life as people unsuccessfully interact with family and friends. Listening, talking, and watching are the primary ways in which people maintain contact with their environment. Every effort should be made to diagnose specific hearing, speech, and language disorders and to treat them to the maximal extent.

Hearing aids and possibly even speech rehabilitation are important for the patient with dementia. Even in otherwise normal people, hearing loss causes misunderstandings and arguments and leads to accusations of mumbling or forgetting. Therefore, when the patient has suffered some hearing loss, it can make the dementia seem far worse than it really is. Because the perception of high frequencies is often lost, particularly among older men, certain consonants, especially the silent ones, are not heard well. For example, "thin" may be heard as "sin" and "fat" as "hat." Indeed, entire sentences may be heard incorrectly as a result of hearing problems, but too often the consequent lack of understanding is mistakenly attributed to the dementia. A hearing aid, and in certain instances surgery, not only will improve the patient's understanding but also will augment the entire family's enjoyment of one another.

Speech impairments like dysarthria and apraxia are common in dementia. Dysarthria may occur in people who have Alzheimer's disease and in those who have had a stroke with or without dementia. The term *dysarthria* refers to speech that is slurred, slow, and therefore distorted. It is the result of weakness in the nerves and muscles needed to produce speech sounds. Speech therapy can be very helpful. The goal in the treatment of dysarthria is to increase the strength and coordination of the muscles used to produce speech.

Unlike persons with dysarthria, those with apraxia are able to produce speech sounds clearly. However, they often say a single sound or word over and over again. Although many are able to produce entire sentences, they speak slowly and with great difficulty. They substitute one sound for another or omit sounds. The speech muscles are not weak in persons with apraxia. The problem results from their inability to consciously use their muscles to make the right sound in a word at the correct time. In some cases speech therapy may be effective. The goal is to increase conscious control as patients initiate and organize their speech production. When speech becomes too impaired, some patients, depending on the severity of the dementia, may be able to communicate by writing or typing out their messages.

Other language problems occur frequently. Patients may have difficulty understanding what certain words mean, or they may not be able to find the correct words to express a thought or identify an object or person. These impairments in language are known as *aphasia*. Persons with aphasia usually hear speech well but have difficulty finding the correct word for a person, object, or idea. They will speak a sentence smoothly but stop when they cannot remember the word they want to use. In many instances, they cannot combine words in the correct order to make a sentence. Depending on the nature of the aphasia, the persons may be able to correctly describe or use the object without remembering its name. They can even make good associations. For example, individuals may lose the ability to say "key" but make motions of turning a key in a lock, or they may repeat "write" for pen and pencil.

Speech therapy has limited effectiveness when aphasia occurs in Alzheimer's disease or related disorders. The therapeutic goals are to help the patient learn cognitive strategies to use the remaining language functions to compensate for the losses. It is often possible to teach the individual to ask for the word or to say, "I cannot remember the word I want," or to use associated terms. Usually, the most effective technique is to make the patient comfortable in accepting help from others, who will often be able to supply the missing word or words that can be correctly identified by the patient.

Even when specific disorders are not present, patients change their styles of communication as the disease progresses. Although it may seem simplistic, it can be helpful to recognize at least two phases of expression during the course of the illness. The first is seen after the diagnosis is established. Many patients are capable of making themselves understood with a minimum of help. This phase may last for a long time; it is characterized by powerful emotions as well as the desire for active and truthful communication. During this phase patients can often remain an active participant in family affairs.

During the middle and later stages of the disorder, communication becomes difficult, partly because the individual is less competent cognitively and verbally, and partly because many family members do not have a clear understanding of the patient's remaining strengths. Despite the cognitive impairment, there are strong needs for comfort, intimacy, and assurances of continued involvement. Families should be alert to the messages and to the changes in style of communication. In the later stages there is less use of words and more use of body language and behavioral change to convey needs.

Verbal and nonverbal acts of care and concern by the family are essential, regardless of the level of dementia. Family members can best help by trying to create an environment that offers the most comfort and warmth. This is not always easy. When a patient loses verbal competence, families tend to talk about the patient less as a person and more as an object, even when the patient is in the same room. Professionals who talk to relatives about the patient in the patient's presence share this tendency. When present, the patient should be acknowledged or involved in conversations. Many patients, even with severe dementia, seem to understand what is said and may react with signs of agitation and uneasiness.

In the later stages of the disease, many patients can convey important needs, and you should be able to deal realistically and supportively with their remarks and behaviors. By responding appropriately to patients' remarks, families can be helpful both directly, in attempting to fulfill specific needs of the patients, and indirectly, by recognizing that the patients have something important to say. Although almost any topic is likely to surface, there are a number of common subjects. The following examples illustrate only a few of the major issues patients raise, and give general suggestions for how to respond to them.

1. "Why Me?"

When bad things happen, it is natural to ask why, and there is no answer to the question. When patients ask the question, do not answer. Pause and wait for the next words to come from their mouths. Nod, and touch a hand or shoulder. Show that you are there and listen to the explanation that comes from them.

This question is not a request for information. It is a cry reflecting sadness, victimization, and an attempt to understand. People express many different reasons and explanations. Jake Eisenberg told his son that he deserved the disease because he had not been a good enough father and husband. People have beliefs and feelings about why they succeed or fail, win or lose, or get sick or stay healthy.

2. "I Wish My Friends Would Still Come to Visit."

It is common for individuals with dementia to feel isolated from others, because they usually are. Many ask whether Alzheimer's disease is contagious, since their friends and relatives seem to shrink from them. Be affirmative that it is not contagious! In the early stages it is helpful for patients and families to make an extra effort to reach out to neighbors. Tell them you need their friendship now more than ever. Even good neighbors and friends may not know what to say or do for you. Let them know. Do not hide behind the anxiety or fears of the diagnosis or anger toward others you thought cared about you and your family.

Some form of replacement is helpful. Start the patient in music, dance, exercise, or art classes to be around other people. Patients can be involved in many social settings, including activities with other patients and families at parties, picnics, and even group meetings. With time, activities with other patients and support groups can become important social events outside the family.

3. "I Couldn't Survive Without My Family."

Patients often find it easy to talk about the importance of their family. Talking with pride about people we love is something that gives all of us pleasure. What patients really need are opportunities to continue to be part of their family, to listen, and occasionally to talk while others listen. Many patients have spoken about how lonely they are because they are cut off. One woman told us she knew she was loved, but she felt like she was the family pet. Her husband and children spoke affectionately to her but in a way showing that they did not expect a verbal response.

4. "I Want to Keep Fighting This Thing as Long as I Can."

It is important to encourage patients to talk about this topic, which may be a reflection of their personality style or of their anger at having the disorder. Praise their courage. We all need encouragement and support from friends and loved ones for our labors, especially when times are difficult. The struggle for survival requires strong positive verbal reinforcement. Since dementia patients have so few rewards or acknowledgments of strength or accomplishment, the families should praise the patients whenever possible. However, this should be done appropriately and realistically, lest the praise become trivialized and lose its value. Praise does not require long or gushy statements. For some achievements this can even be hurtful to patients. A simple "good" or "nice job" or even "thank you" conveys the message.

5. "I Don't Want Help."

This message is very important. It merits a response. Many older people find it very difficult to ask for help, let alone accept assistance for something as personal and seemingly childish to them as dressing, bathing, and toileting. Less personal tasks like driving a car safely, remembering a name, or shopping for groceries are but a few of the myriad familiar things we do throughout the day and take for granted. Yet, these are precisely the types of things basic to our ability to retain our self-esteem.

Dealing with the issue of "help" is often extremely difficult. In general, there are a few guidelines. Try to let the individuals do things for themselves, even when they are sloppy or do not execute the task accurately or capably. When support is needed, avoid using the word *help* as much as possible. Use whatever language is appropriate to communicate effectively, for example, "Let us do this together" or "Can I work with you on this one?"

Emphasize that what was once second nature to them is being changed *by the disease.* Simplify the jobs to be done. Analyze whether certain tasks can be subdivided so that the patient only needs to do a piece at a time. Learn to accommodate the short attention span and the memory deficits and to provide organizing cues in the environment. Color codes in the kitchen or bathroom may make it easier to identify where things belong. It may be helpful to organize the day so that the patient is expected to do the same thing at the same time every day. It often helps to let the patient perform a chore and then later, when the patient is absent, to complete it or correct mistakes.

6. "I Know Nothing Can Be Done to Help Me."

Although this theme is expressed in many different ways, it usually is best accepted and not argued with. It is true that there are currently no cures for Alzheimer's disease, but a great deal can be done. However, little is gained by reasoning with the patients, for it often reinforces their dwelling on the negative side. The appropriate response to such comments is a positive statement about anything. Praise the patients' courage, tell how much the family loves them, or even tell them about a child or grand-child's accomplishment. In essence, change the subject. Later, emphasize that a great deal can be done to help them live as normal a life as possible despite their limitations.

7. "Will This Drug (Any of the New Antidementia Drugs) Make Me Better?"

Many people, especially in the earlier stages of dementia, have great expectations for the antidementia drugs approved by the Food and Drug Administration. Others may be pessimistic. These attitudes and expectations are usually consistent with the individual's personality and world view. Encourage the individual to take the medication and reinforce that you hope it will help them.

8. "I Know I'm Getting Worse" or "I Want to Know What Will Happen. Will I Get Worse?"

Sometimes it helps to quietly acknowledge that, yes, the patient will get worse, and then affectionately emphasize the importance of living "one day at a time" in the "here and now." Identify the patient's strengths and recent times of enjoyment. Be very specific about the joy of everyday life—food and eating, family outings, any and all activities meaningful to the patient. Enrolling your relative in a self-help group with other patients can give him or her an important forum to deal with needs to both reject and accept the reality that the dementia will progress. Perhaps acceptance best evolves as we share our thoughts and fears with others who face the same future. This acceptance also takes time and patience.

9. "Why Was I Not Accepted into the Experimental Drug Study?"

Many mildly impaired individuals are taking part in clinical drug trials to test the efficacy of new medications. It is possible that some may not be accepted, or they may be dropped for medical reasons. To patients in the early phases, explain in simple terms that the drug could seriously harm their health, that the available drug is experimental and may not work.

10. "I Want to Stay Home as Long as I Can. I Don't Want to Go into a Nursing Home."

Many patients say this to their families and others who are caring for them. Institutionalization is a complex issue. It fills some people with anxiety and fear, whereas others find the idea an acceptable and sometimes desirable alternative to a frightening life alone. For some, talking about going "to a nursing home" is another way of expressing a fear of desertion, often coupled with the fear that this is the ultimate in surrendering to the disease. Going to such a place can be symbolic of giving up the fight to remain independent and an ongoing part of the family.

To handle this issue successfully, it is important to know what the statement means to the patient. Often a response like "Don't worry, we'll always care for you" or "We'll keep fighting this together" is the best approach. It probably is best to avoid any promises that you will "never, never, never" use a nursing home as an option, since this is likely to haunt you in the event that institutional placement becomes the best alternative. At such a time the patient may be compatible with the security of an institutional environment while you, as family caregiver, are caught up in guilt and intrafamily conflict stemming from remarks made years before.

11. "Nothing Is Wrong with Me."

Denial is a common reaction to a difficult reality. It is best not to confront patients and argue that indeed they are impaired, when they say, "Nothing is wrong." Unless circumstances force the issue, let the patient talk, and then gently change the subject with a remark like "Let's take a walk." Bringing patients together in groups often helps you understand how to deal with their denial. An environment where patients find a "new family" of other people who are living with the same condition sometimes sets the stage for a careful and supportive confrontation with one's own losses. There is safety and solidarity in a group of patients who

may not be able to state exactly what is on their minds but who by their
presence, composure, or sheer energy speak of their strength to endure.

12. "I Knew There Was Something Wrong Long Before the Doctors Did."

Sometimes statements like this are bravado reflecting a false sense of
knowledge and therefore power. Other times they reflect a self-awareness that is ignored by others. We do not give patients enough credit for
the insights they develop into what is happening to them. It is important to give them the opportunity to tell their story. We all know that
each of us needs to tell what we have done or what has happened to us.
Again, the rule of thumb is to reinforce patients for what they can still
do, to bring out the human gifts of hope and solace, and to strengthen
the sense that they belong to the family, still have something to contribute, and are loved and valued for their own sake.

13. "I'm Going to Beat This Alzheimer's."

It is very common for individuals to speak these words, often with great
passion. The appropriate response is to be supportive, reinforce the patients' determination and not contradict their statements. This attitude of
defiance reinforces a sense of personal control over impossible situations,
and patients with this belief system seem better adjusted and have fewer
behavioral difficulties. Even terminal cancer patients who express this attitude live longer with a higher quality of life.

Other issues and questions will arise. The general rule is to give simple and straightforward answers. Impart information when it is wanted
and convey a sense of support, love, and commitment. The way we respond to each other's questions and carry on conversations is one of the
major ways we create the fabric of human relationships and the home
atmosphere. Talking effectively with patients often requires great patience
and endurance. One wife commented, "Some days it's like trying to
speak Virgil to their Dante. There are also times when we can communicate." It is important to develop confidence in knowing when to respond to the patients' words and when simply to listen, and by doing so
convey the love and support we all need.

Behavioral Problems

Some, but not all, individuals with dementia behave in ways that are disruptive and disturbing to those around them. In many instances, the destruction of the brain is causing changes in eating and sleeping patterns, loss of control of bodily functions, or outbursts of emotions—love, hate, anger, jealousy. Some patients display inappropriate sexual behavior, wander away and get lost, or behave in ways that are improper or offensive without knowing what they are doing.

Anything that could possibly cause physical or emotional discomfort in any human being is a possible precipitant of behavioral disturbances in someone with dementia. Behavioral disturbances usually occur when the patient is thirsty or hungry, tired, bored, or overstimulated. Pain, injuries from a fall, cuts and abrasions, allergies, discomfort from overeating, indigestion, and gas are among the most frequent causes of agitation, upsets, screaming, and wanderings. Side effects from medications, such as dry mouth, blurred vision, or nausea, as well as drug allergies that cause rashes, tingling, or pain can be extremely unsettling to individuals who cannot express their discomfort.

In addition, people with Alzheimer's disease experience many different kinds of failures each day, such as when they forget something, cannot execute a task, or get lost. The reactions to these failures can explain many behavioral disturbances. There are three general reactions to failure—to get depressed, to get angry, or to let it pass—and these three general emotional patterns are seen in people with dementia. Some individuals are sad and depressed and become withdrawn and apathetic. Others become agitated, angry, and sometimes violent. And some individuals just seem to be happy and are not emotionally upset by their failures. These characteristic personality styles in reaction to constant failures, coupled with limited abilities to express anger or sadness, often lead to inappropriate or upsetting behavior.

Strategies to Deal with Behavioral Problems

The first step is to identify exactly what the behavioral problem is. The more clearly you can define the problem, the more success you will have designing an intervention. Gather information about the problem: how often it occurs, when and where it happens, what persons are involved. Think about your observations in relation to patterns of eating, sleeping, dressing, toileting, fatigue, pain and injury, and medications.

Although the range of responses to disturbing behavioral problems is broad, it is a good idea to learn a few general rules to guide your reactions. These rules involve diverting or distracting the patient, rewarding desirable behaviors, ignoring undesirable behaviors, blowing off steam away from the patient, and using specific techniques to control the environment. Finally, it is important to have a fall-back position for emergencies when individuals may be harmful to themselves or others. If your relative becomes paranoid or violent, protect yourself. Repeated violent episodes may be grounds for a serious re-evaluation of your decision to keep a loved one at home.

Diversion

Diversion is often an effective and relatively easy way to eliminate disruptive behaviors. Patients with dementia have a relatively short attention span and as a rule, can be moved to focus on something else without great difficulty. Judy McCormick, the wife of an Alzheimer's victim, was able to calm her husband by saying, "Let's have a cup of coffee, and I'll massage your back." This would often break her husband's angry mood. Caregivers will learn rapidly what diversions work best, and they should share this information with others who spend time with the patient.

It is often difficult for caregivers to remember to distract patients. It takes conscious self-discipline and practice to learn to control the natural inclination to argue or try to reckon with them. Patients do not look impaired and thus often trigger natural responses that are appropriate for cognitively intact individuals. It is a normal part of daily life to ask questions or have disagreements with others. However, many patients have cognitive deficits that preclude having a rational discussion. They may forget immediately or not comprehend what is said. Some patients have a deficit called *perseveration*, which means that they dwell on the same ideas, words, movements, or thoughts. Thus, they may continue to ask the same question over and over or echo the same thought such as "I want to go home." This can drive caregivers to the limits of frustration if they do not know how to respond appropriately, which often means distracting the patients with another topic.

Rewarding Desirable Behaviors and
Ignoring Undesirable Ones

Praising the patient for successes, spending quiet times together, touching, hugging, or giving a kiss all give the same message—"I like you. I enjoy your company." It is important to convey warmth and affection. We are all social beings, and we get satisfaction out of making those close to us happy. For the patients who have so much less to give, the message that they are still giving happiness is a powerful one.

One of our most difficult challenges is the control of our own spontaneous reactions to someone who upsets us. Anger, shouting, and striking out physically are all common responses. What is so difficult to understand is that these reactions often only serve to perpetuate the very behavior we want to eliminate. Years of study have led psychologists to the conclusion that by and large—unless there is some danger involved—ignoring the behavior you want stopped is far more effective than reacting to it. People appreciate any reaction from others. A positive reaction is best. A negative reaction is second best, but even second best is more desirable than being ignored. Behavior that is ignored often stops. A technique called *operant conditioning* systematizes this approach to the changing of specific behaviors. The application of this technique is discussed in the next section.

When patients become repeatedly upset over the same issue, caregivers can often devise an indirect way of calming their underlying fears or frustrations. Olin Wilson dreaded going to bed with his wife. Mona would be fine until he tried to get into the double bed they had shared over three decades. Then she would shout that he was invading her bed. She didn't know who he was and threatened to call the police if he didn't leave. He showed her his driver's license and pictures of their children, to no avail. This happened several times, and Olin became more and more agitated, with the result that Mona grew frightened and even more agitated herself.

Olin finally learned to prevent the situation in an imaginative way. For a few nights he waited for her to calm down and go to sleep before he joined her. A few days later he took out their album of wedding photographs, and he and Mona looked through it before they went to bed. This was a close and quiet time together, and Mona seemed very calm and happy to share her bed with her newly rediscovered husband.

It is common for patients to become angry and frustrated when they are unable to do or say something. Furthermore, they often fear their families will abandon them because they cannot function well. One patient described her situation this way: "I worry that Richard will leave me because I am not perfect anymore. I used to do everything, and now I am no good." Unfortunately, many caregivers have not learned how to deal with patients' fears and anger in a helpful way. In the early stages of dementia it is important to talk with the patients and find ways to work together to compensate for losses. Often it is useful for caregivers to convey the message that they accept the losses and still care for and love the patients.

Hans Dyson, whose wife had been diagnosed with dementia for six months, commented,

> In the beginning Madge and I were both terribly upset. When she would stop in the middle of a sentence, I tried to help her by supplying the words. She would cry, turn away, or storm out of the room. Madge had always been such a self-sufficient individual. With this Alzheimer's disease she needed help, but she simply could not accept help, even from those she loved.
>
> One morning I found her sitting at the kitchen table crying. There was orange juice in the cereal instead of milk. I placed my arms around her and held her in a long embrace. I told her I needed her more than ever. This Alzheimer's disease did not make me love her less.

Ways to Change Behavior: Operant Conditioning

A psychologist or psychiatrist sometimes can help manage patients' incontinence; enhance their ability to dress themselves, exercise, and eat properly; and reduce or eliminate their shrieking and screaming. Behavior can be changed by means of operant conditioning, a type of learning first described by B. F. Skinner. It refers to a strategy in which

rewards are given only when the individual performs specific desirable behaviors, to increase the likelihood that such behaviors will occur and that
undesirable behaviors will stop. For effective operant conditioning, the following principle must be obeyed: ignore undesirable behaviors and pay
attention to desirable ones. Attempting to calm the patient and paying
attention to the patient when he or she is behaving inappropriately is "rewarding" the behavior. A smile, a touch, a conversation, or attention should
only be given during a period of desirable activity as clear "rewards." As
difficult as it may be, leave the room when the patient is behaving inappropriately, for example, yelling, throwing food, or cursing.

Rewards or reinforcers do not have to be given to the patient in the
form of the caregiver's attention or such items as candy, food, drink, or
money. The patient's own behavior can be used to change behavior. For
example, Jackie Needham, aged eighty, lived in a nursing home but refused to attend any therapeutic or recreational activities. Under the supervision of a psychologist, the nurses observed that she spent several
hours of her waking time obsessively cleaning the furniture in her room.
Most of her time was spent sitting mutely by the window; none of it
was spent with other people or in any ward activities. A special program
was designed. Mrs. Needham was allowed to sit by the window only if
she attended an exercise class for five minutes in the morning. Over several weeks she began to spend more time in the exercise class and to attend other activities.

Another important example of a positive-reward strategy is "milieu
therapy." Milieu programs can be very successful in long-term-care settings. They involve the redesign of the institutional social and often physical environment, or "milieu," to make it more compatible with the
functional abilities of the patient with dementia. Rewards are given to
individuals for taking part in specific activities like recreation, maintenance of good personal hygiene, exercise, or attendance at group meetings. Establishing a "happy hour" with small glasses of beer, wine, or
cider before the dinner hour attracts patients, even dementia patients.
One nurse described the changes that took place on her ward: "I could
not believe some of the changes. Even Charlie, who has been here for
four years and seemed so out of it, began to dress up at four. He would
put on his Sunday sweater and wander into the dayroom at four-thirty
to wait. I didn't think he could do anything!"

Operant therapies can successfully change behaviors leading to self-injury. These include such actions as the failure to eat or dress and the ingestion of nonfood objects. For example, it was possible to change Adam Thatcher's behavior of refusing to wear clothing, with the use of beer as the reinforcer. Mr. Thatcher was given small glasses of beer for wearing additional pieces of clothing for longer periods of time. Eventually, he stayed dressed all day and was rewarded with one beer at lunch and one at dinner.

Methods of bowel and bladder training have been applied to incontinent patients with mixed success. Incontinence is a multifaceted problem. Operant techniques are particularly effective when incontinence is an "attention-getting" behavior. A watchful eye on patients will alert the caregiver to indications that signal a need to use the bathroom. Being responsive to nonverbal cues often teaches patients to express their need for help instead of urinating or defecating on the spot. The simple act of allowing people to select and buy their own pajamas has been known to reduce incontinence significantly. It is not always easy to implement operant therapy plans, since it often takes time to "extinguish" or eliminate inappropriate and undesirable behavior. These strategies take professional help, time, and ongoing advice, but they do work. It is also important to monitor medical conditions that affect toileting behaviors, such as urinary tract infections.

Psychosocial Therapies

The capacity for changing behavior in patients with dementia depends on many factors—the degree of cognitive loss, personality traits, motivation to perform, and the ability to communicate. When attentional skills are reasonably intact in patients during the early and middle stages of dementia, they can be appropriate candidates for certain therapeutic approaches.

Supportive psychotherapy and counseling can be effective for many patients in the earlier phases. More and more clinicians are being trained to deal with the problems these patients endure, including that of adjustment to change and loss. Without appropriate intervention, patients' feelings of dependency and helplessness can hasten the impairment process. Unrecognized and untreated emotional distress also can exacerbate the degree of impairment, even in patients with serious cognitive difficulties.

Group psychotherapy or family psychotherapy also can be effective. Groups of patients or patients and family members can successfully confront a range of problems and even help increase the disoriented individual's sense of control over the environment. Groups also seem to facilitate such goals as remotivation, resocialization, and increased activities.

Environmental Strategies

Impaired patients are usually capable of handling a number of changes in their environment if they have some choice or control in those changes. Change, especially a change in residence, often causes a stress reaction, but knowledge and a perception of some control over change decrease the amount of stress impaired patients feel.

Old age coupled with dementia constitutes a period of special vulnerability involving a loss of control over the environment. This sense of helplessness has been implicated in the earlier death of people at home or in nursing homes. One important effect of the operant-conditioning programs discussed earlier is that they not only shape patients' behavior using a system of reinforcements but also give them greater control over what is going to happen to them. This feeling of mastery is itself a very important reward.

A number of therapeutic strategies can be used with the help of professionals to enable the patient to cope as successfully as possible. It is important to shape the physical and social environment to support the patient's strengths and to minimize frustrating situations. This means doing such things as simplifying the daily schedule and providing activities consistent with the patient's memory and learning deficits, sensory acuity, and mobility. It is important to deal clearly and directly with the actions that the patient is simply not able to perform. Caregivers should express understanding and indicate that these actions are not important. New activities should be found to replace those no longer possible.

One crucial factor should guide all psychological interventions. There must be an orientation to the individual as a *person*, not as a patient. Only with this respect for an individual with a past and a future will it be possible to maximize the quality of life. Whatever his or her level of competence, the person with dementia will respond if treated as a human being who is enabled to play an active role in his or her own care within the limits of his or her skills for as long as possible.

Emergencies

Advanced planning is the key. It is important for caregivers to have a well-thought-out plan when emergencies do occur. Who will you contact to calm the patient if he or she becomes extremely agitated, aggressive, or violent? Are neighbors available to come over if the patient gets violent or tries to run away? Is a son or daughter or his or her spouse available to help? When should you call the doctor, police, or sheriff? Is there an agency to turn to, a support group member, an emergency room? The circumstances will vary, but these measures should be examined and realistically checked out. Knowing what to do in an emergency can help reduce your panic should such an emergency occur—in fact, knowing what to do in advance may enable you to solve the problem. Many families have said that just knowing that someone out there was ready to help meant so much to them that they solved the problem themselves. This sort of preparation even has the effect of helping with the decision to keep someone out of a nursing home.

Maintaining Marital and Other Relationships

Alzheimer's disease challenges the intimate bonds between two human beings. For husbands and wives, though, the love may deepen. A special grace and beauty mark those who have learned to live with the disease and continue to find ways to enjoy each other. For most couples, intimacy changes, and in general, the length of the marriage and the quality of the relationship before the diagnosis say a great deal about how well a couple will deal with the serious challenges of Alzheimer's disease. Long-standing marriages do not suddenly collapse even as the dementia takes its course. Recent marriages, particularly second or third marriages, are more vulnerable and may dissolve if the healthy spouse has not developed a loyalty and commitment toward the patient.

The intimacy of most family relationships is likely to change. Any relative—brother, sister, in-law, daughter, son, grandchild, cousin, or parent—involved with the patient must live with a series of emotional reactions. This reality spreads to other relationships between family members. A daughter or son caring for a mother or father may find that these activities strain the relationship with her or his spouse and children, who come to resent the lack of attention and affection paid to them.

The way the family has dealt with conflicts and problem solving in the past predicts how much caregiving will cause strains in relationships. Families who have a history of resolving conflict well with "fair fights" show less strain. Families who have kept busy with a variety of activities appear to deal with caregiving more effectively, and there is less conflict and tension in relationships compared to families who have not been as active.

The nature of the relationship with people outside the family is altered. Friendships wither and often disappear from lack of time given to maintaining them. These losses are among the most difficult for the patient and family to accept. As discussed earlier, consider shuttle diplomacy with the friends who mean the most to you and the patient. Resolve their fears about what to say and do for you, the family, and the patient.

Any caring relationship between persons in or out of a marriage is supported by a history of respect, devotion, and commitment to the well-being of one another. Because marriage embodies the most tender bonds of endearment, over time it forges a strong loyalty between people. The shadow of Alzheimer's disease changes the outlook of a couple's retirement years together, but it also provides opportunities for the dearest expressions of love. It hastens, too, what must sooner or later occur in all human relationships—separation and death. Husbands and wives and often other members of the family must work to enjoy each other—in doing so, they will help overcome some of the tragedy of the dementia.

Husband and Wife—Till Death Do Us Part

Many husbands and wives find the diagnosis a difficult one to accept. For some it becomes a burden of guilt: "I must deserve this for all the bad things I have done." Others see it as a challenge: "We had such a wonderful life together that I should be able to deal with this." For others there is outrage and shock: "Life is cruel. Why did such a wonderful man like my husband get this?"

How do you love someone who begins to change dramatically in front of your eyes and is no longer the person you married? Many family members say that the question never occurs to them and that years of living together have brought them close enough to each other that they can adapt. However, even in the strongest relationships the strain of caring can be significant, especially when opportunities for intimacy are diminished or bizarre behavior is prominent. Many patients may eventually make inappropriate sexual overtures to their spouse, other family members, or friends. One husband exclaimed, "I was shocked. My wife sat out in the lawn chair by the pool—stark naked reading a book!"

Sexuality is an important part of relating to a husband, a wife, or an appropriate partner. Sexuality also has an important impact on the way people feel about themselves. There are many ways to give and receive sexual pleasure, and some couples are able to adjust extremely well to changes in their sexual relationship. They have learned how to engage in a variety of satisfying sexual activities.

Living with Alzheimer's disease challenges the patient and sexual partner to live joyously with one another. Many issues are raised here to help family members at least be able to understand the changing sexuality of the dementia patient and the changes in their personal relationship with the patient. Most of the time sexual difficulties are ignored or not dealt with, because neither partner is comfortable discussing them.

Couples living with Alzheimer's disease face some complex pressures with regard to sexual activity. Unfortunately, most patients and their partners are uncomfortable talking about sex even when they are confronted with a problem. Many individuals are not even comfortable thinking about these issues. They may feel frustrated and upset either because they do not understand what they feel or because they are afraid to talk about their sexual and intimate lives.

Sexual problems should be reviewed with a doctor or knowledgeable health professional. Although this is a sensitive issue, professionals can help enormously in the understanding of the cause of sexual problems and resolving them. Many such difficulties can be treated successfully. Unfortunately, many physicians neglect to ask questions about sexual problems. Although you may be ill at ease, you should take the lead in bringing these issues up when they are a problem. Once you have begun to talk, the discomfort will often disappear. The cooperation of three people—husband, wife, and professional—is often needed to resolve sexual problems. Sometimes the attitudes and beliefs of an entire family need to be confronted.

Joe Tobias was sixty-seven years old, and he had been diagnosed as having Alzheimer's disease approximately six years earlier. His wife of forty-one years had died on his sixtieth birthday, and within the year he was married again. Six months after his second marriage Joe was diagnosed, and within another six months his second wife had left him. She was unable to cope with the changes in his behavior and the grim future facing the two of them.

Joe's children, five sons and two daughters, formed a close-knit family, and everyone, including their wives, husbands, and children, united to do everything possible to keep Joe at home and happy. And they were able to satisfy all of Joe's needs, save one—his need for a sexual partner.

Furthermore, his sexual needs became an embarrassing problem. Each of the women in the family felt uncomfortable around Joe because of the way he stared at them, obviously fixating on their breasts or legs. Although he never harmed anyone, it was not unusual for him to reach over and inappropriately fondle someone's arm, hand, neck, shoulder, or other part of the body.

The incident that galvanized the family occurred one day when the youngest son stopped at his father's house after lunch and found Joe in bed with a young woman who was a waitress at a local restaurant. A family meeting was called that night (without Joe present), and the consensus was that Dad had to be seen by a doctor who would treat his voracious sexual hunger.

The eldest son, Jason, was elected to escort his father to the doctor. Without referring to the incident, Jason insisted that his father keep an appointment with a "specialist." The doctor told Joe that sexual urges were not normal in a man his age and that, fortunately, treatment was available to cure him. The prescription was for a vitamin E shot once every two to three weeks. The family ushered Joe to the doctor religiously. However, his behavior did not change. Joe would sit in the park and watch the girls, sometimes approaching one of them and asking her to have coffee or lunch with him. And, as the family later discovered, he had been having relations with the housekeeper on a regular basis.

Finally, out of frustration the family sent Joe to visit his youngest daughter, Joanne, who lived in another state. The family members had conferred with each other (including Joanne) and had unanimously decided that it was her turn to take care of her father. Within a week trouble began because Joanne's roommate, a young female artist, was afraid to be around Joe. Even Joanne became alarmed by his "unfatherly hugs and kisses." However, Joanne found professional help.

In the very first meeting, which lasted several hours, Joe described as best he could the distress he felt over his sexual urges. He was aware that his behavior was inappropriate, and he was also aware that his need for sexual relief was powerful. The doctor who ordered regular shots had clearly declared his sexual needs to be abnormal, but Joe was confused. The nurse who gave him the injections was beautiful, and he got an erection every time he received a treatment. Furthermore, although the nurse was aware of his reaction, she did not get angry or indeed say a single word to acknowledge what happened. Once Joe even asked her whether she thought that it was abnormal for a man his age to feel romantic and have a relationship with a woman. Her polite answer of no made him feel good, but he still remained confused and concerned.

Having received assurances that sexual urges were indeed normal, Joe seemed greatly relieved. In fact, he then volunteered that he felt that his behavior toward women was not always appropriate. He very much wanted to talk with someone about what he perceived to be a serious problem but one that he hoped could be solved.

He had been happily married to a woman who was the center of his life spiritually and sexually. As long as they had been together, they had intercourse at least once or twice a day. One of the reasons he had married so soon after his wife's death was the need to have the intimacy he craved. When his second wife left him, he had clearly lost a socially acceptable partner in his small town. Furthermore, Janice, his second wife, had not deserted him without trying to make the marriage work. She tried hard, and after several sessions with the minister and Joe, the decision she had to make became clear.

Joe's children clearly loved him, but they also made his life difficult. With all of them "caring" for him, he had absolutely no privacy. He felt guilty about having women in his home. He did not want to embarrass his children or make them ashamed of his behavior. But how could he live his life and have the happiness and satisfaction he wanted?

The solution to Joe's living situation required the sensitive involvement of the entire family. Many meetings were held to help all the family members identify and understand what their father's needs were relative to their own. It was hard work for everyone. Although his sons and daughters were upset about his sexual needs and behaviors, they became more relaxed as they listened to an outsider help them understand how their attitudes and needs had interfered with their father's needs.

With time it was possible to work out an acceptable solution to Joe's dilemma. The family members were able to accept the reality that their father wanted and needed a partner. As it became apparent that Joe had an affectionate and fulfilling relationship with the housekeeper, the family found the affair acceptable. Joe lived another seven years surrounded by his family and the housekeeper-lover, who cared for him until he died.

There exists an extremely sensitive area where husbands and wives report deep feelings of conflict. After a loved one is institutionalized, many individuals describe how their needs for friendships and companionship with the opposite sex cause personal and family distress. Many people are ashamed or embarrassed to be seen together with someone at a restaurant, the theater, a movie, or even on the street for fear of giving rise to hurtful rumors. There is often enormous anxiety about having meaningful affairs or longer-term relationships with a boyfriend or a girlfriend.

Leonard Alexander disclosed his feelings in a group meeting and received support for his desire to ask a friend to spend a weekend with him.

MR. A.: I love my wife, and she has been the emotional center of my life for thirty years. Nothing will change that. My feelings toward my wife have even intensified in a spiritual sort of way. But I have had to admit to myself that I am interested in women now much more than I used to be.

MRS. J.: Explain that, will you?

MR. A.: I was talking to Judy about all the nice women she has introduced me to. When she comes out to the nursing home to visit her husband, she usually brings a friend. It's quite a treat. So when I told her I had an idea about seeing a woman, she encouraged me. I have a friend my age whom I've known for a long time. She was widowed about a year ago, and I thought I would like to invite her for a trip to the islands for a week.

Judy thought it was a great thing to do and encouraged me to ask her. "Lay out the ground rules, split the expenses, and give her a private bedroom. Bring a good book, in case you turn her off that first day, and let things develop slowly."

And frankly, if all I get is some decent companionship, that's fine. But if she wants to seduce me, I don't think I'll protest. I phoned her up, and she was shocked. But she didn't turn me down. She said she would think about it. I told her to take plenty of time, but if she turned me down, she should have some very good reasons why my proposal was not suitable. So it's going to be rather interesting now to see what she comes out with. I hope it's maybe. I don't want it to be no, but if it's no, that's fine. But you know something—I don't give a damn whether it happens or not now—I feel so good about having asked her. I feel alive again knowing that I can plan a little bit in the future. There were some very hard times when I didn't think I could plan anything. Now I feel that I've ventured a little bit. Yet I haven't abandoned my responsibility for my wife, who, incidentally, I'm probably closer to now than I've ever been before, in a strange sort of way.

I'm starting to take care of my own needs. I feel pretty good about everything.

Someone you trust, whether a family member or a confidant, is often extremely valuable to help you evaluate options in difficult life decisions. There are no easy or right answers, and sometimes the answers are very private. Mr. Alexander did plan the trip with his friend, but he had to postpone the trip for a month because he came down with the flu. The illness was fortunate because Mrs. Alexander died on the weekend of the week her husband was originally scheduled to be away on his trip.

For many people, a relationship outside the marriage is neither a desirable nor an acceptable alternative. Lois Barclay Murphy wrote the moving book *The Home Hospital*, which is not only a practical guide to coping with catastrophic illness in a loved one but also the profound love story of her relationship with her husband, Gardner Murphy, who had Parkinson's disease. The two were devoted to each other, and their ability to sustain and nurture one another is a testament to the human spirit and the bond of love that transcends sexuality. Lois Murphy spoke lovingly of their intimate moments together. They lost no opportunity to hug, kiss, or hold each other, even when Gardner was bedridden and nurses were present. Simply holding hands and being close enough to exchange glances carried the strongest message of love and devotion.

A lifetime of emotional investment between husband and wife often cultivates a depth and style of communication that cannot be undone by Alzheimer's disease. The intensity of the human bond is heightened as couples struggle to live together and care for one another.

Lupe Juarez had been diagnosed as having Alzheimer's disease for eight years. Her husband, Mario, had been retired for two years before his wife began having noticeable problems. Both of them found great pleasure in simply being together, as they had for the past fifty-five years. Most of their time was spent at home, in the garden, shopping, and visiting children and grandchildren. During the summer they took to the road in their camper—traveling to new places, fishing, camping, and walking together. The winters were harsh, so they stayed home, quite happy to be together. Meals, family visits, music, and reading were the highlights of the winter days.

Even as Mrs. Juarez deteriorated, Mr. Juarez continued to read to her the newspaper in the morning at breakfast and novels at night after dinner. Although she could not discuss people, events, or issues as the dementia robbed her of speech, memory, and judgment, she sat next to him on the couch, hand on his knee, listening or perhaps only staring into space. No one knew how much she absorbed, but it was clear that a deep love bound them together.

Mr. Juarez managed well until about two years before his wife's death. His children noticed that he was being more irritable and that he was spending more time at the local tavern. The oldest son called for help, and a meeting with us was arranged. During the interview Mr. Juarez sighed and offered some critical information:

> I love my wife more than life itself. It hurts so much to see her wither away. She is like a burning candle which keeps sputtering.

I am afraid of the day the flame dies. She and I have been able to help each other live with this thing. But I am getting tired. She is changing a great deal now and is a shell of the person I married. She is becoming a stranger to me even though I know she is my wife, and, strange as it may seem, I love her more than ever.

Now I have to do everything for her. I just wish there was some little thing she could do for me so I would know that the old Lupe is still there. It would help me go on. Please forgive me. It may sound stupid and selfish, but I even miss her washing my hair in the evenings. She gave a wonderful hair massage, and it helped me relax at the end of a long day.

We then met alone with Mr. and Mrs. Juarez and reviewed with them what they planned to do for the next three months. They held hands as Mr. Juarez spoke openly about his drinking. He enjoyed having a few beers in the tavern with his friends. It was a habit of fifty years. We discussed what might be the cause of his excessive drinking, and he began to express his frustrations. He was angry seeing his wife deteriorate. He was also frustrated sexually. Sometimes at night he would make romantic overtures when the time seemed right and she was willing. However, in the middle of foreplay she would change from a responsive woman to a giggling child. Dealing with these abrupt changes was impossible. His wife was still beautiful and attractive in his eyes, but the "child" in bed was someone else. It broke his heart and made him angry beyond words.

The plan we evolved took patience and personal, careful discussions. Mr. Juarez himself suggested that perhaps they should now sleep in separate beds, which would still be kept close together. It was probably not appropriate, at least in this case, to initiate sex with his wife. It took a long time for Mr. Juarez to digest the reality that the Alzheimer's disease was affecting the part of his wife's brain that helped control sexuality and pleasure. He understood this reality intellectually, but emotionally it was difficult to deal with.

We were lucky enough to find something that Mrs. Juarez could still do for her husband. We encouraged him to reinstate an old tradition— to let his wife wash his hair in the sink several evenings each week. We also suggested that they continue another family tradition—to visit the town diner each Saturday and Sunday morning for breakfast. This was an opportunity to be together and visit other people as they had for so many years.

The strategy was successful. It was a shot in the arm for Mr. Juarez. Hair washing and eating breakfasts out captured the old intimacy and gave him the emotional strength to continue. Mrs. Juarez died several years later, at home, surrounded by her family and friends. Mr. Juarez never remarried. However, he did have a close woman friend, who had also been close to Mrs. Juarez. They met several times a week in the diner for breakfast, lunch, or dinner and enjoyed a healthy intimate relationship. And together with other friends they took day trips around the area.

After Mr. Juarez died, the children found an attic full of letters as they sorted through their parents' belongings. There were many packages of love letters Mr. and Mrs. Juarez had written to each other. The children were surprised at the sheer volume of letters, because their parents had been separated only during World War II, and the correspondence spanned a lifetime together. Through these letters the children came to appreciate even more what a special partnership their parents had enjoyed.

The memory losses in dementia, however, may weaken the bond between two people. The relationship of marriage partners is a complex one. It is sustained by how events were experienced and resolved in the past, by the sense of perceived loyalty and responsibility, by the degree of emotional (and sometimes financial) investment each holds in the other, and by factors outside the relationship. For example, children, family position, or other social and cultural factors affect the way a couple deals with one another over time. Since Alzheimer's disease is one of the most complex challenges an individual will ever face, it would not do justice to the intricacy of human relationships and experience to try to give simple and easy prescriptions for right and wrong behavior.

Anne and Mario Varico had been married fifty-four years before Mario was diagnosed with vascular dementia. For five years Anne cared for him, even though the marriage had not been satisfying for her over the last twenty-five years. Indeed, she had worked up the courage to pursue a divorce just before Mario had the first of three small strokes. After years of caregiving, Anne wanted out:

> I do not want to put Mario in a nursing home. We have enough
> money to pay someone to live with him and do what needs to be

done. He would not do for me what I have done for him. He was a selfish, angry man before the dementia and he is a selfish, angry man now. I have been a caregiver for five years. I have done my duty. I need a life of my own.

Sexual Difficulties in Alzheimer's Disease

Sexual functioning in individuals with Alzheimer's disease and related disorders may be influenced by the physical and emotional effects of the disease. However, there has been little research in this area. It is important to remember that sexual dysfunction is not unique to patients with Alzheimer's disease. Many happily involved or married people have difficulties at some point in their lives together. In many ways the problems of Alzheimer's patients are no different from those of any other human beings who enjoy physical pleasure, the intimacy of another human being, and the success of giving pleasure to another person. Physical illness, medications, depression, feelings of inadequacy, and many other factors can interfere with sexual prowess and satisfaction. In most instances, the condition can be corrected.

Since Alzheimer's disease entails the loss of cells in the central nervous system, many parts of the sexual response can be affected. Alzheimer's disease can affect the ability to become sexually aroused. Many patients have difficulty achieving an erection and complain of a loss of potency. Women with dementia often report a loss of interest and the inability to achieve orgasm. In same-sex relationships, the affected partner may want to have sexual relationships with another person, either of the same sex or of the opposite sex. Increased sexual activity may occur. This hypersexuality may be noticed in many ways, including the heightened desire for sexual intercourse, obvious fondling of one's genitals, masturbation in public or private, and attempts to seduce others.

Self-exposure and masturbation may occur because patients forget where they are, the importance of being dressed, or how to dress themselves. Undressing may also occur if clothes are uncomfortable, and handling genitals may reflect itching and discomfort from urinary tract infections and other problems. If the patient is undressed, calmly and matter-of-factly find a robe and help him or her to put it on. If the patient is exposing himself or herself or masturbating, do not get upset or do or say anything that is critical. Gently guide the patient to a private place. Dress the patient and find another activity.

The short attention span characteristic of the disease also plays a role in sexual activity. Arousal may be short-lived and create frustration in the partner. Childish behavior may emerge, leading to anger and irritability in a spouse who sees the patient as physically intact and, in many instances, no less attractive.

Sexual difficulties in Alzheimer's disease can be divided into five major groups: (1) those resulting from destruction of the brain, (2) those caused by physical illnesses, (3) those that are side effects of medication, (4) those caused by psychological conflicts, and (5) those caused by social pressures and attitudes. The crucial step is to determine to what extent sexual difficulties are the result of structural change in the nervous system or the consequence of psychological factors like anxiety or clinical depression. Several issues are important here. Individuals must be aware of changes in their own body and be able to share this information with their partner. It is also important for partners to tell each other what they do and do not find pleasurable. However, Alzheimer's disease often makes this difficult in later stages or when the dementia is more severe. When the impairment is neurological, several devices may be useful to the male. If prosthetic devices are needed, consult a doctor.

The possible value of medication should not be overlooked. Drugs like Viagra (sildenafil) may be a helpful adjunct to managing the patient. No specific studies have employed Viagra for the sexual problems of dementia patients, but the counsel of a physician and the specific physical condition of the patient can dictate the appropriate use of such medication.

Women having difficulties being aroused or reaching orgasm also should seek professional advice. For problems like decreased vaginal lubrication, an appropriate jelly such as K-Y may be useful. Petroleum jelly (Vaseline) is less desirable because it is not water soluble and often causes vaginal infections.

It helps when sexual partners are able to communicate with one another, but an inability to communicate is precisely the problem in Alzheimer's disease. However, even when the exchange of information is impaired, the healthy spouse can take the initiative. Manual and oral stimulation may become a satisfying sexual outlet or a substitute for intercourse. Not being able to have successful intercourse does not mean that it is no longer possible for an individual to give or receive pleasure.

Husbands and wives have shown the most tender devotion to the other's physical as well as emotional needs. At the age of seventy-five Martin Regan had suffered from Alzheimer's disease for more than seven years. He and his wife, Regina, had weathered the years together surrounded by their two sons and their families. Mr. Regan was hospitalized after a fall in which he broke his hip and also had a subdural hematoma. At that time he could recognize his wife and sister as well as his children, but he could not utter more than a few words. Much of the time he seemed disoriented and confused. He needed assistance with bathing and shaving and was incontinent.

Mrs. Regan's two sons had been urging her to place him in a nursing home. They had become increasingly distressed over her poor health and the strain that caring for him placed on her. Finally, Peter, the older son, and his wife took his mother to lunch to persuade her to put Mr. Regan in a nursing home and not take him home again.

As had been predicted, the lunch was a long and tearful one. Mrs. Regan tried desperately to convince her children that her life revolved around her husband and his care. She would not surrender him to a home because he had made her promise in the early phases that she would never do such a thing. The lunch ended abruptly, but Peter was able to talk his mother into seeing their clergyman. In several sessions with the reverend, she was able to discuss the intensity and richness of her married life even in her husband's deteriorated state. It had a special intimacy that needed to be preserved for her.

Mrs. Regan continued to minister to her husband. She described how she often found him in bed, even in the hospital, starting to get an erection. He would hold himself and look distressed. She did the only thing she could. She gave him the relief he needed, and he would fall asleep holding her hand as she sat by the bed.

This section on intimacy may not have been an easy one to read. Life is very precious, and perhaps nothing is more precious than the shared and private experiences of two people. For some relationships sexuality is a major factor—for others it may have less value. Love is one of the greatest gifts people can give to each other. Sexuality is only one expression of that gift. Intimacy, closeness, familiarity, companionship, and respect are among the other special gifts.

Caring at Home

The next chapter describes the choices families face to keep the patient at home and to provide for his or her long-term-care needs. Most people do not plan for getting Alzheimer's disease, and they do not believe they will need long-term care. However, planning for long-term care is the best way to make appropriate decisions to protect one's resources as well as to make one's preferences known and understood. When Milton Berle said, "I've got enough money for the rest of my life, unless I have to buy something," people laughed. However, the long-term-care challenges of later life are not a laughing matter.

8

Long-Term Care at Home

My friends think that I am a martyr. I feel like both Solomon and Job. Robin has been sick with Alzheimer's disease for less than a year. He has deteriorated very rapidly, and now he just sits much of the day staring out the window. When I talk to him, he may say nothing, smile, or shout nonsense such as "Spitfire! Good! Get them!" I intend to keep him at home as long as I can. That much I know. The children are pressing me, but I will not let him go.

Robin is company to me. Yes, our life is lopsided, but our love is not. He needs so much care, and as long as I can manage him and me, I will. Robin keeps changing and getting worse a little more each day, but I am still able to understand him. He is not the man he used to be, but he needs certain things. And he needs me.

Each morning and evening we keep an important ritual. He sits at the window watching the birds who visit the feeder in our yard. He is not able to put the food out anymore, but he still enjoys sitting for an hour or often more watching the antics of the squirrels and the birds. He was an avid bird-watcher throughout his life. Now the binoculars, the books, and his sketches are meaningless to him, but the birds still bring him pleasure. Yesterday a finch flew into the glass door, breaking its neck instantly. I was on the phone with a friend, but I heard the hard knock against the pane. I walked into the living room, saw the bird on the porch, and saw Robin crying. After checking the bird to make sure it was really dead, I went to the kitchen to find something in which to wrap it. Robin held a brown paper bag while I dropped the bird in. He folded the top down neatly several times and gave it back to me. We buried it in the backyard.

An hour later, I know he did not remember what happened. But for a few minutes that day I had a glimpse of the gentle man who loved the world of nature. Somewhere deep inside, part of him was still there, but I couldn't hold on to it.

Family members have always provided the majority of care over the course of dementia, and today they are providing more care for longer periods of time than ever before. However, caring is not a simple, spontaneous behavior. Caring is a set of technical activities— watching, listening, making decisions, and taking action. Furthermore, you need to be motivated to care, and caring reflects a complex blend of motivations. Different people have different reasons for caring, including love, reciprocity, morality, ethical reasoning, envy, and on occasion even greed. These motivations affect your willingness to do the various tasks associated with caregiving as well as the degree to which you are willing to participate.

You may be influenced by any number of these motivations, depending on your kinship as well as the history and nature of your relationship with the patient. A common belief of many caregivers, especially spouses, is that no one else can provide the optimal level of love, attention, and well-being. If you are an adult child, you may have a strong affection for your parent and want to do more for them compared to other siblings or relatives. Your desire to please your parent may be motivated by the desire to please, by the desire to do the right thing, or even the possibility of being willed the house as an inheritance.

Not all relationships are loving, and over time emotional forces may run counter to each other. You may not like the patient because he or she hurt, abused, or disappointed you, yet you are influenced by the need to respond to the humanity of the moment and do what must be done. Lynn Argo sent us the following e-mail:

I wonder if you could give me some information on social services for elder care in South Carolina—the outskirts of Charleston?

The history is this: My father Larry is eighty-six. His wife Su-
san of thirty years has terminal cancer and is not expected to live
more than a month or so. They live in a mobile home on the
banks of the river outside of Charleston and have been there for
about thirty years. My father is a mess. He has had a stroke, can't
hear (and won't listen if he could), has trouble walking, falls a lot,
etc. and so on.

The problem is what to do when his wife passes on. Her daughters are caring for her now with the help of hospice but definitely
won't be there after she goes. My dad says he won't leave but he
can't take care of himself.

Could you provide names, e-mail addresses of local community services or health care providers?

I am trying to get a handle on the situation but don't know
what to do.

P.S. The irony is that my father walked out on my mother,
brother, sister, and me when I was about 13 years old . . . you
can imagine my feelings about this.

What can I do?

Mrs. Argo wanted nothing to do with her father, and she had had no
communication with him since he had abandoned the family. The two
daughters, Inez and Erin, were taking turns staying with their mother until
she died. As unpleasant as it was, they also had to deal with Larry and cook
and care for him. They also had no love for their stepfather because he had
treated them so badly over the years. After their mother died, Inez and Erin
had no intention of staying in contact with him or helping in any way.

Inez, Erin, and Lynn did decide that they had a moral obligation to inform Larry about his options. Hospice had a caseworker do an evaluation,
and the conclusion was clear: He could not live at home without assistance.
Larry was at high risk for falls, he could not cook or clean, and he could
not dress or bathe without some assistance. With the help of hospice the
family tried to get Larry to accept help in the house or move to a board-
and-care home. He refused to sign a durable power of attorney for health.

The month after his wife died, Larry fell and broke his hip. He was
hospitalized and discharged to a nursing home where he continued to
live until he died a year later.

The Challenge of Long-Term Care

When relationships have been good, family members are often correct in the belief that with assistance and time off, they can take better care of their relative than anyone else can. Familiar faces, sights, smells, and sounds provide valuable reference points for the confused adult. Family members know more about the patient and often understand his or her needs and desires more quickly than others.

Many families find a sense of security in being able to supervise a daily routine and in knowing where the patient is at all times. Indeed, caregivers often feel comfortable only when they know that the patient is being cared for at home, where he or she "belongs." It is the same feeling as not completely trusting a babysitter with your children. The cognitively impaired individual responds well to the love and under-standing attention of the family. But successful caregiving requires de-votion, determination, vigilance, and self-sacrifice. Although family members can often keep the patient at home for years, they need help to protect themselves from burnout and illness.

One of the pitfalls in providing care to someone very close to you is that you may come to believe that you must do everything yourself, and this attitude is a setup for exhaustion, burnout, and health problems. However, in many circumstances there are good reasons for this belief. Caregivers may have experiences with clinics, doctors, and social agen-cies that are not helpful. Over time fewer friends call or visit, and even family members may be less available for assistance when needed. As a result, primary caregivers learn to deal with their problems in isolation with little help, and in these circumstances it is difficult to avoid feeling alone, abandoned, and resentful. Indeed, these feelings may create an emotional armor that isolates the caregiver even more. Thus, when some-one is available to provide needed support and resources, the caregiver is not receptive and may even lash out at the party who wants to be of assistance.

Some caregivers may develop a style of seeing, thinking, and acting that over time becomes quite rigid and isolating. One reaction to the stress of caring is to believe that your way of doing things is the only way that works! This can be beneficial when caregivers reject well-intentioned but ill-advised recommendations to institutionalize the patient as soon as possible. However, in some circumstances, blindly opposing help from others or any course of action recommended by professionals and family members, including respite care, assisted living, or institutionalization, can be detrimental to all parties. Rigidity from the stress of caregiving may create an inflexibility and unwillingess to examine and adapt to the circumstances and available resources. Rigid adherence to any pat formula—"Move them into a home!" or "Never put them into a nursing home!"—paves the way for future difficulties and unhappiness. Such narrow perspectives often prevent family members from examining what resources are available in a changing situation, and how as a result they may not find or accept the help needed from a variety of programs for the aged, disabled, and handicapped.

Alzheimer's disease should be regarded as a management challenge, not an insurmountable tragedy. Although caring can be a source of satisfaction, it also usually becomes a burden to provide for the continuing needs of the patient as the illness progresses into the later stages. Minimal assistance may be needed in the beginning, but problems become more serious with time. Most families are unprepared for the strain of years of long-term caring, and they are caught in a vise of increasing demands and diminishing resources. This is a burden of love, but the enormity of the demands, the stresses, the isolation, and the uncertainty of the future take a toll. In addition, the erratic sleeping patterns, wandering, clinging behavior, and the physical and time demands of caring are a profound challenge. There are fewer opportunities for rest and little time for personal needs and the many problems that exist in any household.

Caregivers must try to be honest with themselves. If the care they are able to provide at home is limited by poor health, financial distress, the need to work, space limitations in the home, or just plain exhaustion, caregivers owe it to themselves and the patient to seek help and consider alternatives. Many relatives who have not helped care for the patient may not accept the idea of an assisted living or nursing-home placement, yet they are not able or may not offer to lend a hand with the around-the-clock care. These discussions often make the primary caregiver(s) feel angry or guilty.

Uninvolved relatives should be given the opportunity to participate in caregiving in some way, and if they choose not to, they should be ignored, as difficult as this may be. Think about your family as a business or corporation. Voting in a corporation is restricted to shareholders, and the relatives who contribute nothing to the care of the patient do not earn the shares required to vote about care decisions. Only the family members caring for the patient's needs on a daily basis know how hard it can be.

Common Family Decisions
Caring for a Relative at Home

Family members caring for a relative at home face many common challenges and decisions. These include providing personal care, negotiating the health care system, accessing community services, limiting the patient's freedom to prevent injury and harm, financial and legal planning, learning to balance caregiving with other work-life roles and family needs, coping with personal and family stress, relocation to senior housing or assisted living, nursing-home placement, and care at the end of life.

Recent research studies have clarified the difficulties involved in decision making. The results of a 1999 survey of caregivers of family members with dementia revealed that the most common decisions involved placement in a nursing home, informing family and friends about the diagnosis, stopping the individual from driving, and seeking a durable power of attorney. Half of the caregivers surveyed who faced the decision to have the patient stop driving considered it challenging, whereas almost all of the caregivers making the decision to provide personal care or place a relative in a nursing home found that decision challenging. Driving cessation was the most frequently made decision limiting the patient's freedom, compared to decisions limiting traveling, cooking, working, smoking, and drinking.

How to Deal with Driving Cessation

Driving requires skills that can become impaired at different rates as the dementia progresses. Safe driving demands sharp hearing and vision; a memory for signs, destinations, locations, and actions; good judgment; quick reaction time; and effective motor skills. However, patients usually have been driving for so many decades that the basic skills of starting, steering, or stopping a car may be intact for years after the disease begins.

Since Alzheimer's disease often impairs individuals' ability to comprehend the full extent of their losses, patients argue that they are competent to drive, and violent arguments erupt when they are challenged. Giving up the car keys is a major loss because driving represents freedom and competence, and so many patients depend on a car to go virtually anywhere. After Alzheimer's disease is diagnosed, the ability to drive is one of the first activities to be questioned because it affects safety. It can be a life-and-death issue not just for the patient but also for any driver or pedestrian in the patient's path.

There are no clear guidelines or criteria for referring patients with Alzheimer's disease and related disorders for a driving evaluation, and there are no precise regulations in most states. States' laws and regulations usually do not provide a supportive political and legal context for decision making by family and friends. If families reach out to the local or state department of motor vehicles, there are no assurances that the reporting procedures in place will support them taking away the license. Most states do not have age-based policies for evaluating and handling at-risk drivers, and age per se is not and should not be the issue. Some states specifically preclude using age as a basis for evaluating at-risk drivers.

As of 1998, at least eight states required physicians to report patients who have a diagnosis of Alzheimer's disease or a related disorder that might affect the safety of drivers in the community. In these instances the physicians are protected from legal action by the family. Yet some physicians may find themselves conflicted about the responsibilities to maintain patient confidentiality and the responsibility to report impaired, dangerous drivers. Indeed, patients may become irate, threaten a lawsuit, and even find a new physician.

Knowing when it is unsafe for the patient to drive is a matter of judgment. Slowed-down cognitive processing and episodes of confusion are the best measures of predicting which older drivers will have crashes. Several researchers developed experimental methods to test driving skills, but no standardized psychological tests are available to determine whether an individual has the coordination and other perceptual and memory skills necessary to drive an automobile safely. The most effective tactic is to go to the local department of motor vehicles and have the patient take a road test.

If the patient fails the test, ask his or her physician or another professional to explain the results of the road test to the patient. Your relative may not like what is said or may not understand, but at least he or she was involved in the decision-making process. Give the patient the benefit of the doubt about what he or she can understand. Involving the patient gives a nonverbal message that he or she is respected and valued as a member of the family. This simple strategy, in contrast to telling the patient outright that he or she cannot drive, may foster an acceptance of driving cessation.

What happens in the physician's office and what happens at home are often quite different things. Patients may concede in the office that driving is dangerous. However, at home they may insist on driving, angrily reject any explanation, and often explode in a violent rage over control of the car keys. One woman told us, "Jack wanted the keys, but I refused to give them to him. He grabbed them from me but held my arm tightly. I was terrified. His eyes were filled with such hate. I never saw such hate. Jack was always such a gentle man. He never even raised his voice to me in all the years we were married."

It is important to remember that you are not talking with a rational person about the right to drive, and arguing only makes the situation worse. Once you make the decision, be firm. Hiding the car keys is probably the most common technique for dealing with the issue of driving. This ploy works well until someone gets into the car with the patient, who then insists on driving. The most useful approach here is to distract the patient with a proposed activity that will be attractive to them, such as "Let's go eat lunch, and then we will go for a drive." The secret to success is distraction with activities the patient enjoys. During the period when driving is an upsetting issue—it will fade with time—it may be helpful to have the patient sit in the backseat with someone else to provide distraction. Refusing to drive with the patient if he or she has the keys and insisting on being the driver can help, as can planning trips when the patient is taking a nap or otherwise distracted.

Give the issue some time to play out while you try to reduce the need for the patient to drive. It is painful for patients to accept the multiple losses that come with dementia, and it is legitimate for them to feel anger, bordering on rage. So much is being taken from them. Patients deserve some time and support to work the anger out of their system. Since they may already have problems in expressing themselves, it is often difficult for the family to know how to help. However, most family members seem to do exactly what must be done without really being aware of it. The love and devotion of caring family members often enable them to endure the greatest hardships, with no professional around to tell them what a great job they are doing.

Although family members report that interventions for driving cessation are difficult, most caregivers are successful. Those who are not successful are those who are reluctant or unable to cope with the consequences of driving cessation. Being too busy to drive the older person and a poor relationship with the older person are barriers to intervention. There are nine characteristics of family and friends who intervene successfully: (1) They have a strong belief that the older driver is a significant danger. (2) They believe that they have a responsibility for the older persons. (3) They are a primary or secondary caregiver. (4) They are able to make the decision and work through the process even when the older person objects. (5) They are able to manage their own frustrations and emotions as well as those of other family members. (6) They have the support or approval of other family members. (7) They are willing to provide or find alternative transportation. (8) They attend support groups. (9) They have the support of a physician, law enforcement officer, or the department of motor vehicles.

Home- and Community-Based Resources for Long-Term Care

With the rapid growth in the numbers of older people with dementia, private and public organizations are offering an increasing number of long-term-care options. Long-term care is different from what most people associate with medical care in a doctor's office or a hospital where diseases and injuries are treated and cured. Long-term care involves helping people to maintain the highest level of functioning for an extended period of time. Because dementia cannot be fixed or cured, support and compassion are key components of quality long-term care.

Long-term care can entail both medical and nonmedical assistance in many settings and with many different caregivers. It can be everything from help with shopping and household chores, to paid in-home care, to supportive living arrangements and skilled nursing care. It can be provided by a nurse, home health aide, a physical therapist, occupational or speech therapist, mental health professional, trained volunteer, or a family member.

Many families find that they can manage home care for years with help from these outside sources. Cooperation between various family members in the care of a patient can strengthen ties and bring family members closer together. Young children will have an opportunity to learn the gentleness and love required in the care of a chronically ill older person. Many people, provided they do have to shoulder the entire burden, find real satisfaction and beauty in the care of their relative, and in turn these feelings strengthen the family.

Fortunately, there have never been more resources in the community to help families. These resources include health care, personal care, transportation, housekeeping, day care, and other services that promote emotional well-being:

Day health and rehabilitation care: These programs offer a range of therapeutic, rehabilitative, and support activities, including nursing, rehabilitation, assistance with life activities, social work services, meals, and transportation. They are provided in a protected setting for a portion of a day, one to five days a week.

Day care: Day-care programs provide supportive but not rehabilitative services in a protected setting for a portion of the day, one to five days a week. Services may include recreational activities, social work services, a hot meal, transportation, and occasionally, health services.

Nutritional programs: Congregate meal programs feed many older adults as a group in a community center, church, or school. Some communities sponsor home-delivered meals to the frail, homebound aged. One noonday meal is provided, containing one-third of the recommended daily dietary allowance for a range of nutrients.

Home health care: These are organized programs of nursing, social work, occupational and physical therapy, and other rehabilitation services to individuals in their homes.

Home health aides: Home health aides provide personal care to individuals at home under the supervision of a health professional. Aides assist with preparing meals, eating, dressing, bathing, administering medications, as well as performing light household tasks.

Homemaker services: Household assistance is provided by professionally supervised and trained homemakers. Services include shopping, laundry, light cleaning, dressing, preparation of meals, and escort services to medical visits.

Housekeeping services: These services usually include cleaning, shopping, laundry, and meal preparation.

Chore workers: Chore-worker services include heavy-duty house-cleaning, minor home repairs, yard work, and pest control.

Companionship services: Companions visit isolated and homebound individuals for conversation, reading, letter writing, and general light errands.

Respite care services: Respite care programs provide temporary twenty-four-hour care to give relief to primary caregivers. The care may be provided in the person's home, an adult care home, or a nursing home.

Hospital and surgical supply services: Supply houses rent or sell medical supplies and equipment like hospital beds, canes, walkers, bath chairs, and oxygen and other equipment.

Transportation: Transportation services provide travel by automobile or specialized vans to and from community agencies and service providers.

Escort services: These services provide personalized accompaniment to service providers as well as personal assistance.

Physical therapy: Physical therapy, or PT, is rehabilitative therapy to maximize mobility. It should be provided by a qualified physical therapist.

Speech therapy: Speech therapy is provided by a qualified speech therapist to overcome certain speech and communication problems.

Occupational therapy: Occupational therapy, or OT, is restorative therapy to enhance or restore the skills necessary for daily living. It should be provided by a qualified occupational therapist.

Skilled nursing services: These nursing services are provided in a person's home or in an outpatient or ambulatory-care setting.

Housing assistance: Housing assistance programs exist in some communities to help in the search for suitable housing, in the moving of personal items, and in the finding of emergency shelters in the event of natural disaster.

Geriatric assessment units and special-care units: Specialized geriatric units, both inpatient and outpatient, exist in many hospitals and medical centers across the country. They usually provide more coordinated multidisciplinary services to older patients.

Finding Help

No matter how educated, experienced, or well-off an individual is, caring for a relative, especially one who lives far away, is very stressful. How do you find out what services are available when your relative lives alone or in a community far away from you? How do you make proper arrangements? How do you juggle career, family, and responsibilities to the patient? How do you deal with your own distress and frustration?

Throughout the country there is a growing network of professionals who offer what is known as case or care management services for a fee. These agencies make referrals for home care attendants, nurses, occupational and physical therapists, homemakers, chore workers, lawyers, financial consultants, and medical and psychiatric specialists. They also may act as your broker, which means that they confer with you about your needs, and then they will arrange for the services you need and take responsibility for monitoring the quality of care.

These care management services, often run by nurses or social workers with a background in aging, can help you when your relative lives far away. For a fee they will find a social worker in any area of the country to assess your relative's needs and arrange for necessary services. In these situations it is important to know that you are getting quality services. Generally, you must rely on your feelings about the responsiveness of the care managers and the quality of the services received. Their willingness to spend the necessary time to answer your questions and the actual help they give you are important criteria by which to judge quality.

The major drawback of care management services is their expense. Many people simply cannot afford this type of help, which should be more available than it is. When care management services are unavailable or unaffordable, family members become the primary managers to coordinate the patient's care. It takes time and the commitment of family members to examine their personal and family resources to decide what can be done.

There are many approaches to help identify and locate services and programs that exist in your or the patient's community. However, it is unlikely that any one resource will have all the information needed to identify the range of services found in the community. Finding long-term-care service takes patience, time, and a lot of detective work. One of the great barriers to finding local agencies in the community is that such agencies cannot afford to invest significantly in advertising and promotion. Since most are nonprofit, they tend to devote what resources they have to services and program development, with little in the budget available for outreach to new cases.

Probably the best starting place is to find the phone number for the state unit on aging. Every state government in the nation has a state unit on aging, usually located in the state capitol, that is required by law to give free information about services for older people. It may be called a department, an office, or a state agency on aging, a division of seniors or senior citizens, or a department of elder affairs. Each state unit oversees a network of what are called area agencies on aging that cover a county or many counties, a parish, or a municipality. Call the state agency and ask about the nearest local Area Agency on Aging to get information about what exists in the community. A local senior center, public library, or a library at a local college or university may have two important directories. One is *A Directory of State and Area Agencies on Aging* and another is the *National Directory for Eldercare Information and Referral.*

An important resource for family members is the Eldercare Locator, which has a toll-free phone number and refers individuals to information, resources, and services. It is supported by the Administration on Aging in the federal government as well as two national organizations, the National Association of Area Agencies and the National Association of State Units on Aging, both of which have headquarters in Washington, D.C. Call 1-800-677-1116 between 9:00 A.M. and 11:00 P.M. EST on weekdays. Be prepared to give the address and zip code for the older person who needs assistance and a short description of the problem.

The Internet is another point of access for information. Start with keywords such as *eldercare, aging,* or *senior services* to locate general sites. The keywords *health* and *health care* will lead to specific disease conditions such as Alzheimer's disease, stroke, and Parkinson's disease. Information on long-term-care insurance can be found using the keywords *health care*, *money and finance*, or *insurance*. Other keywords include *elder law*, *assisted living*, and *specific health problems*.

Librarians at universities, aging centers, senior groups, and aging organizations have created many Internet and e-mail resources on aging. There are several useful federal sites. The Administration on Aging has a home page with information on the administration's programs as well as information for consumers (www.aoa.dhhs.gov). The directory of Web and Gopher Aging Sites lists all area agencies on aging and other Internet sites on aging (www.aoa.dhhs.gov/webres/craig.htm).

A local branch of the Alzheimer's Association can be a valuable resource based on the experiences of individual members who have tried to find help in the community. They can inform you about what needs to be done and how valuable the help is in relation to the efforts necessary to secure it. In the appendices we list the contact points for chapters of the Alzheimer's Association (see Appendix 1) and for a number of national organizations on aging (see Appendix 2).

Other sources of help are local colleges and universities. Many schools have gerontology centers or institutes on aging, and their faculty may be familiar with programs in the community. In an increasing number of instances, a university, medical school, or medical center may itself run such programs for training purposes.

The Department of Veterans Affairs (and in some states the statewide veterans benefits agency) has been interested in the problems of long-term care for years. The veterans department not only has an extensive program of nursing-home care but also has been developing community-based arrangements in certain parts of the country. For qualified veterans, this option may be available. Contact the local veterans administration office or veterans hospital. If that yields nothing, write the Veterans Health Administration in Washington, D.C., which coordinates these activities (see Appendix 2).

Adapting the Home to the Patient

The environment of the home—size, physical design, furniture arrangements, lighting, decorations, colors, number and configuration of rooms, availability and construction of patios, balconies, and other outside areas—can make living safe or unsafe, comfortable or uncomfortable. As patients become progressively impaired and disabled, homes and apartments can be changed in several basic ways, even when financial resources are limited. A number of excellent books describe not only how families can evaluate the home, but also creative affordable ways to change it to make it safe, comfortable, and still attractive. Families can evaluate what can be changed in the home with the following three goals in mind: elimination of barriers, safety, and cognitive support.

Eliminating barriers is very important. For persons with physical impairments stemming from accidents or illness, personal devices like wheelchairs or walkers can make an important difference. However, a number of physical barriers can affect the use of these devices. Narrow doorways or high door sills, loose carpets or throw rugs, narrow passageways between furniture, or the placement of breakable objects in or near places that are heavily trafficked can become serious problems. A positive approach to the elimination of barriers, the addition of a number of such features as grab bars in the bath, and the availability of easily accessible showers with stools and easily reached controls can be helpful.

Most patients do not have physical problems early in their illness. For them other issues are of greater importance. However, as the disease progresses, problems of safety and security need to be addressed. Patients often like to be able to participate in the world by seeing what is going on. Enclosing a porch can serve this purpose, as can allowing access to a window. Ensuring that there are adequate safety devices can also help. The value of internal quiet alarms or door locks, including combination locks with four- or five-button codes, should be examined to help contain the patient who is prone to wandering.

Different rooms of the house have special problems. The kitchen can be a hazardous place. Gas burners without pilot lights are potential dangers for the patient who turns on the gas but forgets to put a match to the burner. The oven is often mistaken for a refrigerator, with the result that it may be turned on while bags of groceries or unwrapped objects are inside. In general, patients in later stages of the illness should not be in the kitchen unsupervised, even if that means controlling access. The use of fireproof burner pads may help. Putting away electrical appliances or unplugging such devices as toasters, mixers, or food processors can eliminate potential problems.

At least one room in the house should be identified as the patient's own space. A safe room, perhaps with an outside view, a television set, a radio, and a source of music, can be a comfort zone. It should be a room where the patient can learn to spend time and feel secure. Time spent there with loved ones can often be a foundation for allowing the patient to be alone while the caregiver performs chores in other rooms. In places like the bedroom it is helpful to organize objects for daily use. Clothing to be worn that day, eyeglasses or hearing aids, or even wallets should go in a regular place or an appropriate shelf or holder. This routine should be started early and maintained over the course of illness.

The Home Care Checklist

The decision whether to keep the patient at home should be based not only on loyalty and commitment but also on a careful and thorough analysis of the physical and emotional resources of the primary care-giver(s). The following list of general questions and suggestions is intended as a guide to help you evaluate your continuing capability to keep the patient at home.

1. *Home Environment: What can you do to make the home safe and comfortable for the patient?*
   - Is the home large enough that the patient can have his or her own room or space on the first floor when a separate sleeping area with a bathroom may be required?
   - Are there ways to rearrange furniture to make the home less cluttered so that the patient can navigate easily around the house?
   - Can you organize the patient's personal belongings so that they are consistently in one place?
   - Can you fix up an area outside of the home that is safe and accessible to the patient, such as an enclosed backyard?
   - Is there a safe place nearby where the patient can walk, jog, or play tennis?
   - If there are stairs outside the home, is it possible to build a ramp if necessary?

- In the event that you decide to hire live-in house help, is there adequate living space for that individual?
- Is it feasible for you and the patient to move to special housing for senior citizens?

2. *Medical Accessibility: Do you have professional help accessible for routine care as well as emergencies?*

- Is a medical center or hospital nearby?
- Do you have the emergency numbers for the doctor and ambulance service?
- Will the patient's doctor help advise you and visit the home?

3. *Finances: Can you afford to pay for attendants, nurses, and special treatments?*

- Analyze your financial assets and those of the patient. Try to estimate the cost of health care—doctors, equipment, procedures—needed each month.
- Talk to an accountant or call the Internal Revenue Service for guidance about what may be deductible on your taxes. Discipline yourself to keep records of your expenditures for the patient.
- Investigate your eligibility for home care benefits from Medicare, Medicaid, and health insurance policies (see Chapter 15).
- Keep a weekly budget and each month examine how you are spending your money.

4. *Transportation: Can you drive or do you have transportation for daily needs?*

- Is the home accessible by means of public transportation if and when home attendants and nurses are necessary?
- What transportation can you use in an emergency?
- Have you made contingency plans to keep your home accessible during bad weather and winter storms?
- Are nearby neighbors who can drive available in the event your car breaks down? Are they willing to help? And are you comfortable asking for help?

5. *Your Health: Are you realistic about your ability to care for the patient at home?*

- Are you strong enough to help the patient in the bathroom, bath, or shower?
- Do you have to make regular medical visits that interfere with your caring responsibilities?

- Can you get away for regular periods of rest and recreation? By regular, we mean daily or at least four to five times a week.

6. *Equipment: What will you need to care for someone in your home?*
   - Canes, walkers, wheelchairs, special hospital beds, and mattresses can be rented. Grab bars and rails may have to be purchased.
   - Can you arrange the house so that it can accommodate a wheelchair?
   - Is there a place in the home for a hospital bed where the patient will have privacy and still be near family activities? Will the floors bear the weight of a heavy bed?
   - What special equipment can you get to help your relative exercise?

7. *Family and Personal Services: Do you have family members who can share the burden or can you afford to hire trained reliable help?*
   - Will those who volunteer fulfill their obligations?
   - Do other family members live close enough to be of assistance?
   - Can the family cooperate in making decisions about the patient's care?
   - If you are the primary caregiver, are you able to share the burden of caring?
   - Can you find qualified nurses and home care attendants?
   - Can the patient participate in decision making or at least be included in family meetings?
   - Have you made neighbors aware of the problem?

8. *General*
   - Are you prepared to care for your relative at home even through the final stages of the dementia, when he or she becomes very sick and bedridden?
   - Are you willing to accept help to keep yourself from becoming burned out?

Choosing a Home Health Care Agency

Home health care includes many types of services, ranging from nursing care and medical procedures such as intravenous and oxygen therapy, to hospice care for those who are dying at home. Home health care also may include visits by appropriate professionals to provide physical therapy, occupational therapy, speech therapy, nutrition, and podiatry care as well as professionals who educate patients and family members to use everything from walkers, wheelchairs, and hospital beds, to prostheses, intravenous setups, and technologically intensive home care procedures. Home health care covered by Medicare and Medicaid must be prescribed by a doctor, and the amount of care is limited. Agencies that provide skilled nursing services must be certified. Agencies that only provide home health aides and homemakers are not certified by Medicare.

Choosing an agency requires some homework. There are no uniform regulations for home health agencies, but most states require agencies to be licensed. Every state has a toll-free hotline to get information about quality of care as well as report problems with agencies. Call the Area Agency on Aging to get the phone number in your state. Some agencies have gone through a process of voluntary accreditation. Contact the Community Health Accreditation Program in New York (1-800-669-1656, ext. 242). The hotline also provides a checklist about quality of home health care and cost. For information on how to choose home care agencies, you can order a free copy of *How to Choose a Home Care Agency: A Consumer's Guide* from the National Association for Home Care, 519 C Street, N.E. Stanton Park, Washington, DC 20002. A *Consumer Guide to Home Health Care* is available from the National Consumers League, 815 15th Street, N.W., Suite 928, Washington, DC 20002, and *Staying at Home* is a guide from the AARP, 601 East Street, N.W., Washington, DC 20041.

Whenever home- or community-based services are needed, a stranger will be coming into the home. There are a number of important items to check before you make any decisions:

- When using an agency for a personal care aide or home health aide, ask for references from the agency. Ask if they are bonded and insured and if they are a member of the Chamber of Commerce or Better Business Bureau.
- Contact references for the aide.
- Check to see that aides have been trained for the duties and responsibilities needed.
- Before the aide begins, agree on all payment arrangements, including travel and Social Security, and put it in writing.

- Prepare a schedule of tasks as well as working hours, and work with the aide to follow that schedule.
- Prepare a list of phone numbers of people who can be called in the event of an emergency.
- Request that the aide's supervisor, if from an agency, visit on some regular basis.
- If an aide is not working out, request another person from the agency or find someone else.

Assisted Living Residences

There are housing alternatives for the patient when caring is a strain or hurting the health and well-being of the caregivers. Assisted living facilities, also known as personal care or board-and-care homes, are one of the fastest-growing housing markets for older people with dementia. They are for people who need assistance and cannot live independently but who are not sick enough for nursing-home care. Assisted living residences provide a full range of assistive supports and services with trained staff. They are a new model for providing residential rather than institutional long-term care. The focus is on a home environment where supportive services are specialized, health care is designed to maximize functioning, and the involvement of family and friends is encouraged. Some assisted living companies specialize in the care of older persons with Alzheimer's disease and related dementias.

There are at least eight issues to consider in the choice of an assisted living residence. Overall, the residence should be attractive, safe, and comfortable and should respect the rights and dignity of all residents. Tour the home and look carefully at the residence. First, pay attention to the sights, sounds, and smells as well as the location and outward appearance, the homelike quality of the inside areas, and the appearance and behaviors of the residents. Watch how warmly the staff interact with residents, with each other, and with you. Think about whether the residents are appropriate housemates for your relative.

Second, evaluate how well designed the environment is for older persons. Look for elevators; handrails; nonskid floors; easy-to-reach bathrooms, beds, shelves, and cupboards; and good temperature control.

Third, ask questions about how residents are evaluated as well as costs and finances. Is there a written care plan for each resident? How often are residents re-evaluated for changing needs? What are the circumstances when a contract can be cancelled, and what are the refund policies? Are there different costs for different levels of care and services, and what are the billing, payment, and credit policies? What are the policies for insurance and personal property?

Fourth, evaluate the health care and medication procedures. How are drugs stored, administered, and tracked? How knowledgeable are staff about the main effects and side effects? Can residents take their own medication? Who arranges therapeutic consults and services such as podiatry, physical therapy, and so on? Do physicians and nurses provide regular examinations? What is the procedure for medical emergencies?

Fifth, determine whether the staff are trained to provide twenty-four-hour assistance with the full scope of activities of daily living and other personal activities. These include dressing, eating, grooming, toileting, bathing, and ambulating, as well as cleaning, laundry, using the telephone, shopping, housekeeping, and transportation for physician appointments.

The sixth issue involves social and recreational activities. Find out what organized activities exist, whether residents go out into the community for some activities, and whether pets are allowed or whether the residence has its own pets.

Food is an important issue for well-being. Does the residence provide three nutritious meals a day every day of the week, as well as snacks? Are meal hours flexible, can residents eat in their rooms, and are there common dining areas? Would you eat the food?

The final area targets features of the individual units or rooms. Are different types and sizes of rooms available? Do residents have personal locked doors? Is there a personal emergency response system in each room? How is billing handled for televisions and telephones in residential rooms? What personal items can residents bring with them? Is smoking allowed and if so, where?

When assisted living communities offer specialized care for Alzheimer's disease and related disorders, there are three major issues to target. First, does the community have a written mission statement or philosophy of special care? Second, what specialized training do the staff have? Third, does the local or state Alzheimer's Association rank the community as having quality care?

In the long run, planning and decision making, based on good information rather than beliefs, enhance the quality of life for everyone. The patient, his or her environment, and your own ability to deal with the inevitable changes are areas about which you need information. There are opportunities for getting help from others, be they community services, health care agencies, or senior housing facilities.

9

Coping with the Stress of Caring

We had spent two days with an attorney and friend to do financial plan-
ning with Mom. He patiently explained everything to her, and we thought
we had her complete approval. Mom wanted me to have power of attorney,
and she agreed that we should retitle some of her accounts.

I can still see her the day we went to the bank to make the changes. She
was adorable with her freshly coifed hair, warm-up suit, and Nike walking shoes.
She was the picture of a refined, dignified "with-it" older lady. I, on the other
hand, was in a hurry, because I was due back at school before twelve, and I
probably seemed to be rushing this dear lady into something she was not sure of.

Seated in the conference room with several bank executives, we began
the task. My mother had forgotten the discussions of the past two days, and
suddenly this was all new to her. When asked to sign a document trans-
ferring some assets, she looked at the gentleman and said, "This is the first
time I've heard of this! You know it would be different if I only had one
child, but I have three of them."

I'm almost as embarrassed now as I was then. Here I appeared to not
only be taking advantage of my poor defenseless mother but also cheating
my brother and sister out of their inheritance.

C aring for someone with Alzheimer's disease is a task as complicated as any we face. Over time the needs of the patient over-
shadow everything else, and inevitably the pattern of daily life
changes. Since the dementia usually progresses slowly, family life is trans-

formed gradually, but the changes can last for years. If the caregiving goes on long enough, it inevitably interferes with healthy family functioning, even in the most resourceful families. The illness creates both expected and unexpected transitions for family members, and the greatest challenges are not the specific tasks of caregiving, but the new roles the illness imposes on everyone.

Those who have a caregiving role face the constant task of balancing the needs of the patient with their own needs, and often those of other members of the family. Tension, anger, frustration, guilt, and sadness are all normal responses to the strain of living with and caring for any individual with a prolonged or chronic illness. The constant demands of caring can and do lead to emotional and physical fatigue. It is easy to feel overwhelmed and helpless in the situation. The single most important principle for successful coping is to recognize that the caregiver role is impossible and then to try to do the best you can.

Most family routines eventually are disrupted when patients become unable to carry out their usual responsibilities. Family members report becoming isolated from the mainstream as patients can no longer participate in recreational activities, hobbies, and social engagements that were once pleasurable. Isolation from neighbors and friends leads to feelings of being trapped. As tension increases, family members may quarrel with each other. Financial problems may mount as the expenses of the illness accumulate. Important needs of children and other family members that require money are frequently postponed.

The behaviors of patients are frustrating to live with, and it is normal to feel irritation and even rage. For example, many patients ask the same questions continually, even when the answer is given over and over. This trivial manifestation of the memory loss of dementia becomes a stressful daily occurrence. Family members, especially spouses, express enormous sadness at the loss of someone in whom they confided and with whom they shared the ups and downs of everyday living. Some family members report being enraged at the dementia itself. One middle-aged man expressed appropriate frustration at his loss: "Why did it have to affect my father? I have been robbed of the chance to be a son and enjoy him."

It is the number and range of problems that often prove to be overwhelming for caregivers. Many family members suffer from physical as well as psychological health problems, insomnia, irritability, and physical exhaustion. In order to watch over an individual, it is often necessary to quit a job or at the very least lose time at work. Perhaps the most frequent consequence of the stresses of caregiving is depression. At least half of all caregivers living at home with the patient have a clinical depression. Thus, family members often become unrecognized patients themselves, and as a result lose the capacity to provide the best care for their loved ones and for themselves.

Successful coping involves first identifying your problems and then, most important, recognizing which ones you can do something about and which are beyond your control or anyone else's. Many practical ways to help the patient keep active and feel secure and comfortable are discussed in this book. Friends, self-help groups, and professionals can be enormously helpful. Without outside assistance, it is often hard to keep a healthy perspective on the limits of caregiving as the dementia progresses. If you lose your objectivity, you can become overwhelmed and sick and cease to be in a position to care for the patient effectively.

The question then is "How do you cope?" or "How do you know if you are coping well or not?" There are several answers. Regardless of how competent, experienced, or sophisticated an individual is, the dementia changes everything, from the most routine daily events to special ceremonies like birthdays and anniversaries. There are ways to cope with the stresses, and specific strategies to monitor yourself and determine how well you are doing. These are the focus of this chapter.

Dealing with Feelings

Emotions are complex. The way you respond emotionally depends on your personality, your mental and physical health, your stage of life, the particular situation you are in, and your previous experience with similar circumstances. The feelings of a caregiver are also affected by the nature of the established relationship and style of communication between the caregiver and the patient. Although some people will feel little anger toward the patient, others will experience a great deal. However, feeling anger does not mean that you love the patient less than someone who does not seem to feel it. In fact, for some it is helpful to feel the anger and then express it in an appropriate way. Furthermore, there are periods in your life when times are rough, and you are simply more vulnerable. The ability to care for anybody when you are hurting and vulnerable is severely compromised.

An especially important determinant of how you feel about the caregiving role lies in the balance between a sense of satisfaction with what you are doing for the patient, and the frustration of caring for someone who is continuing to deteriorate despite your efforts. This equilibrium can be affected by the severity of the dementia, the intimacy of family relationships, and the types of resources and support available to caregivers. The pain of watching a loved one in the later stages of dementia, when he or she becomes incontinent or cannot eat, or when pneumonia or contractures develop, is often overwhelming. One woman exclaimed, "I am blinded by my sadness now. My Louie always did for others, and now nobody can do for him. I could handle everything until they put the tube in his stomach. There is nothing but oblivion for him and me now."

It is not always the dramatic, heartbreaking events that upset the emotional balance of caregivers. The many years of living with the progressive changes exact a heavy toll. Elmira Jones, whose husband had Alzheimer's disease, told us, "I talk to my pillow each night and cry myself to sleep. Willie still sleeps with me, and I take him everywhere—shopping, church, choir, my bridge club, everything. During the day I am okay. It's the nights when I break down. My tears over the past eight years would fill the house."

Personal history plays an important role in the way people adapt or do not adapt. Individuals who have lived through major crises and stressful life events tend to have developed emotional resilience and more effective coping skills. Some people simply have adaptive personalities and can handle themselves well in most situations. However, even the most experienced or composed individuals will experience feelings of sadness, anger, frustration, and resentment.

The crucial question is, how do you deal with the feelings? The answers are personal ones. You may have to hide more negative feelings from the patient, depending on the severity of the dementia. Many patients react strongly to anger, with everything from anxiety to violence. In general, it is wise to protect them as much as possible from explosive outbursts, noisy arguments among family members, and strong emotions. It is important to judge an individual's ability to respond to expressions of legitimate emotions and when possible to present concerns lovingly and honestly. Some patients can handle feelings reasonably well if they are not too impaired.

However, it is crucial that honest feelings not be bottled up inside you. There are many ways to relieve such pressure. First, look inside yourself and admit that you are angry, afraid, or upset. Next, do something about it and get the feelings out of your system. Writing letters to family or close friends, telephone conversations, and long discussions with a supportive individual are often helpful. Exercise vigorously. Throw pillows on the floor. Find safe ways to vent. Be open and get your feelings out where you can recognize them.

Pat Conroy wrote several letters each week to her daughter. Even though they spoke often on the telephone, Mrs. Conroy reported that the letters helped her "package her feelings" each day.

> My dearest daughter,
> I have just finished writing in your father's journal tonight. Jim is asleep now on the couch beside me. Even though he is changing as the Alzheimer's takes its course, he is still the most precious and dearest of beings to me.
> I am writing to you now to try and shed my feelings of aloneness and sadness. I know we have done everything possible for Jim, but tonight I feel overwhelmed by my love and my anguish.
> Today your father seemed more like himself. He went shopping with me, and we even met friends for lunch at our favorite Italian restaurant. Jim seemed especially happy. He smiled and laughed. Tonight the laughter is a fading memory, but I am fighting to cling to that memory. I need the good times to live through the bad days.

What do you do when frustrations seem to swell uncontrollably inside of you? It may not be easy, but try to take several deep breaths and compose your thoughts. It is helpful to write down exactly what is bothering you. The next step is to do something constructive about it. If you are upset with the patient, talk to someone about it. If your relative is in the early stages, explain to him or her, when possible, what is annoying you. If you are angry with a nurse, aide, or attendant who has committed an error or been lax or careless, be pleasant but firm in your criticisms. You have a responsibility to inform such persons that you expect them to be more sensitive and caring with your relative. If they do not correct their mistake or change their behavior, you may need to dismiss them if they are in your employ. Or if the individual is on the staff of a nursing home, you should report your continued dissatisfaction to one of the administrators.

Dealing with your general anger at the illness is a more complicated matter. If you cannot alleviate your distress at the sad plight of your relative, you may rage with blind fury at yourself and the patient and only end up physically and mentally exhausted. However, there are ways to lessen the frustrations of living with dementia. It is important to learn how to do three things.

First, reframe the way you think about your family. A family can be thought of as a long running play on Broadway or the London stage or a well-established sports team like the New York Yankees or Chicago Bears. This means that you and your family, like all families, have spent a long time together, developed an identity and pattern of interacting with each other, and have already adjusted to many changes, such as birth, marriages, in-laws, new jobs, illness, and death. And with all of these changes, family members have developed new roles and responsibilities.

When someone in the family is diagnosed with dementia, it also changes the way every player acts. Change is difficult because the rhythm of working together that the team or cast has developed is disrupted. Accommodating to change is emotional business. Anger, hurt, and sadness are normal reactions that must be dealt with in the process of reorganizing the situation. Change is a continuing process as the dementia progresses. It causes turmoil and conflict in the family as everyone struggles to find new ways of coping.

Second, focus on ways to enjoy as many activities as possible, with and without the patient. Al Rogers cared for his wife for over fifteen years: "Jill and I went everywhere together for many years. Even though she could do very little, she seemed content just to be near me. Indeed, she seemed happiest when surrounded by her entire family." Lorraine Thomas remembered the two years she cared for her husband: "Roger went downhill so fast. It was hard to accept that he wasn't my husband anymore. I did everything I could to care for him, but I had to get out of the house every day to rejuvenate myself. I had to do things I enjoyed, or I would have gone crazy."

Third, cultivate a philosophy of "living one day at a time." One way to cope with catastrophic events of all kinds—war, natural disasters, terminal illness—is to live day by day, focusing your energy on survival. June Anatole said it this way:

> Bart has been dead two years, but I still think of him every day. I remember the five years of hope and suffering. Yes, we had both. For most of our married life, Bart would get out of bed each morning, extend his hand to me, and say, "Come on Mama, we have another day ahead of us. Let's not waste it." It was a simple ritual in our lives, but it was the way I loved to start my day.
>
> I remember the awful loneliness I felt the morning Bart forgot our ritual. It was about a year after the doctor had told us that Bart had Alzheimer's disease. He simply got out of bed, went into the bathroom, and called out to me that he wanted breakfast. I remember how afraid I was. This Alzheimer's problem was getting worse, and Bart was changing.
>
> The days took on a special meaning after that. It wasn't easy, but we changed roles. I was the one who got up first and extended my hand, "Pop, it's time to spend another day together."
>
> Bart lived another four years; no, not years, more than 1,400 days. And each day carries a special memory for me. I know we did everything we could.

People handle their emotions in many different ways during the long months and years of caring. Some individuals are stoic and are able to deal quietly with the sorrow and sense of loss, while others enlist the active support of friends and family. The capacity of family members to care and cope are often profound testaments to the love individuals feel for each other.

Samuel Jackson took care of his wife, Lily, for eighteen years with the support of his daughter and two sons. Their daughter had never married and continued to live with them, which proved to be enormously helpful during the long period Lily had been ill. Sam cared for Lily tenderly morning and night, day after day. They continued to go out and do many things together. Around the house Lily was on the move constantly. When she tired Sam out, he would ask her to sit on the couch so that he could lay his head on her lap to rest. No matter how agitated or active Lily was throughout the entire course of her dementia, she would sit quietly stroking his hair while he rested. If anyone walked in, she would raise her finger to her lips: "Shh! Sam is sleeping!"

The bonds between people are of many types. Not all relationships are characterized by such devotion, but that does not mean that other people do not love as well or as much. Many good and stable relationships are hard-pressed by the demands of caring. Indeed, there are many situations in which family members should, in the best interests of everyone involved, find a nursing home for the patient. Caring is hard work, physically and emotionally. Amanda Potter finally let her son make the arrangements for her husband, Albert, to go into a nursing home. She simply wasn't physically strong enough to care for her husband after he was bedridden, and she could no longer afford home help. Amanda told her son, "Your father and I lived through the concentration camps, but I never expected another Holocaust! I love your father, and I am powerless to protect him from this."

Who Takes Care of the Caregiver?

The primary caregiver, usually the spouse, may find it very hard to accept the reality that Alzheimer's disease or a related disorder cannot be managed without help. Over the years of living together, husbands and wives develop unique patterns of caring for each other's needs and desires. Indeed, what makes entire families special is the way different members relate to one another with various degrees of loyalty, obligation, and commitment. Families are often able to meet many of the complex personal and social needs of their members. However, Alzheimer's disease is akin to a major catastrophe or a natural disaster. Responding to it requires a lot of individual effort, but it cannot be handled alone. Other people are necessary, and by working together and sharing responsibilities, you and they can do a great deal. You will find it easier to cope if you let yourself accept help when you need it.

The availability of a people support system is one of the most important resources anyone can have. It is common for a husband or wife to feel he or she can do everything necessary to care for their spouse. However, even though a spouse may have the yeoman's job, it is important, even lifesaving, to share the responsibility of caring.

Children, grandchildren, brothers, sisters, in-laws, friends, neighbors, and other important individuals can provide much needed assistance if you will let them.

Hugo and Alicia Prado had been married forty years and had raised five children. Two daughters, Anne and Jean-Marie, had started their own families and lived within ten miles of their parents. The eldest son, Jacques, who was divorced, also lived in the same town and ran his father's business. The other two sons were still single and lived in other states: George was in law school, and Bryan worked for an insurance company.

Hugo had been diagnosed as having Alzheimer's disease a year and a half earlier. Indeed, it was on their fortieth wedding anniversary that Alicia knew she could no longer delay taking her husband to a doctor. Their five children threw a surprise party, at which Hugo, in making a toast, stunned everyone by wishing his wife a happy birthday!

Mrs. Prado reminisced about the past several years:

My family has been my anchor. I would not have been able to handle myself without them. There were so many days when I felt completely lost and helpless. The pain welled up inside me, and I . . . I wanted to die. The children surrounded me and gave me the strength to face Hugo's illness. There is no greater agony than to see the one you love obliterated, and without the kids I would have fallen apart.

It is also important to find ways to get away from caregiving responsibilities on a regular basis. However, this goes against natural instincts and desires. Ordinarily, someone caring for another looks for ways for them to be together, but the toll that dementia extracts is a high one. Even people with normal routines need vacations and breaks during the day and week. Alzheimer's disease and related disorders are extremely demanding, and if caregivers are not able to refresh themselves, there is a danger that their energies will be depleted and that they will have less to give.

Depression: A Danger for Caregivers

Depression is not a rare condition in caregivers, and sometimes it can become quite serious. If clinical depression goes unrecognized and untreated, it can worsen and become deadly. It is a complex emotion, spanning the continuum from normal and appropriate feelings of sadness and despair to any one of several major clinical disorders. The first question is, how do you recognize when you or someone you love is in danger of becoming seriously depressed? The next is, what can you do about it? We discuss depression generally in this chapter and then devote the entire next chapter to depression because it occurs so frequently in caregivers.

In order to develop some insight, it may be helpful to examine the many faces of depression. All of us have felt despondent, gloomy, despairing, helpless, and hopeless at some time in our life. Sadness is a normal and appropriate response to an illness. Death, the anniversary of a loved one's death, a financial loss, a personal failure, or any one of many life stresses can cause such feelings. Sometimes we get the blues when we have been working too hard and are simply overtired.

Living with and caring for a relative with dementia can bring on great sadness. Some of the emotions become overwhelming, and help for those feelings is warranted. Unfortunately, depression is not always easy to recognize and diagnose. There are many different symptoms. Some of them are psychological, and others are physical. You do not have to look and feel consciously sad to have a clinical depression, and this is one of the most difficult things for nonprofessionals to understand.

Problems with memory and with concentration are often characteristics of depression. Many caregivers complain that they have a memory problem. It is common to hear, "I must be getting demented myself. I cannot seem to remember things any better than my husband." Depression contributes to slower thinking, feelings of confusion, and real memory losses. Making the simplest decisions becomes difficult. One husband described his situation:

> I sat in my office and worried. I could not get any work done. I would read a report and would reread the same paragraphs over again. At the end of the day, I knew I had accomplished nothing.

I had paced around the office, shuffled piles of paper, and stared at the walls. I felt impotent—psychologically impotent.

Depression can also be a psychological state characterized as the blahs—your zest for life is gone, you feel low and empty. You may also think about your life and feel guilty about all the mistakes you have made. In a clinical depression people often dislike themselves and feel like failures. They may see themselves as incompetent and unworthy—even unworthy of the time and help of a professional.

The depressed person is often pessimistic and convinced that things can only get worse. The future seems bleak and hopeless. Their feelings of oppression are so strong that others become depressed from being around them. Depressed people also may talk and act more slowly. The answers to even simple questions may be accompanied by empty silences and long sighs.

Pain is a prominent symptom of depression. The presence of depression in a caregiver may exaggerate the pain of arthritis and other chronic illnesses. Indeed, the combination of emotional distress and physical illness in the long run may seriously disable caregivers and compromise the quality of care they can render.

Depression shows itself in bodily functions. Not only is it visible in one's face and posture, but also other changes occur. The sleep cycle is altered. Although the ability to fall asleep may be relatively unchanged, people who are depressed often awaken in the early hours of the morning and cannot fall asleep again. This condition is also known as *terminal insomnia*, that is, insomnia at the end of the sleep cycle. Sometimes people stay in bed and sleep many hours. When awake, they complain of being tired all of the time. Appetite changes. Most people lose their appetite, eat far less than usual, and lose weight. Others eat more and gain weight. Constipation also occurs as a result of depression.

Be on the alert for the signs of serious depression, and if and when you see them, seek help as described in the next chapter. You are doing yourself and the patient an important favor. If something is wrong, the longer the depression lasts, the harder it is to treat. Often a friend or relative first suggests to the caregiver that he or she should see someone. Try not to be angry or defensive if persons you trust say that they are worried about you and that perhaps you need help. It is often sound advice. At least give yourself the benefit of a checkup.

Untreated depression can affect the way you treat the patient. Husbands, wives, children, or whoever the primary caregivers are may become so angry or depressed that they neglect or physically abuse the patient. Seemingly uncontrollable emotions and actions impair the caregiver's thinking and ability to care for the patient. These circumstances should be openly discussed, and the conditions treated. Sadly, neglect and abuse of a patient do not usually come to anybody's attention until the patient is hospitalized and medical staff become suspicious of the patient's injuries and circumstances.

Hope Conti had been married to her husband, William, for over forty years. William had been diagnosed with Alzheimer's disease at the age of sixty-four. Eight years into the Alzheimer's disease, Hope hired a home care attendant to help with bathing, dressing, feeding, and light cleaning around the house. She and her husband continued to do as much as his strength permitted. Each day they would drive somewhere for lunch and later take a walk or go shopping. During the summer they drove to the country with the attendant every weekend; there she and her husband would hike in the woods, swim in the pool, and go boating on the lake. William enjoyed the exercise and seemed to continue to take pride in his athletic prowess.

One afternoon while William was napping, the home care attendant announced that she was quitting. She accused Hope of beating her husband. There were large bruises on William's chest, shoulders, and arms. Hope was horrified at the accusation and angrily told the woman to leave.

The next weekend the Contis drove to the mountains for a weekend with friends. Sunday afternoon William lost his balance and struck his head on the rocks. With the help of her friends and of a local ranger, Hope was able to get her husband to the car. They drove to the local hospital, where William was admitted.

William was hospitalized five days before being transferred to a university hospital in his hometown. He stayed there another three weeks before being sent home. He had sustained a subdural hematoma, but he also was anemic, malnourished, and had a urinary tract infection.

Hope's daughter Carol had successfully persuaded her mother to talk with one of the doctors at the hospital. During the interview Hope described her firm desire to take her husband home and not place him in an institution, as everyone on the hospital team had recommended. Staff and family were united in their concern about Hope's health and her continued ability to care for her husband. She had lost twenty pounds in the last month, was waking up every morning at five, and even admitted to having thoughts of wanting to die. She also conceded that she was extremely frustrated with her husband and that she sometimes wanted to hit him when she couldn't understand what he wanted or needed. In the intimacy of the conversation, she gradually admitted her shame and embarrassment that she had struck her husband on a few occasions. The few turned out to be many.

The doctors conferred with Carol to share their concern that Hope had been abusing her husband. For his own safety William needed to be institutionalized. And just as important, Hope was suffering from a severe depression and needed help.

Placing William in a nursing home could be a temporary placement until Hope felt well enough to assume his care again. Depending on how she felt after her depression was treated, she might also decide that institutionalization was an acceptable solution. Caring for William, as much as she deeply loved him, had become an overwhelming task for Hope. The physical exertion of turning him in bed, helping him to the toilet or with his bath, even with home help, was akin to an Olympic decathlon for Hope, who herself had multiple health problems.

Hope responded to the antidepressant treatment. She retained a deep regret and shame over her behavior, and her family also had difficulty accepting what they perceived as her cruelty. However, after several family sessions they were able to understand how the situation had become so toxic. They also saw ways to help one another prevent such a problem from recurring. The entire family was enormously relieved to understand the cause of Hope's actions and was prepared to support her in the future.

Dealing with Ambivalence toward the Patient

The very nature of dementia causes ambivalent or confused emotional reactions in caregivers. If you are unsure about an individual's competence and safety, you will find yourself vacillating between wanting to help the patient maintain independence and forcing him or her to accept help. It is emotionally confusing to live with an individual who looks like the human being you knew yet who has lost the capacity to carry out the simplest actions. Everyday situations may generate powerful mixed feelings of love and anger, tenderness and rejection. The need to come to grips with these ambivalent feelings is extremely important. The consequences of not recognizing them are inevitably reflected in unnecessary anguish and a poorer quality of caring.

Alexander Frishman lived at home with his wife Betty, who had been diagnosed as having dementia two years earlier. He explained how he tried to maintain a normal life:

> Betty tries to do many things around the house—set the table, wash the dishes, dust the furniture, and little things like that. She is always eager to help, but she gets confused and doesn't finish anything. That's what gets me so upset. I get so frustrated sometimes that I want to lash out. For example, she will get the silverware out of the drawer, walk to the table, pick up the napkins, and walk back to the drawer with both silverware and napkins. I know that the Alzheimer's is causing her to act this way, but little things like this happen every day. She seems so normal in many ways, but it's like only half of her mind is working.

Coping successfully with the stress of caring requires improved insight into your own behavior. However, it is often difficult to recognize what you are doing wrong unless someone points it out to you. Alex Frishman responded to the advice of his daughter to take Betty for a psychological evaluation. After the testing was completed, the psychologist met with the entire family. He identified the types of tasks Betty could do and gave the family explicit instructions on how to respond when she made mistakes. Alex was upset about Betty's confused behavior, and his anger and frustration actually made Betty anxious and tense. When she insisted on doing the smallest task, Alex would often become so frustrated that he would shout, "Go ahead and do it if you can." This would only aggravate the situation. Alex eventually learned to deal with his own anxiety about her mistakes. Even if Betty would stand for twenty minutes fumbling with the silverware, she was not hurting anyone. Indeed, she seemed to be happy to be doing something, even though it made no sense to anyone else.

There are many constructive ways to deal with ambivalence, but usually this can be done only with help. Unfortunately, many people are afraid to seek help, and the results can be dangerous to the patient or the family. Mrs. Grace Arrow became increasingly frustrated about attempts to keep her husband, Ronald, in bed at night. After retiring, he would get up and walk into the kitchen eight or ten times, try to remove his pajama bottoms, and hold them over the stove burners. On several nights he turned the burners on, igniting his pajamas. This routine went on for several weeks before Mrs. Arrow, becoming increasingly agitated, took her husband back to the doctor. The visit was precipitated when Mr. Arrow screamed at his wife and struck her in the face while she was trying to prevent him from repeating this dangerous activity.

Everyone was baffled by his ritualistic behavior, and Mrs. Arrow was weary from lack of sleep. She was legitimately upset and angry not only because she was tired but also because she did not understand her husband's unusual actions. They had been married over fifty years, and she had prided herself on her ability to care for her husband's needs. During the daytime he seemed quite content. However, his "craziness" and violence at night were devastating because Mr. Arrow had never raised his voice to her in all the years they had been married. She loved him deeply but could not understand the action of this man, who seemed to be someone else. She was so upset about her feelings of anger and guilt that she endured his behavior, as dangerous as it was, until his blow appeared to snap her out of her conflict and led her to seek help.

It was possible to make sense of his actions. It was the middle of winter, and to conserve fuel and money Mrs. Arrow kept the thermostat at sixty-six degrees. This had been their custom for as long as they had lived in the Northeast. Since it was possible that Mr. Arrow was trying to communicate that he was cold, the doctor suggested an experiment. Raise the thermostat to seventy degrees and observe whether there was any change in his behavior. The very first night, Mr. Arrow slept soundly and did not get out of bed except to go to the bathroom.

It is often difficult for spouses and other family members to reconcile their ambivalence toward a loved one. Furthermore, patients themselves are capable of experiencing ambivalent feelings. Mrs. Abigail Truman lived with her husband, Dale, aged sixty-nine, who had been diagnosed as having Alzheimer's disease more than three years earlier. This was the second marriage for Mrs. Truman and the third for her husband. They were a handsome couple who enjoyed each other's company and were devoted to one another's happiness. The marriage had lasted twenty-two years, and although they had no children, Mr. Truman's three daughters from his second marriage were devoted to both of them.

The oldest daughter, Mary Jane, became deeply concerned about a growing depression in both parents. Her father had begun to deteriorate. His memory was worsening, and he napped more often during the day. It required three or more hours for her stepmother to get him out of bed, dress him, and feed him in the morning. Mr. Truman claimed he was too tired and simply did not want to leave his bed.

Mrs. Truman was a strong, beautiful woman determined to keep her husband active. Having become distressed by his inability to rise in the morning, she was increasingly frustrated and tired. Once he was out of bed and dressed, she kept him active in the afternoon and evenings. The ceaseless hours of caring, however, were taking their toll on her, and with time she found herself averting her husband's romantic advances. He, in turn, became irritable and began to withdraw from her. Mr. Truman ate and slept more and began to put on excess weight. It was at this point that Mary Jane invited her parents to visit with her for a few weeks. She also persuaded them to see a specialist in Alzheimer's disease to see whether anything might be done for Mr. Truman.

Several discussions with Mr. and Mrs. Truman, together and separately, were revealing. It was clear that the marriage of twenty-two years was a solid one and that despite the dementia there were several areas of mutual pleasure. Both were gourmet cooks, and although Mr. Truman could no longer cook, he could still enjoy his wife's special meals. Although both also had enjoyed collecting stamps and building miniature furniture, these hobbies had been among the first pleasures to be dropped as expenses mounted. Finally, it was clear that sexual relations were extremely important to both of them.

The couple were approaching a crisis during the visit to their daughter's home. They had not had sex in the past month. Mrs. Truman cried frequently but was unable to confide in her daughter, and both she and her husband were trying to act as if nothing were wrong.

Mr. Truman was greatly distressed about what he perceived as his wife's rejection and withdrawal. He knew that the Alzheimer's disease was progressive, and his greatest fear was that his wife would reject him and abandon him as the disease destroyed him. He described how his wife refused to discuss the future with him. She would hide articles on dementia, and she even tried to keep him from watching a television special on the topic. He knew that his future was a grim one, but he also wanted dearly to talk with his family and help prepare them emotionally. He was becoming increasingly angry that his wife would not cooperate. He felt excluded, and he was also afraid that the disease would rob him of his senses before he could complete his preparation.

His wife's sexual withdrawal was the ultimate rejection. He was ashamed that the Alzheimer's had deprived him not only of his manhood and dignity but also of the woman he loved. He wanted to die and often said so to his wife.

Mrs. Truman was deeply troubled by her husband's wish to die. In fact, she was so overwhelmed by the situation that she felt she would soon be on the verge of a breakdown. She was adamant that her husband must not know about the final stages of Alzheimer's disease, and it took time to convince her that he already knew. Indeed, the two of them had been so busy protecting each other that neither had any sense of the other's real thoughts or feelings.

Mrs. Truman understood the possible effect of her sexual withdrawal. She loved her husband but was exhausted from the long hours. She had no energy and was depressed and angry. She did not know how to deal with her confused feelings of love and anger and sadness.

After several meetings it was possible to help Mr. and Mrs. Truman communicate with one another and to understand how this situation had evolved. Mr. Truman was relieved that his wife was not rejecting or leaving him. And at first Mrs. Truman found her husband's fears unbelievable. As his loneliness became clearer to her and as the two began to see how each was torn by ambivalence, it became easier to plan the future together. Mr. Truman responded well to antidepressant medications, and both he and his wife participated in several therapy sessions. Eventually, they re-established their former intimacy and trust.

Maintaining Balance in the Family

Changes in the patients threaten everyone's ability to sustain a rewarding and loving relationship. At some point in the course of the disorder, patients may no longer understand what is happening around them or be able to share experiences with family members. Some patients become so belligerent and unpleasant that it is easy to see why even close relatives and friends become resentful and upset. Even when families understand that brain damage is causing the irritating, unreasonable, or violent behavior in their loved ones, it is still difficult for them to tolerate the upsetting behavior. Feelings of hurt, anger, and frustration may become so unbearable that family members isolate themselves from friends. In some families this isolation only further increases the emotional turmoil and leads to a premature decision to institutionalize the patients. Other families may refuse to institutionalize their relatives regardless of the disruption in the family.

Even families that have coped well for years may find they need help as the dementia worsens. Alice Chen and her husband, Frank, accompanied Alice's mother, Mei, and father, Hong, to see a physician. Hong was seventy-two and had been diagnosed as having Alzheimer's disease approximately six years earlier. The entire family was involved in the decision as to whether Hong should be moved to a nursing home. Mei and Hong had three other daughters (and sons-in-law) who could not be present for the meeting because they either lived too far away or because work responsibilities prevented their attendance. However, all of them had reached the consensus that if their mother could not accept the help of a home care attendant, then perhaps it was time to think about an institution.

Over the past years the children had become more concerned about their parents. Their father had changed very gradually through the first five years, but in the past year he had begun to deteriorate more rapidly. Hong required more help with dressing, feeding, and other personal activities. Mei managed well for a while, but she gradually became overwhelmed, as his nightly wanderings interrupted her ability to rest.

Family and close friends would visit and offer to schedule time to be with Hong and give her the opportunity to get away, sleep, sew, and resume her volunteer work at the local hospital. Mei had been very active raising funds for her church. Even while her husband was sick, at least until the last six months, she had been on the phone and at meetings night and day to raise money. However, she refused help and took great pride in caring for Hong by herself.

At the same time Mei refused help, she also placed her daughters in a double bind. She called them daily to ask them to visit her and keep her company, but then she withdrew and even asked them not to visit. She was a proud woman and embarrassed by her husband's behavior. He would shout obscenities, undress himself, or pace restlessly around the house throughout the day. It was the children's concern with this situation that precipitated a visit to us for professional assistance. They could not deal with repeated cries for help followed by rejection.

Mei submitted to the children's demands to have a home care attendant. However, as might be expected, she had great difficulty surrendering the responsibilities of caring to anyone else. She refused to leave her husband alone with the attendant, Bertha, and insisted on helping with every single task. Even though Bertha was a well-trained, bright, and sensitive individual who understood Mei's feelings, she was becoming increasingly frustrated. Mei was not just stubborn in her determination to care for her husband; she also interfered with everything and was unfairly critical of everything Bertha attempted. Mei would ask Bertha to feed her husband and in the middle of lunch would take over the feeding and criticize Bertha without cause. She would ask Bertha to bathe her husband and within minutes send her away, accusing her of being too rough. Or she would ask Bertha to accompany Hong on a walk, only to change her mind and insist that the two of them must help him to prevent him from falling.

In desperation Bertha called the oldest daughter, Lois, to plead for their intervention, or she would have to quit. She could not do her job with Mei's interference. Bertha understood Mei's suffering but sensed that she was in a serious emotional state and needed help.

With great difficulty the children persuaded Mei to see a counselor. After she was treated successfully for a severe depression, the entire family agreed to several family therapy sessions to develop a plan for working together to care for Hong. Even though Mei felt better, she resumed her old pattern of demanding and rejecting help from her family. This became one of several important family problems to be resolved.

Mei described how she had cared for both of her parents when she was only a teenager. She nursed her mother for three years and her father for five years before they both died. Her brothers and sisters were all younger, and that left her with the burden of supporting the family and physically ministering to her parents. In the course of several discussions, Mei's children learned a part of their mother's history that was new to them. They began to understand the basis for her double-bind behavior in regard to caregiving.

Mei also was able to relive painful memories and share her frustration that she had had no help in caring for her parents. She even believed that had she been able to do more, her parents might have lived. She wanted her children to care for their father (and her) with the same intense devotion she had rendered to her parents. At the same time she sheltered them the same way she had protected her own brothers and sisters. She was the oldest, and therefore it was her responsibility to do what needed to be done. This, too, was part of her culture. In the context of family discussions, Mei and her family were able to understand each other better; they learned to collaborate in such a way as to share in the decisions and in the hands-on caring of Hong.

When families are in trouble, they can benefit a great deal from meeting together (if necessary with professionals) to discuss the needs, hurts, and rights of various family members, including those of the patient. Negotiations may unearth the various problems of all family members involved and lead to a plan of action to balance needs and responsibilities. Furthermore, as was evident in the foregoing description of the Chens, family interventions can bring to the surface those intergenerational and cultural issues that help explain an individual's behavior.

Continuous family negotiations are needed to help everyone decide what must be done to balance the needs of various family members with those of the patient. Since the patient is changing, however slowly, the delicate balance of family relationships is threatened, and family members must re-evaluate what they are doing. Some family members may not be able to cope well, and if it is not possible to restore equilibrium to the family system, it is likely that some of its members, including the patient, will suffer. When serious conflicts between family members exist, a patient's care may be seriously jeopardized.

Sue Ellen Grant was a seventy-seven-year-old widow. She had lived alone in her apartment for more than ten years since the death of her husband. According to her family she never seemed to recover from his death, and over the years she socially isolated herself from everyone, including her family. Mrs. Grant had three married sons, all of whom lived far away from her. The youngest, Teddy, was stationed in Europe. Richard, the oldest, was a minister whose parish was several hundred miles away, and although Todd lived the closest, he was still more than a two-hour drive away. Teddy had joined the armed forces at an early age and was estranged from his brothers. However, each month he sent his mother short letters with a check. Todd was a successful banker who had little time for his family, and it was Todd's wife who called Mrs. Grant several times a week. Richard was very attached to his mother. He called her daily and visited at least once a month with his family. In the last year he had noticed that she had some mild memory problems and often forgot what she was saying or repeated stories over and over.

Several events caused Richard to become greatly distressed. His mother called him several times with complaints that her landlord was trying to poison her and that men in dark hoods entered her home at night. Richard visited her to investigate, and it was clear that she was very paranoid and needed help. There was rotten food in the refrigerator, piles of newspapers were stacked throughout the house, and she was very forgetful.

When Richard tried to arrange to have his mother see a doctor, Todd objected violently, insisting that she was only old and a little eccentric, just as she had been for her entire life. When Richard argued that she was quite sick and that Todd should see for himself, Todd did visit and promptly took his mother home with him. However, within three days Mrs. Grant was back in her apartment, and Todd was more insistent than ever that nothing was wrong with her.

Mrs. Grant immediately began to call Richard at all hours of the day and night. She was afraid to be alone because her neighbors were plotting to kidnap her or poison her with gas. Once she claimed to have been raped by several of the hooded men. Sometimes she would call in the middle of the night, thinking it was morning.

Richard contacted several doctors and with their assistance persuaded his mother to check into the hospital for a complete examination. Although Todd objected, the rest of the family, including his own wife, insisted that she get help. Mrs. Grant's paranoia was successfully treated, and she even seemed to enjoy the experience of being in the hospital. However, the results of the medical, neurological, psychiatric, and psychological evaluations suggested Alzheimer's disease. She had serious memory deficits and would not be able to live safely in her home.

The medical team insisted that Richard, Todd, and their wives meet together with them to discuss discharge options. Todd dominated the discussion. He was angry throughout the conference, insisting that his mother had been taken to the hospital against her will, that she was old enough to be a little senile, and that there was no good reason for her to need any additional medical help. He refused to talk directly with his brother and would speak only with his wife.

The meeting concluded with everyone tired and angry, except for Mrs. Grant, who was present for part of the conference. She felt that she was ready to go home and live by herself as before. She admitted to being a little afraid but thought all would be well once she was settled in her apartment. Todd insisted that he would take his mother home with him for a few weeks and then find another apartment for her close to them. Richard protested vigorously, but he was exhausted from caring for his mother as well as from his demanding duties at the parish. He and his wife had also suffered a major tragedy. Their eighteen-year-old son had been killed in a car accident two months earlier.

Within a week of discharge, Mrs. Grant was again alone in her home, calling Richard day and night. She was confused and paranoid. Richard began to search for alternative housing arrangements for his mother, since it was clear she could not live alone. Todd called Richard several times, accusing Richard of trying to take his mother away from him. The bitterness of Todd's sibling rivalry tortured Richard. He wanted to help his mother, and he was angered and hurt by Todd's lack of cooperation and angry assaults, which impeded all of his efforts.

On the same day Richard had completed arrangements for his mother to move into a health-related facility, Todd "kidnapped" her. He told the family that he had taken her away to care for her, but he would not tell anyone, not even his own wife, of her whereabouts. Richard called a close friend of his brother to use whatever influence he had with Todd to bring him to the discussion table. The talks began but broke off many times over a period of a month, before the "mediator" asked to remove himself from the emotional deadlock.

Richard made the difficult decision to call the police. Todd was forced to divulge his mother's location. The police found her locked in Todd's country home, malnourished and extremely confused. Todd had hired someone to look after her, but the attendant had visited her only once a day to bring food. Mrs. Grant was hospitalized, her physical health was restored, and she moved into a nursing home near Richard. Richard refused to press charges against his brother.

Family dynamics are extremely complex. Powerful loyalties bind family members together, and although many of these forces are nurturing, others are destructive. Mrs. Grant's son Todd interfered with her care, despite his perception that he was helping her. If circumstances had been different, Richard might have been able to work around Todd. However, in this situation Todd's denial of the reality of his mother's problem, coupled with his own psychopathology, created trouble.

This sad family saga is clearly an extreme example of how an older parent with Alzheimer's disease further unbalances the complex relationships among family members. Unless significant disruption exists in a family, regular meetings are an effective way to minimize family conflict, to anticipate future problems, and to develop alternative solutions in order to care effectively for the patient. The process of developing contingency plans is one of the most effective means of minimizing stress. It also provides opportunities for family members to examine how they can best cooperate with each other in various situations.

In preparing for family meetings, each member would do well to prepare a list of issues, as is done in labor management negotiations. Identify the important issues, write down the steps needed for a solution, and specify exactly what you will do and what you expect others to contribute. Clearly, this analogy is a limited one because of the special nature of family commitments, but the approach has real merit as a way of discussing problems and solutions. If you become deadlocked, bring in a mediator, who can be a trusted friend, a clergyman, or a health professional. Mediators can help identify the loyalties and obligations people feel toward each other and get family members to deal with each other's needs. Some conflict is normal in this process. The discovery and ventilation of angry feelings are healthy coping mechanisms and pave the way for constructive actions to help correct the situation.

Talking about feelings and difficulties associated with caring may sometimes be done productively with the patient present. Great caution needs to be exercised to avoid the mistake of blaming the patient. When the focus of the meeting is planning, however, it is valuable to have the patient share in the experience.

The Effects of Dementia on Young Children

Young children and adolescents may find it extremely difficult to accept that a parent or grandparent has dementia. They may not understand the strange behavior of someone they love and admire even when they are aware that something is wrong, and for some the explanation that the behavior is due to an illness seems to have no meaning. They may withdraw from friends and family or become angry and rebellious. Children vary in the way they cope, and many factors are important—the child's age, the number of other children in the family, the closeness of the relationship between the child and the patient, the culture the child lives in, and the availability of other family members. Some children assume the role of a caregiver in the household, whereas others are unable to deal with a "changed" parent and become more childlike in dealing with the healthy parent. Occasionally, young children and even teenagers who cannot understand what they interpret as a loss of interest or of love by a patient may act out, becoming demanding and rebellious, or show violent outbursts and generally misbehave at home and school. Clearly, these behaviors create even more stress in the family.

Some children seem unaware of their parent's suffering or seem to adapt to it. Others become preoccupied with worries about parental loss or about the possibility that they will become sick like their mother or father. Dr. James Turner was a young, respected surgeon in his late thirties whose father, uncles, and grandfather had developed Alzheimer's disease sometime between the ages of sixty and sixty-five. He was married and the father of a three-year-old girl, Beth. Both he and his wife, Ann, talked openly with each other, and once in a while consulted their clergyman, about the possibility that he would someday get the disease. Both were actively involved in the care of Jim's father, and everyone, including their young daughter, frequently visited the nursing home.

Jim had two wisdom teeth extracted and spent several days at home recovering from the oral surgery. The first afternoon, Beth crawled next to him on the couch and asked, "Daddy, is this the beginning? Are you starting to get Grandpa's disease? . . . I have a toothache too. Will I lose my memory before I have a chance to grow up?"

There are several guidelines for dealing with younger children. First, it is important to involve children at a level appropriate to their ability to understand and participate in family activities. In the earlier phase of dementia and when the patient is not aggressive or violent, the presence of infant grandchildren can bring laughter and smiles. For the most part, young children should not be kept away from the patient. Hiding a relative with dementia only makes the person and situation more difficult for a child to understand. Even two- and three-year-old children are able to sense their parents' anxieties and fears. Children learn many of their fears from others. Involve them with you and the patient, and let them see and feel your comfort. Whenever possible, find time to be alone with your children. Talk simply and directly. Provide opportunities for them to be around the patient and to do even simple tasks like carrying food and drink or playing in the same room with the patient.

Children often give us valuable insights into our own attitudes and behaviors. Sometimes another person, usually an outsider, is necessary to help us see accurately what is actually happening. Robert Blanc, a fifty-two-year-old retired mechanic. had been diagnosed as having Alzheimer's disease more than three years earlier. His wife, Louise, and two daughters, Cindy and Marjorie, had been doing well until Mr. Blanc started to become more agitated and combative. The younger daughter, Cindy, aged seventeen, whom everyone reported to be a great deal like her father, had a rebellious relationship with her father prior to the diagnosis. Following his diagnosis Cindy withdrew from everyone and became sullen. The arguments with her father intensified, and within six months Cindy angrily moved out of the house. She refused to confide in her sister or her mother. She spoke of her father as an arrogant, stubborn, unfair person, and the anger spilled out into all of her relationships, with girlfriends at school as well as with her boyfriend.

One of the teachers at the high school finally called Mrs. Blanc to arrange a meeting. Irene Dalton had been Cindy's student adviser and teacher. Irene had also been Cindy's hockey coach for several years and had become a special person in Cindy's life. In the course of the meeting, Irene relayed what Cindy had confided to her over the past several months.

Cindy was angry not only with her father but also with her mother. She resented the fact that no one had told her about the seriousness of her father's memory problems or the many doctor appointments that led to the diagnosis. Her response to her anger was to cut the family out of her life. The only person she had been able to talk to for any length of time was her father, and now she was so blinded by her anger that she could not accept his illness. Instead of dealing effectively with her hurt, she lashed out against all of her family. She rejected them because she felt that they had rejected her. She also had deep feelings of rejection by her father because he was not the father she knew. He was there and not there at the same time.

Irene recommended that Mrs. Blanc take a brief weekend trip with both her daughters. She thought that the lack of communication between then could be repaired. The relationship between Cindy and her father could also be improved but would probably be handled best with some professional help.

Guidelines for Families to Evaluate Coping Skills

Is there a healthy family response to caring? Yes, the healthy family is one that is able to cope with change, becoming flexible and resilient. Is there one right way to cope with change? No. There are no easy prescriptions, and there is no prototype for the healthy family. There are many different ways to successfully respond to the challenge of caring for a relative with dementia. Families differ in numerous ways, and the history of what happens to every person within and across generations and different cultures affects how each responds as an individual and as a member of the family.

There are several questions family members can ask themselves to evaluate their coping skills as a family unit. Asking questions and searching for answers helps caregivers adapt to the challenge of caring.

1. What was the patient like before the disease? Was he or she open and sharing with the family or aloof? Did he or she have close friends

or keep counsel only to himself or herself? Did he or she express anger or happiness easily, or was he or she emotionally controlled? Family expectations for the patient's behavior must be consistent with the individual's previous personality style. There are no "gold standards" for how a patient should behave throughout the course of the illness.

2. Who is providing most of the care—husband or wife, children, brothers or sisters, in-laws, fictive kin (important and valued people in the family who are not blood relatives), or perhaps a parent? Is there a natural leader in the family to whom everyone looks for decision making? Do several members of the family share the burden of caring? If one person such as a spouse dominates the caring, does he or she know how to ask for help or let others help? Solving problems together and sharing the burden of caring is a continuing challenge to the family.

3. How did the patient relate to other members of the family prior to the diagnosis? If relationships were ruptured or if conflict was prominent, is it feasible to repair the relationships before the patient deteriorates, or is it better to leave things alone? If the patient was married several times, is it possible for the different families to relate to each other, if only around the care of the patient?

4. If the patient is married, is the relationship a stable one? If long-standing disruptive marital conflict preceded the diagnosis, it will probably continue or worsen. What steps, if any, can children or other family members take to ensure the safety and care of the patient and still respect the autonomy of the couple? Is professional help useful?

5. How close do family members live to the patient or to the patient and spouse? What plans can be made to allow distant family members to participate in caring? If geographically close relatives feel overburdened, what steps can be taken to remedy imbalances or perceived imbalances?

6. How well are different family members accepting the diagnosis? Does anyone need professional help?

7. What are the cultural norms and expectations for caregiving in the family?

8. Does anyone else in the immediate family suffer from a major physical or emotional illness? When several people are sick, the family's

emotional and financial resources are strained. It is not uncommon for family members to feel that a child with leukemia, an adult with multiple sclerosis, or a younger paraplegic relative is "more deserving" of family resources. Families often face difficult decisions that need to be made carefully, and often with help.

9. Have any recent life crises affected other members in the family? Did someone die, lose a job, get married and move away, or have legal or criminal problems? Many major as well as minor unpleasant life events can disrupt families. The family's ability to deal both with the stresses of everyday life and with major crises potentially jeopardizes the balance of care for the patient.

10. How well informed is everyone in the family about dementia and the problems of caring?

11. How well do family members cooperate with each other to solve problems around the patient's care? It is sometimes useful to get outside help to improve the communication patterns among family members. It is often possible to find solutions to a problem if individuals are able to avoid conflicts of style and personality. Sometimes the way people talk interferes with the message. Anxiety, anger, and other emotions often color a conversation and precipitate unnecessary arguments.

12. Do family members take responsibility for what they do and say, or do they blame others? When things go wrong, it is easy to say it is the other person's fault. It is important to have family meetings not only to focus on the patient's problems, but also to examine problems family members experience.

13. Do family members listen to one another and are they sensitive to each other? Do people speak for one another rather than let the other individuals speak for themselves? Do family members let the patient speak up or do they "bury" the patient? It is important to give the patient time to talk. It often takes the patient longer to make a response, and this may be difficult to do in a group where people tend to interact quickly with one another. Remember, the patient often experiences the world differently. His or her world may be slower, less coherent, and less organized.

14. Have financial matters been addressed? Unless these issues are being solved, anxiety about money may color discussions about everything

else. This is not unusual. Throughout the lives of most people, financial transactions have been known to cause many domestic arguments.

15. Are there irresolvable conflicts in the family? If so, seek help. Families are complex systems, and it is not legitimate to expect to change an entire family. However, it is realistic to focus the family on the needs of the patient as a member of the family.

There are many ways you can cope successfully with the demands and challenges of caregiving. However, even the most resourceful, adaptive family members are vulnerable to the most common negative consequence of the strains of caring—depression. The next chapter is devoted entirely to a discussion of depression—how to recognize it and what to do about it.

10

Depression

Getting the Help You Need

Depression is a medical disorder that occurs in about half of family members caring for a relative with dementia. Spouses are the most vulnerable, especially wives. As many as a third of adult daughters and daughters-in-law and about one-fourth of adult sons become depressed.

Depression cannot be ignored. It interferes with your ability to feel good about yourself, the world you live in, and your future. It affects your desire to care for the patient, take medications, follow health care regimens, relate to other people, and live a healthy lifestyle.

Depression can happen to anyone. When you are depressed, you feel bad. Mike Wallace, the news correspondent of "60 Minutes," described his depression as an "endless darkness." In testimony to Congress about depression, Mr. Wallace said: "Sunshine means nothing to you. The seasons, friends, or good food mean nothing. All you focus on is yourself and how badly you feel."

It is also not easy to live with and love someone who is depressed. Stress, arguments, and misunderstandings are common. When someone you love is depressed, you may feel angry, lost, frustrated, or frail. You can feel shut out and drained.

This chapter on depression is meant to help you deal with depression, because it is treatable! It describes what you and your family need to know about depression. It discusses the different forms of depression, how to recognize depression, when and where to get help, what causes depression, the different forms of treatment, and many other important topics. Recognizing and dealing with depression is essential not only for your health but also for that of the patient and the rest of the family.

The Many Faces of Depression

Depression has many faces, ranging from brief feelings of sadness to a serious medical condition. Most people feel sad and worried many times throughout life. Feelings of depression and sadness are normal reactions to hard times, disappointments, losses, illness, or death. These events take the joy out of life, and it is natural to feel sad, lose interest in people and things, have sleep problems, and feel tired. These are all common expressions of what is a normal reaction to loss. The problems causing a reactive depression may or may not go away, but you find ways to accept or deal with your losses or problems. You bounce back and start to feel better in a few days or weeks.

When sadness persists or keeps returning, when the things you do every day like eating, sleeping, working, and enjoying life continue to be difficult, you are dealing with something more than just "feeling down" or "feeling blue." You are dealing with a clinical depression, an illness that requires treatment. Many people wrongly believe that depression is normal in older adults. It is not! Clinical depression is a medical illness, and biological, psychological, social, and existential factors can interact to cause depression.

Fortunately, most depressive disorders are treatable. However, if undetected and untreated, clinical depression worsens health problems and destroys the quality of life. It can lead to personal suffering, withdrawal from others, family disruption and conflict, and sometimes suicide. And because of the potential for suicide, depression is a life-threatening illness.

Types of Depression

There are several types of clinical depression. The most common forms include major depressive disorders or unipolar disorders, dysthymia, and bipolar disorders, also known as manic-depressive disorders.

A *major depressive disorder* is characterized by a sadness, helplessness, and hopelessness that does not go away, as well as altered patterns of eating and sleeping, weight loss or weight gain, and loss of interest in sex, friends, and other pleasures. Major depressive disorders differ from a normal reactive sadness in many ways, including the number of symptoms, how severe they are, and how long they last. Major depressive disorders are not just mood changes. They are truly debilitating and may be incapacitating. Life feels overwhelming and miserable. William Styron, a Pulitzer Prize–winning author, described his depression as feeling "condemned" to life, where "the entire body and spirit of a person is in a state of shipwreck."

Some people with severe depression may have hallucinations, where they believe they hear voices or music, see lights or images, taste or smell things, or have the sensation of being touched. Others may experience delusions, where beliefs about who they are or what is happening are not true. Voices condemning them for failings may trouble them, and the utter futility of life weighs them down like a millstone around their neck.

Dysthymia is similar to a major depressive disorder, but it is characterized by chronic mild depressive symptoms that last at least two years. This is in contrast to a major depressive disorder, for which there are one or more distinct episodes of depression. Some people have described living with dysthymia as seeing the world through dark glasses. They are able to function and get on with life, but they do not feel happy. One woman described her dysthymia this way: "I do what I have to do but I feel like all my lights are out." Dysthymia also can occur with major depression, and this condition is known as a *double depression*.

Bipolar disorder is the medical name for manic depressive disorder. The hallmark of bipolar depression is that in addition to the depression there are one or more episodes of mania. *Mania* is the occurrence of symptoms at some point in a person's illness that are the opposite of depression. These include elation, pressured speech, hyperactivity, a belief in one's ability to do great and important things, reckless spending, and the inability to sleep. Bipolar disorder is characterized by mood swings of both depressive and manic behavior. Although the shifts from one state to the other are usually gradual, they can occur suddenly. The rapid-cycling form of bipolar disorder involves four or more complete mood cycles in a year.

Since clinical depression is not always associated with feeling depressed but rather increased sensitivity to pain, feeling tired, and general malaise or "having the blahs," many people and even physicians mistakenly attribute these symptoms to age or physical health problems. When depression occurs, it will make anyone who already has health problems feel worse. Most depressed persons also lose interest in caring for themselves, ignore good health care, fail to take medications, and as a result may get sicker.

The Signs of Depression

Clinical depression affects the body and the mind. It causes changes in thinking, mood, behavior, and bodily functions. The key to detecting signs of depression is "change."

Thinking

Depressed individuals often feel inadequate or overwhelmed. Even easy tasks seem impossible. Concentration is difficult, disrupting activities from reading to driving. Making decisions is burdensome, from deciding what clothes to wear or making business decisions. The world appears bleak, and feelings of pessimism color the perception of self-worth. Even successes are interpreted as failures. Thoughts of suicide may occur when the depression is severe.

People with bipolar depression are usually distracted very easily. They think and talk very quickly, often without making much sense. Judgment is impaired such that they do not recognize the hurtful consequences of inappropriate sexual behaviors, poor financial investments, or extravagant spending. They often have grandiose thoughts of being the world's best lover, authority, or business person.

Mood

Depressed individuals feel empty, helpless, hopeless, and worthless, or they may report overwhelming pain and despair. Individuals may cry a great deal, often for little or no reason. Many people with depression often experience symptoms of anxiety such as agitation and excessive worry.

It is also common to feel anger or even rage, irritation, frustration, and anxiety in addition to the sadness and despair. Depressed moods are pervasive and persistent and do not lift even when good things happen.

During manic episodes individuals may feel on top of the world, so much so that they believe there is nothing they cannot do. Excitability and irritability at the slightest change are common. Individuals may be paranoid and have delusions of being followed or persecuted for their religious beliefs. Hostility and violent behavior may also occur.

Behavior

Many behavioral changes are a signal of depression. These include restlessness, hand-wringing, pacing, the inability to meet deadlines and complete projects, withdrawal from friends, staying in bed most of the day, and loss of interest in sex. Depressive behaviors can be destructive and hasten death. It is not uncommon for individuals to self-medicate, by drinking alcohol or taking sedatives, in an attempt to make the depression go away.

Many behavioral changes signal bipolar depression. These include restlessness, increased talkativeness, laughing inappropriately or inappropriate humor, increased sexuality and impulsive behaviors such as buying someone twenty pairs of red shoes, selling or buying a new business, or arranging to take friends or strangers on an expensive trip.

Bodily Functions

Depression is a disease affecting the entire body. Individuals report any number of physical pains such as headaches, backaches, joint pain, stomach problems, chest pain, and gastrointestinal distress. Individuals with bipolar depression usually sleep very little, have little or no appetite, and lose a great deal of weight.

Test Your Depression

Do you want to know how depressed you are? The test in Table 1, developed by Dr. Leonora Radloff at the National Institute of Mental Health, may help clarify what you are feeling. A high score on this ques-

Table 1. Center for Epidemiological Studies—Depression Test

Select the answer that best describes your situation over the past week, and circle the corresponding number.

0 = Rarely or none of the time (less than 1 day)
1 = Some or little of the time (1–2 days)
2 = Occasionally or a moderate amount of the time (3–4 days)
3 = Most or all of the time (5–7 days)

During the Past Week:

1. I was bothered by things that usually don't bother me.	0 1 2 3
2. I did not feel like eating; my appetite was poor.	0 1 2 3
3. I felt that I could not shake off the blues even with help from my family or friends.	0 1 2 3
4. I felt that I was not as good as other people.	0 1 2 3
5. I had trouble keeping my mind on what I was doing.	0 1 2 3
6. I felt depressed.	0 1 2 3
7. I felt that everything I did was an effort.	0 1 2 3
8. I felt hopeless about the future.	0 1 2 3
9. I thought my life had been a failure.	0 1 2 3
10. I felt fearful.	0 1 2 3
11. My sleep was restless.	0 1 2 3
12. I was unhappy.	0 1 2 3
13. I talked less than usual.	0 1 2 3
14. I felt lonely.	0 1 2 3
15. People were unfriendly.	0 1 2 3
16. I did not enjoy life.	0 1 2 3
17. I had crying spells.	0 1 2 3
18. I felt sad.	0 1 2 3
19. I felt people disliked me.	0 1 2 3
20. I could not get going.	0 1 2 3

To determine your score, add up the numbers you circled for each question or statement. Your total will be between 0 and 60. If you scored from 0 to 9, you are in a nondepressed range. You are also below the average score of adults in the United States. A score of 10 to 15 places you in the mildly depressed range, and a score of 16 to 24 in the moderately depressed range. If you scored over 24, you may be showing the signs of severe depression.

tionnaire is not the same as a diagnosis of depression. However, if you do score high or regardless of your score, if you have thoughts about suicide, reach out to someone as soon as possible, ideally a professional with mental health training.

If your score falls in the moderately depressed range, take the test again in two weeks. If you still score in that range, please call your physician or a crisis hot line in your community.

Testing for Mania

Impaired judgment is as much a part of mania as it is of depression. It is usually more obvious to friends and family. The scale in Table 2 is designed to help you determine the severity of manic symptoms and decide whether you should get professional help. It was developed by Dr. Ivan Goldberg.

Getting Help

It is not a sign of weakness to see a doctor when you are depressed. The very nature of depressive symptoms drains you of the desire and energy to talk with family or seek professional help. Yet the most courageous and important thing you can do is to get help. It is the first step to feeling better.

Both men and women get depression. There is a widespread myth that depression is a woman's disease. It is not "unmanly" or "wimpy" to admit feeling depressed. Unfortunately, men are reluctant to seek treatment and instead become irritable or angry, drink or use drugs, withdraw from loved ones, or act irresponsibly. Depression increases in older men. Older men have the highest suicide rate of any age group, and most of them have a recent history of depression.

Because depressed people often feel like failures, many feel they are not worthy of help. They also may feel hopeless to the point of not wanting to get out of bed or to ask for help from a professional or the family. Individuals with manic-depressive illness may deny that they have a problem and feel that getting help is a preposterous idea because they know more than the professionals do.

Table 2. Goldberg Mania Scale

The items below refer to how you have felt and behaved during the past week. For each item, circle the appropriate number.

0 = Not at all
1 = Just a little
2 = Somewhat
3 = Moderately
4 = Quite a lot
5 = Very much

During the Past Week:

1. My mind has never been sharper.	0 1 2 3 4 5
2. I need less sleep than usual.	0 1 2 3 4 5
3. I have so many plans and new ideas that it is hard for me to work.	0 1 2 3 4 5
4. I feel a pressure to talk and talk.	0 1 2 3 4 5
5. I have been particularly happy.	0 1 2 3 4 5
6. I have been more active than usual.	0 1 2 3 4 5
7. I talk so fast that people have a hard time keeping up with me.	0 1 2 3 4 5
8. I have more new ideas than I can handle.	0 1 2 3 4 5
9. I have been irritable.	0 1 2 3 4 5
10. It's easy for me to think of jokes and funny stories.	0 1 2 3 4 5
11. I have been feeling like "the life of the party."	0 1 2 3 4 5
12. I have been full of energy.	0 1 2 3 4 5
13. I have been thinking about sex.	0 1 2 3 4 5
14. I have been feeling particularly playful.	0 1 2 3 4 5
15. I have special plans for the world.	0 1 2 3 4 5
16. I have been spending too much money.	0 1 2 3 4 5
17. My attention keeps jumping from one idea to another.	0 1 2 3 4 5
18. I find it hard to slow down and stay in one place.	0 1 2 3 4 5

To determine your score, add up the numbers you circled for each statement. A score of 20 or higher suggests that you should see a professional.

It is not unusual to resist getting help, but telling someone how badly you feel is the first step to feeling better. A physician or another mental health professional is the best person to contact. If you are resistant to seeing a physician, ask a friend, member of the clergy, nurse, or other confidant to make the appointment. Some of the resistance is really an overwhelming fatigue and feeling that nothing can be done. A helpful family member or friend can be a lifesaver for someone who is immobilized by depression.

Clinical depression is a medical illness that can be treated. Depressive disorders are diseases of the brain, just as cardiovascular diseases are diseases of the heart and circulatory system. Depressive disorders are not the result of character flaws, bad parenting, divine punishment, or personal weaknesses. They are nothing to be ashamed of or embarrassed to have.

Indeed, you should feel just the opposite. Learning to spot the signs of depression is like learning to spot signs of cancer. It can save your life! Being proactive, learning to detect the signs of depression, and getting help are essential steps to good health!

The Diagnosis of Depressive Disorders

To be diagnosed with a *major depressive disorder* using current diagnostic criteria, you must display at least five of the following nine symptoms:

1. Depressed mood most of the day, nearly every day
2. Loss of interest or pleasure in most or all usual activities, nearly every day
3. Loss of appetite with associated weight loss or overeating with sudden weight gain (this means a gain or loss of more than 5 percent of your body weight in a month)
4. Insomnia or sleeping a lot nearly every day
5. Agitated behavior or slowed thoughts and movement nearly every day
6. Loss of energy or tiredness nearly every day
7. Feelings of worthlessness or excessive guilt nearly every day
8. Decreased ability to concentrate, think, and make decisions nearly every day
9. Ongoing thoughts of death, or suicidal thoughts or actions

This list of symptoms is not intended as a way for you to diagnose yourself, but rather to educate you about the dimensions of depression. It also gives you a sense of the areas about which your physician may interview you.

Symptoms of major depression usually develop over days to weeks. In the months before these symptoms become serious, you may have anxiety or even panic attacks. It is also possible for a major depression to develop suddenly under severe stress, such as a major life crisis or change in your health.

The features of *dysthymic disorder* are similar to those of major depression. Dysthymic disorder usually begins in childhood or adolescence. To be diagnosed with a dysthymic disorder, you must have a depressed mood most of the day, more days than not, for at least two years and have at least two of the following symptoms:

1. Poor appetite or overeating
2. Insomnia or sleeping too much
3. Low energy and fatigue
4. Poor self-esteem
5. Difficulty with concentration or decision making
6. Feelings of hopelessness

To be diagnosed with *bipolar disorder*, you must have at least one episode of mania. There are two types of mania, euphoric and dysphoric, and a person can experience both types when they have bipolar disorder. A person who is euphoric is on a high, in love with themselves and the world. They are full of energy, talk a mile a minute, and are full of grandiose thoughts. A person who is dysphoric is experiencing a different kind of high. They talk fast and have grandiose thoughts, but they are agitated, angry, destructive, and often paranoid.

Some people may have had previous episodes of depression as well as subsequent cycles of mania and depression. To be diagnosed with a manic episode using current diagnostic criteria, you must have a noticeable period of persistently elevated, expansive, or irritable mood lasting at least one week, and three or more of the following symptoms in the same period:

1. Inappropriate grandiosity or inflated self-esteem
2. Significant decrease in the need for sleep (feel rested after only 2 to 3 hours of sleep)
3. Unusually talkative with pressured speech
4. Rapidly racing thoughts
5. Very distractable
6. Increased agitation and goal-directed activities
7. Excessive time spent in pleasurable activities without awareness of negative consequences (sexual indiscretions, excessive shopping, or foolish investments)

Bipolar disorder is a chronic illness. It cannot be cured, but it can be managed effectively. Bipolar illness usually causes substantial problems that affect marriage, work, and family life. Individuals with bipolar disorder need to be protected from the likely negative consequences of poor judgment and excessive activity. Over time, even in periods of remission, the chronicity and unpredictability can lead not only to legal, marital, and job problems, but also to medical complications as well as suicide.

Tips for Coping with Mild Depression

There are a number of things you can do to cope with mild depression. The following tips are helpful for everyone who experiences a normal reactive depression.

1. *Try not to focus on yourself too much.* You perpetuate your own depression when you think and talk about yourself and your problems too much. Be aware of this focus on yourself. Do not brood and mope around. Find other people and events to focus on, such as a family holiday or a friend's birthday. Reach out to other people and talk about their activities.

2. *Try not to use words like* can't *and* shouldn't. Instead, use words such as *can* and *want to*. Think in the positive: "I can do something, I will go out. I will call somebody." When you are depressed, the ten-

dency is to think negative thoughts. Practice thinking positive. It is not easy at first, but be persistent.

3. *Get involved in a project.* If you are depressed, you need to find ways to get out of yourself. Being with children or other people or reaching out to others by volunteering in some activity will help you get your mind off yourself.

4. *Talk.* Keeping your feelings bottled up inside only increases your tension. Talking with someone may help you get a new perspective on yourself. Reaching out and talking to others will also stop the cycle of introspection, brooding, and self-pity that is characteristic of depression.

5. *Know your limits and limitations.* You need to come to grips with what you can and cannot do. Know how much you can do before you get tired. Pace yourself.

6. *Rethink your need to be right all the time.* There are many people who always need to be right, dominate the conversation, or win every argument. Your depression may be caused by your need to be right or be in control when you are with your doctor, friends, parents, and other family members. When you do not win, you feel let down and rejected, which leads to anger and depression. Learn to give in once in a while.

7. *Exercise.* Physical activity is a great way to blow off steam and release your tension and frustration. This is one of the most important things you can do to lift your mood. Walk, ride a bike, swim, or join an athletic club, spa, or local recreation center.

8. *Find activities that give you pleasure.* Spending time in a club or group or starting a new hobby can be therapeutic. Stop sitting around. Get out and do things. Replace your feelings of sadness and self-pity with joy, happiness, and humor. See a funny movie, read the comics, and make it a point to laugh every day.

9. *Think about positive things.* Focus on what you have accomplished, not what you did not or could not do. Use your talents and skills, and think about your successes!

10. *Develop good nutritional habits, and get enough rest.* Depression can be aggravated by not eating properly or by not getting the rest you need. Don't eat alone. It's more fun to eat with others. Also, do not take naps during the day. Stay active and you will sleep better at night.

11. *Don't let life overwhelm you. Take one day at a time.* Figure out what is most important, and do it. If you let yourself be overwhelmed, you can become paralyzed and unable to function, which makes your depression worse. Write down what you think all of your problems are. Then look at the list and prioritize the problems. Choose the most important one, and list your options for dealing with it. Then devise your plan and list the steps to carry it out. Give yourself a deadline and meet it!

Effective Treatments for Clinical Depression

Most individuals with depression respond to treatment. Available treatments include antidepressant medications, psychotherapy, and when necessary for seriously depressed individuals, electroconvulsive therapy (ECT).

Antidepressant medications correct imbalances of certain chemicals in the brain that cause depression. These chemicals are known as neurotransmitters. Depression involves changes in two major neurotransmitters, serotonin and norepinephrine, that play an important role regulating mood, sleep, eating, sexual activity, thinking, and motor activity (see Chapter 6).

If you are prescribed an antidepressant, ask your doctor, nurse, or pharmacist to explain how the drug will affect the neurotransmitters in your brain. Understanding the biochemical changes associated with depression can help you get better. Knowing the effect of the treatment plan should reinforce the sense that you are in control of changing the chemicals in your brain.

There are more than three-dozen different kinds of antidepressants. Four major classes of antidepressants are used to treat major depressive disorder: tricyclic antidepressants (TCAs); monoamine oxidase (MAO) inhibitors; selective serotonin reuptake inhibitors (SSRIs); and other new atypical compounds including venlafaxine (Effexor), bupropion (Wellbutrin), and nefazodone (Serzone).

All antidepressant drugs available in the United States have been demonstrated to be effective in treating major depression, but no single antidepressant medication has been demonstrated to be significantly more effective than another. Furthermore, no single drug results in success for all patients. The selection of a specific drug depends on many factors, such as side effects, whether the drug was effective for you in the past, other co-existing medical illnesses, other medications you are taking, the type of depression, and how much the drug could interfere with your lifestyle. Ask your physician to explain why he or she chose the specific drug for you.

Side effects occur in a certain number of patients taking any medication, and they usually are dependent on the dose and the level of drug in your blood. Many side effects are more likely to occur at the beginning of treatment or for a short time after the dosage is increased. Many patients adapt to most side effects over time. However, if you experience significant side effects, let your doctor know. If you cannot tolerate a certain drug, there are others to try.

Most SSRIs take several weeks before there is noticeable improvement. Reach out to others to help you until the symptoms improve. Sleep is one of the first changes you will notice as the depression responds to treatment. Improved energy will follow, but improvements in mood may take a while. Side effects need to be monitored closely, and medications changed when the side effects are intrusive.

The newer SSRIs are usually prescribed as the first-line treatment of depression. They are equally effective in treating depression per se, but they vary in their effect on different individuals. Furthermore, the drugs have differing side effects, the most common of which are gastrointestinal such as nausea or diarrhea, agitation, trouble sleeping, and decreased sexual activity. About half of people who take SSRIs do not have side effects, and those who do can usually tolerate them. There are subtle differences in the side effects so it is important to ask your doctor to explain them to you.

Prior to the SSRIs, TCAs were considered the standard treatment for depressive illness. These drugs are equally effective, but their side effects differ. They can cause dry mouth, blurred vision, sweating, urinary retention, a speeded heart rate, and a tendency for a drop in blood pressure when rising from a sitting or reclining position, known as orthostatic hypotension. Tricyclics are less expensive than the SSRIs, but their side effects and toxicity make them less desirable for many people, particularly those with a history of cardiac problems.

MAO inhibitors usually are used only after other drugs have not worked. MAO inhibitors are effective, but because they have bad effects if you eat foods that have a protein called tyramine, dietary caution is important. A partial list of foods to avoid include cheese, yogurt, smoked foods, soy sauce, bananas, caffeine, and chocolate. Medications that contain norepinephrine can also be dangerous when used with MAO inhibitors, causing a dangerous rise in blood pressure with the risk of stroke. Drugs to avoid include antihistamines, decongestants, any cold medication, codeine, narcotic pain relievers, and some anesthetics. Talk with your physician and pharmacist.

Three types of psychotherapy can be especially helpful, often when used in conjunction with drugs. These include cognitive-behavioral, behavioral, and interpersonal psychotherapy. If there are marital difficulties, couples behavioral therapy can be very effective.

Cognitive therapy is a short-term therapy. It is designed to change your negative views of yourself, the world, and the future. Behavioral therapy focuses largely on improving social skills and communication skills to change certain behaviors. You learn to monitor daily activities, schedule pleasurable activities to counter depression, and review activities that are difficult for you and find ways to master them. Interpersonal psychotherapy is based on research findings that interpersonal relationships play a significant role in depression. You learn how to resolve difficulties in interpersonal functioning, such as how not to isolate yourself and how to deal with grief, with role changes, and with your health problems.

No one therapy is more effective than the other. However, different people may get more benefit from one or another. When your doctor suggests psychotherapy without drug therapy for your depression, make sure your doctor or the therapist has experience. If there is no improvement in six weeks and no significant improvement in twelve weeks, ask your doctor about starting a drug as well. It is important that you consider yourself in a partnership with your doctor. Each of you contribute special knowledge and skills to the treatment of your depression.

ECT can be extremely effective when an individual has a psychotic depression or is severely depressed and has not responded to antidepressant drugs. ECT works rapidly and can literally save a person's life, allowing him or her to return to a productive life. It can be administered in a hospital or initiated in the hospital and continued on an outpatient basis. Most people tolerate ECT very well and recover from their depression.

Effective Treatments for Bipolar Disorder

Three types of drugs are commonly used to treat bipolar disorders: mood stabilizers, antidepressants, and antipsychotics. Mood stabilizers are the primary treatment for most people. Lithium is the oldest and most common mood stabilizer, and it is usually the first drug you will be given after the diagnosis of bipolar disorder. Most people tolerate lithium well; it is effective in more than half of all patients. More recent mood stabilizers are described in Chapter 6.

Some people have side effects to lithium that may include nausea, fatigue, diarrhea, weight gain, tremors, or having to go to the bathroom frequently. The blood level needs to be monitored regularly to avoid lithium toxicity and ensure that the drug is at an appropriate level.

Appropriate antipsychotic medications may be prescribed for bipolar illness to calm the patient down during an acute manic phase while waiting for the mood stabilizer to take effect. Again, as with all drugs, these medications need to be monitored for side effects, which can include slowed speech and thinking, sleepiness, restlessness, confusion, stiffness, or twitching.

Finding the right combination of drugs and dosages may take a long time. If the first medication does not work, do not give up. It is very important to work with your physician to find out what works for you. If the drugs are causing side effects that make you uncomfortable, do not be afraid to complain to your doctor and ask him or her to lower the dosage or try something else. You may find that you will have to balance the complete elimination of symptoms with a level of side effects you can handle. It is essential that you and your doctor communicate and be patient.

Although drug therapy is the primary treatment for bipolar depression, psychosocial treatments are effective to increase compliance with drug regimens, decrease the number and length of hospitalizations and relapses, improve quality of life, and help cope with stress. Bipolar patients and often families express frustration and resentment because they receive so little information about the disorder and their medications. Education about the complexities of bipolar illness and its successful treatment is highly effective.

Family Can Help

Depression affects the entire family. Depressed individuals can make other family members as well as friends feel angry, frustrated, and guilty. These negative reactions can occur when family members do not understand that a relative is depressed. They also occur when the depressed person denies the problem and other family members become frustrated with the deepening depression as well as the helplessness of not being able to overcome the resistance to seeing a professional. More than half of depressed adults report that their family members do not understand them. A vicious cycle can evolve when the negative emotional reactions of family members aggravate the sadness, hopelessness, and low self-esteem of the depressed person.

It is not easy to live with and love someone who is depressed. Chronic depression makes life tough. Arguments and misunderstandings are common in close relationships. Sexual problems often lead to distancing, stress, conflict, and even divorce. Children and grandchildren also are affected when a parent or grandparent is critical, easily irritated, angered, or emotionally distant.

There are many ways for family members to help and support a depressed relative. Knowledge about depression, patience, and persistence are the keys. It is important for family members to learn as much as they can about depression—what causes it and how the disease affects a person's thinking, world view, ability to function, and ability to communicate.

It is also essential to learn how to communicate with the depressed person. Learn how to be an active listener and ask your depressed relative what he or she hears you saying. If you think your relative has misunderstood, say, "I don't think I made myself clear," and explain yourself in a different way. Try not to be angry and accuse the depressed patient of not listening. This is not an easy task. The goal is to ask your relative to help you understand him or her.

Tips for family members to cope constructively with a depressed relative include the following:

- Do not think about depression or manic-depression as a family skeleton. Depression is a disease just like diabetes and cancer.

- Do not expect the depressed person to snap out of it. The depressed relative would if he or she could. No one enjoys being depressed.
- Try to maintain a normal relationship and do not act as if only you know what is best.
- Accept that a relative is suffering and encourage him or her to get help. Reinforce how much you care and value your relative and how help will ease the pain and distress.
- Involve the depressed person in as many activities as possible.
- Don't criticize or blame the person for depressed behavior. It is likely he or she has already told himself or herself everything you want to tell him or her.
- Do not use the phrase "if you loved me." The depressed person is not in control of the disorder, and this approach increases guilt. It is the same as saying "If you loved me, you would not have diabetes."
- Avoid threats unless you have thought about them carefully and are ready to carry them out. There may be times when actions are necessary to protect children or other vulnerable members of the household.
- Do not take alcohol or drugs away or hide them from the depressed person. This only increases the anger, depression, and desperation, and the person will find ways to get all the drugs or alcohol he or she wants. If excessive drug or alcohol use is a significant problem, do not let the person persuade you to join him or her as a way to help him or her cut back.
- Do not be jealous of the therapy a person chooses. It is normal to feel left out when a relative turns to someone else for support.
- Do not expect an immediate recovery. Depression requires a period of convalescence just as for other illnesses. There may also be relapses where family tension and resentment are normal.
- Do not protect the depressed person from situations that you think will be stressful and upsetting. Making your depressed relative feel dependent on you guarantees that he or she will pull away from you.
- Do not shy away from questions about the illness, treatments, drugs, and other issues. Let your relative decide whether he or she wants to talk about the depression or not.
- Be supportive during the recovery process. Disapproval will only increase the feeling that anything the depressed person does is wrong.
- Find ways to take time out and enjoy yourself. Time away doing plea-

surable activities gives you the strength to live through the recovery process. Remember you and your family are important too!

- Notify a physician immediately when there is any talk about suicide.

It is not uncommon for depressed people to resist or refuse going for treatment. They frequently deny having a problem. Feelings of fatigue, helplessness, and hopelessness immobilize and paralyze them from taking action. Some depressed people resist asking for help because they feel guilty for causing trouble. And if the physician is uncomfortable or embarrassed dealing with depression, this will reinforce the denial or make the patient resist help even more. If there is concern that the physician will not take the time to discuss depression matter-of-factly and sympathetically, family members should find another one.

Family members should reassure the depressed patient that depression is not a sign of weakness. It is an illness like heart disease, arthritis, or the flu, and it can be treated. The family should ask the physician to explain to the depressed relative in detail, even using pictures, what parts of the brain are involved. This reinforces that depression is a "real" disease and the brain is affected. The doctor can link specific symptoms to chemical changes in the brain, and later continue to reinforce this in discussions with the depressed relative.

Education, understanding, patient persistence, and reaching out to allies such as clergy, significant kin, or friends are the keys to success. Relatives should assure the depressed person that they are concerned and willing to be there. They should take everything one day at a time. Remember that living with and caring for someone with depression is impossible, so family members can only do their best. They can focus on being there until the depressed person reaches the "light at the end of the tunnel." The agony, torture, and bleakness can be erased and a joy of living and togetherness restored.

11

Rehabilitation

A Focus on Function

"You have a beautiful chapel. Will you let me visit sometime?" Shirley Everitt, a victim of Alzheimer's disease, spoke those words as she and her attendant, Henrik, took their morning walk. Before Henrik could answer, Shirley darted into the dark room, walked to the front row, and sat down. He followed and sat down next to her. Shirley turned and whispered quietly, "Follow those trees up the hill to the stone wall and push open the gate. You will see my house in front of you."

Henrik placed his hand on hers and replied, "I don't think we will find your house there. But we are in a house now . . . a house of God, the chapel. Do you want to stay here awhile?" Shirley nodded and said, "I wonder if we have gone out of our minds. I want to go home, but I can't find it. This place looks familiar. But there is no chandelier, no fountain, no furniture. I will sit here and wait for it to change. We can read this book."

Henrik opened a prayer book and gave it to her. Shirley sat holding the book for several minutes. She then stood and circled the room as if looking for something. She touched each of the colored glass windows and said, "This glass will have to be replaced. I want new ones. We have to keep this place in shape. This house is messy, and people will be here soon. We can't have people see it this way."

Henrik agreed with her. She was right. The chapel was in a state of disarray, and the windows were dirty. The two of them spent about an hour cleaning things up. They stacked the prayer books, moved tables and chairs, and even dusted the altar. When they were finished, Shirley wanted to sit down again. "The windows are still dirty," she said, "but you'll do that later, Henrik, won't you? I like my house. You may call me at my house anytime now."

As long as Shirley could walk or be pushed in a wheelchair, Henrik would take her to the chapel regularly. On some days she enjoyed simple cleaning tasks, but most of the time she seemed happy to spend time there—sometimes it was minutes, sometimes hours. Although Shirley deteriorated quickly and became increasingly confused and unable to express herself clearly, Henrik could understand her needs most of the time, keep her occupied, and make her comfortable. Up until the last few months of her life, when Shirley was confined to bed, the chapel retained its special meaning.

During her last months Henrik arranged for students from a nearby divinity school to visit Shirley regularly. Several of the young men even set up a small altar in her room. After that, other nursing-home residents would gather in her room when the priests visited to pray or talk. Even though Shirley was dying, she was continually surrounded by the people who cared for her.

Several weeks before her death a young priest was playing his guitar in her room. More than twenty residents and staff spilled out of her room into the hall listening. After an hour the priest finally placed his guitar in its case. As he bent over Shirley's bed to say good-bye, she reached for his hand and kissed it. Only the priest and Henrik could see the tears in her eyes. Even though Alzheimer's disease had rendered her frail, helpless, and unable to speak, Shirley Everitt could still communicate with others.

Shirley Everitt and others like her are evidence that dementia is not a hopeless condition for which little can be done. Patients are human beings first, last, and always. Many individuals live for years with the disease, and they are long and difficult years. The challenge over the course of the illness is to maximize an individual's ability to function at the highest possible level.

Rehabilitation is an important concept in the care of dementia victims. It is both a philosophy and a technology. As a philosophy, rehabilitation is the way we think about people's problems and make decisions about what we do or do not do to increase their ability to function. For example, if a severely impaired dementia patient develops a disease of the hip, the response may be a wheelchair and institutionalization after hospitalization rather than orthopedic surgery and physical rehabilitation, with walking as a reasonable goal. Surgical decisions should be based on information about a person's physical health and orthopedic status, as well as the likely outcome of the surgery, given all the medical issues. The *severity* of the dementia is a factor too, but the *presence* of dementia per se should not be a deterrent to appropriate treatment. When a child, young adult, or middle-aged person sustains a disability, parents and family members as well as doctors are usually aggressive in finding ways to reduce the degree of handicap. This usually includes some form of rehabilitation. Unfortunately, a diagnosis of dementia often leads to professional nihilism toward the patient—an attitude of "Why do anything? The patient has Alzheimer's disease."

Intellectual decline should not by itself be a barrier to rehabilitation. Cognitively impaired older persons deserve to be treated as people. Patients often develop a number of such disabling conditions and disorders as arthritis, osteoporosis, immobilization, fractures, incontinence, and infections. It is important to do everything possible to rehabilitate the patient and restore function when possible. What you learn here, from other medical sources, and from your doctor will not only help you maintain your relative's comfort and mobility but also lessen the need for hospitalization or premature institutionalization.

Even when patients are living in a nursing home, a great deal can be done to keep them mobile and active. Many nursing homes have active rehabilitation or restorative programs for residents, and family members should become vigorous advocates for their relative to have this care. Families have an important responsibility to work with nursing-home staff and often need to be aggressive with administrators and other staff. Being aggressive here means taking time to meet with the medical director and other professionals; asking questions about realistic expectations for a program of care, including rehabilitation; and teaching staff what you would like them to know about your relative. Tell them what he or she was like before the dementia. Help them see the human side of the patient and let them know your expectations. When there are discrepancies in what you expect and what the medical director or other professionals expect, ask them to clarify their conclusions in ways you understand.

The first week after Rachel Breton had moved her husband, Jean, into the nursing home, she made appointments with everyone on the staff, including all the administrators, the nurses and nurse's aides, the director of social services and the social workers assigned to her husband, the medical director, the dietician, and the recreational, occupational, and rehabilitation therapists. She wanted them to know a little about him as the man she had lived with, not just the frail, angry, agitated figure who had been wasted by Alzheimer's disease for the past seven years.

She began each talk the same way:

I know you are terribly busy. I will only stay a short while. Here I have a few photographs of Jean taken at different times in his life. He was born in 1893 to a poor Parisian family. His father died when he was fourteen, and in 1909 he moved his mother and his four brothers and sisters to the United States. He worked very hard to support them.

We met in 1915 and were married within the year. We had no children and have spent the past sixty years together. He was a good man and spent his life helping others.

I know his condition is getting worse, but I want him to be as comfortable and happy as possible. He can still walk, and he enjoys other people when he is not in one of his angry moods. I know some ways to control them. He needs to have regular exercise several times a day. I do not want him to be in a wheelchair all the time. What will you do to help him live out the rest of his days? I wish I could keep him at home. Since that is impossible, I will do what I can to help you here.

The staff members were receptive to Mrs. Breton's questions and desire to help with her husband. She was pleasant yet persistent. She wanted to know what could be done as well as what she could do. Needless to say, there were times when the staff felt Mrs. Breton was making unrealistic demands on them; likewise, there were situations in which she was legitimately upset with his care. She was an aggressive, loving advocate for her husband, just as she had been throughout their life.

Not all nursing homes have administrators and staff as receptive to family involvement as the last example indicates. Some staff regard families as troublesome and do not understand family desires. There are many reasons for this, but whatever the reasons, families have the right to see that a relative is receiving optimal care. Do not let staff brush you aside. The director of volunteer services, a clergyman, or a patient advocate can be valuable informants to help you understand and deal with the various personalities in a nursing home. Remember that staff may not always be the obstacles. Your own anger, sadness, or guilt may be so great as to interfere with your ability to deal with other people. Even when your message is legitimate—"I want the proper therapy for my relative"—it may not be heard if the staff react to your anger. These emotions are natural reactions in caregivers who have moved someone into an institution, but it is futile to take your anger out on those who could be your allies. If you are having difficulties with staff over care issues, ask a friend or clergyman to accompany you and observe what happens when you talk with staff. It usually takes an outside observer to help see that your emotions are alienating staff or to confirm that staff behaviors are the problem.

Families and professionals have an important responsibility to work together as a team. Goals need to be established and plans implemented to keep patients healthy, active, and comfortable. The mandate for everyone involved with patients is to have a realistic set of expectations based on assessments of the patients' physical cognitive and emotional status. It is also important to understand the personality of the patients prior to their illness. Who were they? What were their accomplishments in life? What were they like before the dementia? Knowing the persons behind the mask of dementia is often the first step to successful rehabilitation. "Rehab" embodies the principle that each individual patient has a distinctive personality with specific physical and emotional needs and the potential to restore functioning.

Identifying and Stabilizing Treatable Disabilities

Over the course of illness, when is it realistic to attempt to restore physical, mental, and social functioning? How are decisions made to help individuals overcome their limitations and disabilities to the fullest extent possible? Before answering these questions, we first will identify the different treatable problem areas: (1) chronic diseases, (2) conditions that reduce mobility, (3) psychiatric illness accompanying the dementia, (4) social rehabilitation, and (5) rehabilitation of life skills.

Very specific rehabilitation goals in each of these areas can be defined if the patient is evaluated properly. Family members should search carefully for the right team of people to help them. The list of selected readings at the back of this book provides suggestions for user-friendly references. This chapter is intended to serve as a checklist to review ways to ensure the highest level of functioning.

Rehabilitation is a necessary process throughout the course of dementia. In early dementia, we sometimes refer to *re-enablement* or *reactivation* rather than *rehabilitation* per se. These concepts also embody a philosophy and technology for maximizing functioning, emotional well-being, and health. In early dementia when cognitive impairments are mild and less disruptive to lifestyle activities, the goals of reactivation or re-enablement are to help the affected individual cope with the illness and deal with some of his or her problems.

When the patient is living at home, it takes time and effort to find health professionals who will come to the home unless a good home care agency is available. Rehabilitation specialists are available in most nursing homes. In addition to rehabilitation specialists, the people to look for include physicians who specialize in chronic conditions, psychologists, nurses, social workers, physical and occupational therapists, audiologists, speech therapists, podiatrists, and where available, dance therapists and exercise specialists.

Recognizing and Stabilizing Chronic Conditions

If your relative has one of the chronic conditions briefly described in this section, ask the doctors about treatment strategies. Families that want to learn more can consult the references in the back of this book or search for reading materials in medical libraries.

Osteoarthritis

Osteoarthritis is a condition in which the cartilage of the joints degenerates and inflammatory reactions occur in the surrounding tissue. Physical therapy combined with anti-inflammatory drugs is often an effective means of improving mobility and easing pain.

Rheumatoid Arthritis

Rheumatoid arthritis can occur suddenly, with severe inflammation in the joints, or it can progress for years and gradually incapacitate the individual. Anti-inflammatory medications are the treatment of choice. Question the doctor carefully about anti-inflammatory therapy and especially about the side effects of these medications. Enteric-coated salicylate drugs like diclofenac sodium (Voltaren) and ibuprofen (Advil, Nuprin) are often effective and have few side effects. Naproxen (Naprosyn) is another drug that can reduce inflammation. Small doses of steroids may be effective when the objective is to keep the patient comfortable during later stages of the illness.

All anti-inflammatory drugs should be given with food. The patient should be monitored very carefully, because side effects are very common in the aged and because patients with dementia living at home may take them more frequently than is safe for them.

Pain

Rheumatoid disease, osteoporosis, and many other conditions as well as bruises, fractures, and other injuries are all painful. Treating pain in people with dementia requires careful observation. Often we do not know how much pain they experience because of language and cognitive losses. Poor memory tends to prevent them from describing the onset or exacerbation of symptoms.

Drugs should be used carefully, with administration of the smallest dose possible to achieve pain relief with the fewest side effects. When the patient is in constant or extreme pain, drugs should be given on a regular schedule. This may sound simple, but in the best hospitals and nursing homes the need to care for many patients or staff shortages may disrupt these simple routines. Certain drugs, such as meperidine (Demerol), are not recommended for severe pain because they cause delirium, making the dementia even worse; they can even cause permanent damage.

Morphine and addictive medications should be avoided whenever possible. However, in the later stages of dementia, near the end of the patient's life, the use of these agents should be considered. They may provide comfort for whatever limited time remains. Since we know so little about the world of the late-stage patient, because of an inability to communicate, regular physical examinations and careful monitoring are essential.

Musculoskeletal Disorders

Osteoporosis, progressive bone loss, causes significant disability, especially when there is a history of fractures of the spine, hips, arms, and legs. The most important treatment is to keep the individual active. Walking as much as possible, simple stretching exercises, and light weight-bearing exercises are important. Bed rest leads not only to more immobility but also to more bone loss.

Consult a physician about other forms of treatment. Calcium supplements and vitamin D, when prescribed by the doctor, may be useful. Three eight-ounce glasses of milk contain the daily requirement of 1.5 grams of calcium. Orange or grapefruit juices and milk substitutes are available for patients who are allergic to the lactose in milk. The use of estrogens and sodium fluoride must be carefully justified by the treating physician.

Multiple Chronic Diseases

Older patients with dementia often have multiple disabling conditions known as comorbidities. Diabetes, heart disease, respiratory disease, and many other disorders are severe problems by themselves; when they exist together, especially in very old impaired patients, they can be profoundly disabling and painful. How do we understand impaired patients' needs when they are withdrawn, agitated, or violent, when they talk and act as if in another world? How do we measure their discomfort? Severely demented patients who are living their last years in the nursing home pose an enormous and complex challenge to staff members and family. A thorough knowledge of patients' medical conditions, the potential for pain, and astute observation of their behavior are crucial. Family members can make a considerable difference by working closely with professionals to monitor the patients.

The Eyes and Vision

Seeing well is essential to one's quality of life. The external structures of the eye should be examined. For example, older persons commonly have dry eyes, which puts the conjunctiva or lining of the eye at risk for inflammation or infection. A thorough ophthalmoscopic examination of each eye should be done, starting with the lens and working back toward the retina. Corrective adjustments in glasses can make a significant difference in the comfort of the patient as well as facilitating activity and safety. Regular testing for glaucoma is a must.

The Ears and Hearing

Loss of hearing can be due to several causes, some of which are correctable. Hearing loss may be caused by excess wax in the external ear, external otitis due to allergic reactions, or irritation due to hearing aids or foreign bodies in the ear. Wax or cerumen in the ear canal is usually the primary cause of hearing problems, and it is easily dealt with. Men, particularly those with a history of working in a noisy environment, may show high-tone hearing loss, which in and of itself can compromise communication.

The combination of hearing loss and dementia can lead to social isolation and paranoia. Hearing loss can be evaluated simply by whispering in the person's ear. In addition, several clinical tests using a tuning fork can be done to determine whether the deafness or hearing losses are due to a conduction problem in the ears or sensorineural changes. Professional audiologists also can ascertain severe hearing loss, even in the patient with dementia. If the patient wears hearing aids, a regular check of the batteries is essential—the hearing aid with a dead battery acts simply as a plug, diminishing what hearing is available.

Surgery

When is corrective orthopedic surgery helpful to the older dementia patient? This is an important and sometimes difficult question to answer. Family members should get several medical opinions when patients have peripheral vascular disease, soft-tissue contractures, or a wide variety of other anatomical impairments. Dementia patients should not be denied appropriate corrective surgery and therapies. However, the decision for surgery requires a careful evaluation of the medical risks as well as the potential benefits to the patient, given all the other issues involved.

Maximizing Movement and Mobility in Frail Dementia Patients

Although keeping patients active is relatively easy in the earlier stages of dementia, keeping them active and mobile in the later phases becomes more difficult. But physical activity during the later stages is vital. Bed and chair rest and prolonged immobility usually lead to even more immobilization. Rehabilitation efforts should focus on walking, where possible, and appropriate nonimpact exercises to limber up stiff limbs.

Therapeutic massage simulates some aspects of exercise by stimulating the lymph system as well as stretching and working muscle groups. Massage is also therapeutic touch that relaxes and comforts the confused. Massage triggers the release of chemicals in the brain that cause feelings of well-being.

There are many profound disabling consequences when even the frail older patient is kept active within the safe limits of his or her condition. Read the list below carefully and ask your doctor what is being done to ensure that your relative is being cared for in ways that protect him or her from these disabling conditions:

- Loss of muscle tone and strength
- Stiffness and contractures
- Accelerated osteoporosis
- Thrombosis in arteries or veins
- Pressure sores, known as decubiti
- Dehydration and malnutrition
- Urinary tract infections, incontinence, urinary retention
- Constipation, impaction, incontinence
- Chest infections
- Hemorrhoids
- Corns and other foot problems

Although there are limits on what can be done to mobilize the patient as the dementia progresses, families should discuss these issues with health professionals to feel confident that appropriate decisions are being made to care for their relative's comfort and well-being.

Dehydration

Many dementia patients do not have an adequate intake of liquids. At the very minimum eight glasses of water and other liquids are required daily. Dehydration causes fatigue, apathy, constipation, and abdominal discomfort because the concentrated urine irritates the bladder.

Incontinence

There are many different causes of incontinence, but in most instances it can be prevented. During aging, the bladder becomes smaller and more insensitive to stretching. The result is that the urge to empty the bladder comes when the bladder is almost full. In men, prostate problems can cause retention of urine, resulting in "overflow incontinence." In women, constipation can block the bladder so that urine leaks past the blockage point when the pressure has increased sufficiently.

The more immobilized the patient, the greater the risk of incontinence. Simply being in a bed with guard rails, restraints, and anything that causes immobility increases the risk. The absence of a commode near the bed may make it impossible for the individual to go to the bathroom.

In many cases, getting the patient to the bathroom regularly will prevent incontinence. In the more cognitively impaired patient it may be necessary to schedule trips to the bathroom every two hours and be watchful for warning signs. Although language is impaired, the patient may hold the stomach, reach for the belt or groin, and look distressed.

When incontinence cannot be controlled, diapering the patient becomes necessary. An indwelling catheter is hardly ever recommended because infections are inevitable and lead to other problems. Catheters are necessary only when the patient has significant skin sores or when there are other compelling medical reasons.

A thorough diagnostic evaluation of incontinence is important because there are so many possible causes. Make sure the doctors conduct a thorough history and physical examination, including laboratory analysis of a urine specimen, if "bladder training" does not work. If the cause of the incontinence is still unknown, a series of urodynamic tests can determine how well the urinary system is functioning. This may also include cystoscopy, a procedure for directly observing the bladder. These procedures are uncomfortable, involve the risks of repeated catheterization, and are expensive. They may or may not be practical and beneficial with the dementia patient. Caring for the patient requires continual decisions about what helps and what hurts.

Constipation and Impaction

An adequate diet of fluids and fiber is needed to prevent fecal incontinence. To maintain regular, comfortable bowel movements, the patient should eat cereals with bran, whole-grain breads, and high-fiber fruits and vegetables; drink at least six to eight glasses of fluid; and get adequate exercise. Sometimes it is necessary to use stool softeners when the patient has a history of constipation. Many physicians recommend adding fiber in the form of Metamucil, Citracel, or similar drinks or wafers to develop regularity and avoid the need for laxatives.

Untreated constipation leads to fecal impaction—hard feces that block the rectum. This not only is a serious physical problem but also tends to be associated with very agitated behavior. A rectal examination is necessary to diagnose the problem; once it is discovered, the bowels must be cleaned.

Pressure Sores

For the bedridden patient, bed sores can be a very serious problem leading to severe, even lethal infection. Pressure sores, or decubiti, can be prevented by turning the bedridden patient every two hours and using special egg-crate or other mattresses to prevent the pressure from reducing local circulation. Pressure sores start as red irritated areas with reduced blood circulation and proceed to become ulcers, which may spread deep and wide. They are extremely painful and can take months to control and heal. Wound-healing techniques and even plastic surgery may be required. Prevention is by far the best approach.

Bedridden dementia patients are vulnerable, especially if they are frail and malnourished or have diabetes. Individuals at risk should be examined daily and have a carefully monitored food program, including nutritional supplements. Ask the doctor to do blood tests to see if your relative has protein malnutrition. The key to prevention is early recognition of red skin areas and shifting the body to avoid impeding circulation in any one area for too long.

Thrombosis

Confinement to bed impedes the return of blood from the legs to the heart. In normal circumstances the blood is moved through the veins by one-way valves in the vessels and by the movement of the leg muscles. Thrombophlebitis occurs when a clot forms, most commonly in the legs or pelvic area. If a clot breaks off, is passed through the circulation, and is caught in the lungs, this condition is called *pulmonary embolism*. Nothing may happen, or the patient may die suddenly. These individuals are at high risk for chest infections. If pulmonary embolism persists, the patient may develop progressive breathing problems.

Activity and adequate intake of fluids will often prevent thrombosis. When patients with dementia have had hip surgery, low doses of a heparin anticoagulant, or a blood-thinning agent, may be helpful for certain patients. Discuss this with the doctor. Even in severely impaired patients, massage and passive range-of-motion exercises help ward off circulation problems. Automated massage devices are expensive but effective in patients at high risk for embolism.

Poor Nutrition

Malnutrition is a common problem for the frail older person with dementia because many eat improperly. Dietary consultation is a crucial aspect of rehabilitation. If poor nutrition is not detected and corrected, there will be significant consequences for health and well-being. Wounds will not heal, teeth and gums will decay, muscles will atrophy and waste away, and weakness and apathy result. This is an area in which families can educate themselves by consulting the references listed at the end of this book. Guidelines for nutritional screening, evaluation, and intervention have been published.

In early dementia, eating patterns are not usually affected. As cognitive impairment progresses, people forget to eat, eat several meals because they forget, eat inedible items, refuse to eat, or develop problematic behaviors. Some may have trouble chewing and swallowing, and the avoidance of choking is a priority.

Here are a few general guidelines. Offer small servings of fewer items at meals. Provide nutritious between-meal snacks so the patients can graze through the day and maximize intake. Reduce the noise level and minimize distractions at meals by turning off the television or stereo. Give patients supplemental nutritional products in liquid forms when they are agitated or pacing. These behaviors make feeding difficult and they use up calories. Interventions for behavioral problems are covered in Chapter 7.

In the later phases, the challenges of nutritional care are to make eating a pleasurable experience and to meet calorie, protein, carbohydrate, fat, fiber, and vitamin requirements. Nutritional supplements often taste like chalk, and people refuse them. Experiment until you find one that is more palatable. Often just serving it at a colder temperature is helpful. Changing the texture, flavor, volume, and temperature of any foods can make them more attractive and enjoyable.

The use of more invasive feeding procedures, such as tube feeding, in advanced dementia should be discussed with a geriatric specialist. The best evidence suggests that gastrostomy feeding probably does not improve survival or quality of life, but in the absence of controlled clinical trials we do not know.

Cardiovascular Disease

Diet and exercise are important factors in the reduction of vascular disease, even in the older cognitively impaired patient. High blood pressure should be controlled and the patient monitored carefully. Spend time with the doctors to understand the impact of different vascular diseases on the dementia. Ask them to explain to you what is being done if the patient has congestive heart failure, arteriosclerotic heart disease, high blood pressure, arrhythmias, diabetes, or any other cardiovascular condition.

Oral Hygiene

Regular dental care is essential, as are regular brushing, flossing, adequate hydration, and a nutritious, balanced diet. Eating is one of the great pleasures of life for many people. Rotting teeth and sore gums make eating difficult, unpleasant, and often painful.

Foot Care

A good podiatrist will help prevent many foot problems. It is difficult to walk when the feet are swollen and cracked, toenails are long and thick, and fungal infections are present. Regular care and properly fitting shoes are essential.

Infections

The patient with advanced dementia appears to be extremely vulnerable to infections. Regular, thorough physical examinations and immunization are important. Pneumonia and influenza vaccines should be given each year. Also check to see that the patient has had diphtheria and tetanus shots.

Urinary tract infections can be prevented by appropriate exercise, adequate intake of fluids, and avoidance of catheterization. The frail dementia patient is at high risk for pneumonia, a common cause of death. Mobilizing the patient as much as possible, proper hydration, and chest therapy go a long way toward helping prevent pneumonia.

Falls

Keeping patients mobile and active carries the risk that they will fall. However, in many instances the consequences of not moving around may be more serious than the degree of risk from falling. Falling is an issue that must be considered carefully. When the risk is high for certain patients, careful management with appropriate and supervised exercise patterns is important.

Many factors increase the likelihood that patients will fall. Work with the doctor and other professionals to evaluate the following problems:

- Poor vision
- Loss of peripheral vision

- Poor night vision
- Unstable walk and swaying
- Coordination problems
- Muscular stiffness
- Osteoporosis
- Postural hypotension (dizziness caused when people stand up quickly)
- Medication dosages and side effects, particularly psychoactive medications
- Alcohol use

The more problems the patient has in the above list, the higher the risk of falling. However, a few practical environmental alterations can be made to help the patient compensate for some problem areas. Canes, walkers, and wall handrails help the patient get around. Low tables and chairs and uneven floors are hazardous. Carpeting and throw rugs should be secured. Chairs should be solid, with arms but no rollers, and should bear the weight of a person sitting down or standing up.

Certain conditions seem to cause repeated falls. These include irregular heart rhythm, epilepsy, cerebrovascular disease, heart failure, and diseases causing dizziness or vertigo. A number of medications can cause dizziness, increasing the likelihood of falls. The internist, psychiatrist, and neurologist should regularly evaluate dementia patients for their risk of falling so that caregivers can plan accordingly.

Recognizing and Treating Psychiatric Disturbances

See Chapter 6, which discusses the recognition and treatment of psychiatric conditions that can coexist with the dementia, such as depression, anxiety, paranoia, and sleep disorders.

Social Rehabilitation

Family, friends, acquaintances, social and professional contacts, coworkers, and other people are an important part of anyone's life. One of the greatest challenges to those involved with the dementia patient is to keep him or her socially engaged. Working with the patient's social network is often an effective means of reinforcing feelings of independence and self-worth, which can lead to improved health and satisfaction with life. Thus, people close to the patient are important resources for reinforcing the patient's motivation to continue to live and feel wanted.

Scientists have long known that social ties have a profound impact on physical and mental health, but they do not know exactly how they do so. One theory is that social relationships give people a feeling of support that in turn leads to a sense of control, which is important for health. Another theory suggests that family and friends help individuals stay healthy and force them to seek medical help when they need it. Still other scientists propose that support from family and friends helps people adapt to stress and that this in turn prevents illness.

Occupational Therapy and Rehabilitation of Life Skills

Occupational therapy is a profession in which registered and trained occupational therapists teach patients the skills necessary for the activities of daily living. During the course of dementia, individuals gradually develop more difficulties in taking care of themselves—in dressing, bathing, eating, going to the toilet, grooming, getting around, working, and playing.

Although cognitive losses affect many things the patients try to do, occupational therapists can help the family and patients understand what the limitations imposed by the dementia are and what can be remedied. Occupational therapists help patients learn to use strategies and techniques to compensate for losses.

Special attention should be paid to ensure that patients are doing the appropriate exercises to strengthen muscles and restore maximum function. It is common to find that even patients who have access to good medical care are not doing what they should to rehabilitate themselves.

Occupational therapists examine social and physical barriers in the home or institutional environment that impede the individuals' ability to do for themselves. Family members may insist on dressing patients because it seems simpler, when patients can in fact do much of it themselves if some accommodations are made. In the later stages of dementia, if patients are confined to a wheelchair, the clothes rack in the closet may be too high for them to reach. Lower racks can be built or purchased. If motor dexterity or hand impairments make buttoning difficult, clothes with larger buttons or Velcro fasteners or pullover clothes should be substituted. Families need to understand and distinguish when memory losses are the problem and when other problems inhibit patients from helping themselves.

Many patients in long-term-care institutions have coexisting problems like Parkinson's disease or other physical diseases that further reduce their functional abilities. Many specialized devices are available, and the books listed under selected readings have addresses. Eating utensils and cups come in many different sizes, weights, and shapes. A weighted spoon may help patients who have hand tremors eat by themselves. Spoons with long handles are useful when arm range is restricted.

Patients also may need special equipment to participate in leisure-time activities. Many types of specialized equipment are available. There are devices that enable individuals with a paralyzed arm to hold playing cards or books. There are ways to help people write letters, knit, crochet, build furniture, and do many other tasks. Some of the equipment is expensive and should be purchased only after a thorough professional evaluation indicates that such devices will be helpful.

The Courage to Live

Much of what occupies daily life is very ordinary and task oriented—shutting off the alarm clock, getting out of bed, walking to the bathroom, bathing, preparing coffee and breakfast, turning on the television or radio for the morning news, and so forth. It is difficult to imagine not being able to hold a fork or spoon and to move it to your mouth, not being able to swallow juice from a straw, or not being able to move your own body out of bed and to the bathroom.

The losses of dementia tear the family fabric. However, the family can triumph over dementia if everything has been done to prevent physical deterioration, to rehabilitate patients as much as possible, and to keep them active. Even the most impaired patients can be active if the tasks are simple enough. Seeing and smelling flowers, watching people and traffic on the street, watching children play ball, walking through a park, sitting on a dock watching boats, walking along a beach collecting shells, drinking a beer or a glass of wine or cider, listening to music, or having a photograph taken. All these things and many more can be done to stimulate life.

One patient's husband brought a mocha cake and a bottle of champagne to the nursing home for his wife's eighty-fifth birthday. Lucinda Kerns had been a victim of Alzheimer's disease for thirteen years and was now confined to a wheelchair or bed for most of the day. She did not speak except for incoherent sentences or an occasional yes or no. Mrs. Kerns enjoyed the cake but refused the champagne. However, when her husband and the staff raised their glasses to toast her, she smiled and clutched her glass. After the party Mrs. Kerns quietly watched her aide clean the room, but she cried out when the aide went to throw the champagne bottle in the wastebasket. The aide heard her and placed the magnum on the window where she could see it. Even after her husband left that day, Mrs. Kerns would not let go of her glass. How many of you have saved matches from a restaurant, a wine label or bottle, or pressed flowers to remember a special occasion? Simple pleasures are often available even to the most impaired.

The Future

With continuing research, more techniques and devices will be developed to help rehabilitate and reactivate patients, helping them cope with losses and live life to its fullest. Rehabilitation research is a focus of many federal agencies and institutes. Write to the Administration on Aging, the Rehabilitation Services Administration, and the Alzheimer's Disease Education and Referral Center for information they may have about new procedures, devices, and equipment to help Alzheimer's patients (see Appendices 2 and 3).

It is hoped that someday technology ranging from computers to robots will be available to meet a portion of the needs of the aged who are cognitively impaired. Several rehabilitation research centers across the country are attempting to develop devices to improve mobility and communication and compensate for sensory and motor losses in the disabled, including patients with Alzheimer's disease and related disorders. In the future, robots may carry out home tasks by voice command and help patients communicate their needs more effectively. Currently, telephones with computer memories can help patients place phone calls; eventually, other memory computer aids may be invented.

The challenge to the family is to search for information and trained help to rehabilitate the patient. Several books listed in the back of this volume are valuable references containing helpful ideas for families that do not have easy access to health professionals. Rehabilitation is a philosophy and a set of strategies and techniques to maintain the self, even when the disease disabling the individual leads to the loss of self.

12

Choosing a Nursing Home
If the Time Comes

I will never forget the day we brought Dad to the manor. He slept later than usual, and he refused breakfast. Dad and Mom stayed in their bedroom with the door closed for more than an hour. The rest of us waited in the kitchen. It was a strange morning. This was the first time all of us kids had been together at home except for Christmas and Thanksgiving holidays, and even then one of us was often missing.

Sitting around the table together stirred childhood ghosts and memories. Mickey, Joe, Ellen, and I each felt transformed to our childhood selves. We also felt inadequate and scared of the task ahead of us that day. How could the four of us move Dad from the home in which he had raised us and take him to a strange place—a nursing home? We felt guilty and nervous.

Mickey was the oldest, and she finally stood up and walked to the window. With her back turned to all of us she spoke slowly and solemnly: "I feel very empty inside. There is no justice in a world where we must move those who gave us life into a house of death."

E ach year thousands of families make the difficult decision to place someone they love in a nursing home. It is often a heartbreaking and painful decision. Unfortunately, in most instances institutionalization in a nursing home is seen as a tragic defeat rather than as a natural transition to the best possible care for someone with dementia. Mickey's lament reflects the overwhelming grief of a daughter grappling with what were irreconcilable feelings. Her guilt and that of the rest of the family were real and unavoidable. Mr. Ascot needed a nursing home, yet they abhorred surrendering him. It was a cruel defeat for them to have to cast him out of his home. Even though they had done everything possible to meet his needs over nine years, he had deteriorated considerably and required constant nursing care. Mrs. Ascot was eighty-six and frail herself. Each of the children lived in a different state, and to transport Mr. Ascot in his present condition would be difficult and uncomfortable for him. Moving would also take Mrs. Ascot away from her friends and the home she loved dearly.

Moving the person with dementia out of the home is agonizing for many reasons. First, it is a major life change that disrupts the fabric of relationships woven over many years of being together and depending on one another. Second, moving to a nursing home is not seen as a natural part of the family life cycle. Whereas people anticipate going to school, getting jobs, leaving their parents' home, marrying, having children, and going through many other life transitions, moving to a nursing home is not something people plan for in later life. Third, institutionalization confuses the bonds of loyalty, commitment, and justice between children and parents, brothers and sisters, husbands and wives. Placing a parent in a nursing home, under the care of others, arouses guilt in children who once were the beneficiaries of parental investment for many years.

One woman cried, "How can I live with myself if I cast off my mother in her old age? She and Dad did so much over the past seventy years. Mom never abandoned us kids—how can we abandon her?" Fortunately, her own son answered her:

> You are not casting her off, Mom. That is what you may think that you are doing. I wish there was some way I could help you understand how I see what is happening. You will never stop loving Nana. None of us will. And you do not love her less by moving her to a home. You are spending every minute of the day with Nana, and it is taking its toll. You must care for yourself as much as you care for her.

Several important messages lie in this son's response to his own mother. Caring for persons with dementia does not mean that their needs must dominate the lives of every other member of the family. As discussed in earlier chapters, optimal caring is achieved with a balance between responding to the needs of the patient and those of the family members. Dementia requires a long-term emotional investment, and the well-being of many people is important. Family members are interdependent on each other. It is absurd to think that the price a wife should pay to care for a cognitively impaired husband is her own poor health, impoverishment, and perhaps death! It is also wrong to think that the bond between a child and parent can be repaid by total devotion between an adult child and parent to the exclusion of everyone else in the family.

Making the decision to institutionalize a relative is difficult for all the reasons stated. However, there is another important factor. Nursing homes have become emotionally loaded symbols. Many individuals see them as houses of death or warehouses for the sick and dying, and the thought of moving a family member into one often ranges from unacceptable to repulsive.

Nursing homes were created as a societal response to a need. Although they may be regarded as a less-than-ideal solution to the problem of caring for the increasing numbers of frail older persons with dementia, or with any other disorder that impairs individuals' ability to care for themselves, nursing homes have their place in the continuum of care. The quality of care many such facilities provide may be much better than what many families are able to offer at home.

At present, nursing-home beds are more common alternatives in most communities than are the options of day care, home care, respite care, or other long-term-care services. As we will discuss in Chapter 15, the current policies for financing health care encourage institutionalization rather than other options.

Searching for the Right Facility

When making the decision to use a nursing home, it is important to invest time searching for the right facility. After admission most patients are likely to remain there for months or years. Therefore, selecting the right place is as important as choosing one's own home. Unfortunately, most people postpone the decision and prefer not to think about it until the last possible moment. The problem then is that the family has to decide in a time of crisis, when it is under intense pressure and must act quickly. Many new and different problems emerge.

First, in most places nursing-home beds are not easily available on very short notice, and some of the better-rated facilities have waiting lists that are months long. As a result families may have to accept the first place available. There is also little time to prepare the patient for the move, since beds that become available may have to be filled "immediately," at least according to the hospital discharge planner or nursing-home admission worker. The tragedy is that decisions are thus made precipitously, and patients are often placed in inappropriate or inadequate facilities.

Second, nursing-home care is expensive. People may live in a nursing home for several years, and the average cost of staying in a long-term-care facility is $150 or more per day. Therefore, costs of $54,000 a year or higher are not rare. As we will discuss in Chapter 15, it is important to know that Medicare, which pays most hospital costs for older Americans, does not pay for nursing-home care except in rare instances. Medicare coverage of skilled nursing services in a subacute-care center or a long-term care skilled nursing center is limited to a total of 100 days during the same bout of illness. This means that if the patient with dementia broke a hip, Medicare would only pay for up to 100 days of skilled nursing care after discharge from the hospital. Some hospitals also have skilled nursing centers so the patient can be transferred to that unit in the hospital, if space is available, rather than discharged to a nursing home.

Increasingly long-term-care insurance is becoming an option, but a phase-in period is required. You would be well served to investigate the various types of long-term-care insurance shortly after the diagnosis. It may also be wise to examine long-term-care insurance options as part of an overall health insurance plan for your future, regardless of your age.

Most of the costs for nursing homes are a private matter unless (or until) the patient's and the family's resources are reduced to such a level that they are eligible for state financial aid through Medicaid. Each state has different financial requirements for Medicaid eligibility, but all states have a "means test," which requires that the patient must be "medically indigent" to qualify. The specific financial levels, how poor you have to be, vary from state to state, and many states are changing their eligibility criteria as they try to meet the rising costs of long-term care. This shifts even more of the burden onto the family. Even with these additional problems, however, the main question remains, How does one choose a suitable nursing home?

Types of Facilities

There are about 17,000 nursing homes across the country, for a total of about 1.8 million beds. About 92 percent are privately owned, with 66 percent being for-profit and 26 percent nonprofit. The remaining 8 percent are owned by federal, state, or local governments. Of the for-profit, or proprietary, nursing homes, nearly 70 percent are owned and operated as chains and managed by employees of larger corporate groups. Less than 30 percent of nonprofit and religious institutions have such an affiliation in an effort to reduce operating costs through larger-scale purchasing.

It is worth remembering that long-term-care institutions are a profit-making business for some and that the quality of their product, caring, may be tempered by the profitability factor on the one hand and the marketing strategy on the other. This does not necessarily mean that facilities run for-profit are worse or better than those in the not-for-profit sector. Large chains may have more capital to invest in the physical plant and more efficient operations and programs. On the other hand, the corporation, individual managers, and regions may be driven more by the fiscal "bottom line" than by their role as service providers. Not-for-profit facilities also have financial incentives and may minimize or reduce the quality of programs to meet fiscal constraints, the needs of the local sponsoring group, legislated budget cuts, and bureaucratic controls.

What the family must know is that although long-term-care facilities are among the most regulated enterprises in the country, there are significant differences in the quality of care found in individual homes. The old adage "Let the buyer beware!" must certainly be applied to the choice of a nursing home at the present time. Some are outstanding caring settings, while others leave much to be desired. In recent years many nursing homes have marketed themselves to have Alzheimer's disease special care units. Again, be careful. It is not uncommon for homes to talk a good line where the only thing specified about the unit is the signage.

How to Locate a Good Nursing Home

The first step is to identify a selection of facilities in a location relatively convenient to you. The physician may know of some fine nursing homes, but it is a good idea to inquire whether he or she has an ownership interest in these facilities. If so, and if you are satisfied with the doctor's care, ask him or her to personally guide you through the facility. Ministers, especially hospital chaplains, may be knowledgeable about facilities where they have visited patients or facilities related to their church. It is also helpful to contact the state health or welfare department to obtain a list of nursing homes licensed by the state, names of administrators, and the level of care offered in each facility. Hospital discharge planners and social workers are also excellent sources of information. It is then up to you to find out as much as you can about specific nursing homes using as many sources as possible:

- Other patients and their relatives
- Your rabbi, priest, or minister, who may have parishioners in these facilities
- Your family physician
- Friends
- Local chapters of the AARP (see Appendix 2)
- Your Area Agency on Aging
- Other nursing homes
- Ombudsman nursing-home organizations
- National Citizens Coalition for Nursing Home Reform (see Appendix 2)
- Local chapters of the Alzheimer's Association

Directories of nursing homes also can be obtained from state nursing-home associations, which usually have their offices in the state capital. Every state also has affiliates of the American Association of Homes and Services for the Aging, representing nonprofit or church-sponsored homes. The American Health Care Association, which has its national office in Washington, D.C., represents for-profit homes (refer to Appendix 2).

Guidelines for Determining
the Quality of Long-Term Care

Once you have identified one or more facilities, what should you look for to ensure that the institution is a suitable environment for your relative? There are at least eleven areas to examine closely in your investigation of nursing-home options. Each is discussed briefly in the remainder of this chapter.

- Philosophy and conduct of ownership and management
- Quality of professional staff and management of patient care
- Special care units
- Range of activities and programs
- Patients' rights and daily life, and resident-staff relationships
- Physical plant and housekeeping
- Food services
- Physical design and accessibility
- Community ties
- Professional affiliations
- Cost

The next important step is to call and visit the nursing homes you have selected. It is a good sign if you are welcome to visit them at any time. You may see the real flavor of the home if you time your visit to occur on weekends and during the change of shifts, between seven and eight in the morning (when breakfast is served), between eleven and one (when lunch is served), or at night. The more open the facility, usually the better the care.

Ownership and Philosophy of Management

Does the ownership have a philosophy of care? You may be assured that places are run with a specific orientation in mind, and that orientation, whether expressed or left unsaid, should be clear to you. If you cannot get this senior administrator or intake worker to articulate the facility's approach, you may have to get it indirectly, by interviewing patients, families, or other staff. If this is the case, think twice.

There are several questions to keep in mind. Is the point of view of the staff similar to yours with respect to the use of medications, the sedation of agitated patients, resident participation in the nursing-home community, the care of the dying, the role of staff, family involvement, and other aspects of care? Is there a special ward for patients with dementia? Are less deteriorated patients integrated with other patients? The more satisfied you become initially, the easier it will be for you in the months and years to come. Having once settled your relative in a nursing home, you should avoid moving him or her to another. The longer patients reside in a home, the more disturbing any move is likely to be for them. Therefore, choose carefully and deliberately.

- Interview the administrator. Ask to see the nursing-home license and the administrator's license. In most instances they are required to be posted by law. Is the administrator the owner? What is his or her educational and employment history? Does he or she have any other business interests? Is the administration on the premises? Is it easily reached during normal working hours, on weekends, and in emergencies?
- Inquire about the number of nurses—full-time and part-time. Who is the nursing director? Take down the names and check them against the nursing registry in your state.
- Make sure there is a registered nurse (RN) in charge of all three shifts of nurses.
- Since most employees are nurse's aides, find out whether the home provides in-service training for aides.
- Check to see that only licensed personnel set up and give medications.
- Discuss whether the registered nurses really spend most of the time with the patients or on administrative work.
- Ask how much nurse's aides are paid and how many there are. Do they know what to do in an emergency? What is the turnover rate?
- Inquire whether patients can bring personal furniture and belongings.
- Do the administrators seem to know patients and their families? Do they spend time on the floors, or do they seem aloof from the resident population?

- What is the ratio of personnel to patients? Nursing homes should have roughly the same number of employees as patients.
- If you are shown cards on a time clock as evidence of the number of employees, check to see how many are either blank or for part-time employees.
- Ask the administrator how many full-time and part-time therapists are available. Good homes provide speech therapy, occupational therapy, and physical therapy. Write down the names of these employees and check their credentials with the appropriate professional associations.

Professional Staff and Care Management

The quality of professional staff is not always easy to judge without your spending time getting to know them. As a minimum, however, you can judge the credentials of the medical and nursing directors and of the chief of social services. Along with the administrator, they set the professional climate of caring, and you should try to meet with them and learn as much as you can about them. The following questions may be helpful:

- Is the medical director the house doctor who treats patients who have no personal physician, or does he or she care for all the residents? Most nursing homes expect the patients' personal physician to continue to care for them in the home.
- Will your physician continue to provide care in the nursing home?
- Are medical specialists available?
- Are psychiatrists with expertise in geriatrics and the special problems of residents in long-term care available?
- Are there any specialists connected with the nursing home who are interested in patients with Alzheimer's disease and related dementias?
- Who is responsible in an emergency?
- What procedures are followed when a patient is admitted to the nursing home?
- Are all patients given a complete medical and psychiatric examination on admission?
- Does the home have the services of dentists or podiatrists, and how often do they visit the facility?

- How many incontinent or nonambulatory patients does the home have? The way these patients are treated often tells you a great deal.
- Do the patients have bedsores?
- Are they left sitting in their own waste? Turn down a few made-up beds and look for stains or worse.
- Are many patients restrained? If so, how long are they restrained? Are they sitting in adult high chairs? Is there a physician's note to justify restraints?
- Do patients look sedated, or attentive and happy? Are their feet swollen from constant sitting? Is there evidence that they get exercise? Can they walk on the grounds?
- Check the nursing stations. Narcotics should be kept in special locked areas within the locked medications room.
- Can the nurse see down the corridors from the nursing station? Do the drugs appear to be kept in a neat fashion? Beware of boxes full of drugs on the floor.
- Do over-the-counter medications have prescription labels on them? Are all drugs supplied by the same pharmacy? Patients may have the right to retain their own pharmacy. Check on this. Denial of this right often leads to inflated prices.
- What agreements does the nursing home have with nearby hospitals if the patient becomes acutely ill?
- Are there trained, caring social workers available to help patients and families?

Special Care Units

Many nursing homes have designated special care units (SCUs) for people with Alzheimer's disease and related dementias. The number of SCUs has grown significantly. The rationale for SCUs has been to provide an environment that enhances comfort, safety, individualized care, and staff who are trained to deal effectively with behavioral problems, nutritional needs, and falls. Carefully interview the administrator and director of nursing about what makes the unit special.

- Does the home have several dementia SCUs for persons at different levels of functioning?

- Are these real SCUs where the home has articulated a philosophy of dementia care and an enriched program of activities, rather than an empty title for a wing of the facility?
- Are residents separated into high- and low-functioning groups?
- Is there a program of activities throughout the day and night to appropriately keep patients active?
- Are finger foods and snacks made available?
- Are the staff trained to communicate with the residents?
- Do staff receive special training on a regular basis?
- Do the staff take time to get to know you and make you feel welcome?
- Has the environment been modified to make residents feel secure and comfortable?

At this time Texas and Iowa are the only states that have regulatory policies about SCUs. The Joint Commission on Accreditation of Healthcare Organizations (JCAHO), a private, not-for-profit organization in Chicago has developed a set of quality standards for SCUs. Since 1994 nursing homes have been able to voluntarily ask for a survey by the JCAHO. Only a small percentage of homes have asked for accreditation. You can write the JCAHO (see Appendix 2) and ask for the survey standards.

Activities and Programs

Just as activities are the backbone of family life at home, so should programs and activities be available for nursing-home residents. Games, social engagements, clubs, organizations, musical events, classes and lectures, and crafts and hobbies are only a few of the innumerable opportunities people have to enjoy the company of others. Not only should there be a wide variety of programs, but also options should be meaningful and available to even the most impaired residents.

- Is there an activities director?
- What activities are available? How are they conducted, and how are they received by patients?
- Is there evidence that activities actually take place?
- Is there an active volunteer program?

- Do patients have a wide choice of activities?
- Are the activities and programs appropriate to the cultural background and previous experiences of the residents?
- Are there religious services?
- Are there efforts to involve patients who are withdrawn and uninterested in activities?
- Are volunteers available to help patients? Talk to volunteers and find out how they feel about the home.
- Are there special programs for patients with dementia?
- Are there physical exercise programs for the severely disabled?
- Are there appropriate activities for men as well as women?
- Are there trips away from the home?
- Are there activities where residents can be of service or help to others? Older adults often can give a great deal of emotional support to children, especially to those who are mentally retarded or physically handicapped.
- Are family members encouraged to participate in activities?

Patients' Rights and Daily Life, and Resident-Staff Relationships

The challenge of long-term-care institutions is to provide a homelike environment along with a range of health services to a chronically ill population. People have many needs—for privacy, accomplishment, independence, self-identity, and self-determination. Unfortunately, institutions can be dehumanizing environments. It takes administrative leadership and a compassionate staff to create an environment that is pleasurable, comfortable, and stimulating for the people who must live there.

- Become familiar with the Patients' Bill of Rights set forth by the Department of Health, Education, and Welfare in 1974. Copies should be available in the nursing home.
- Are there combined patient-staff meetings?
- Observe staff and patients together. Do people seem particularly sad, angry, or irritable? Is morale high?
- Observe how patients are treated by staff (from housekeepers to administrators).

- Is there kindness and respect?
- How do staff respond to requests for help?
- Can patients come and go as they please?
- Can patients have pets?
- Are rooms personalized?
- Do patients have any areas for privacy?
- Can husbands and wives share a room?
- Are patients clean?
- Do patients seem happy?
- What opportunities do patients have for decision making? What choices do they have?
- Is there a residents' council or some other mechanism for involving patients in decision making? Do they meet with the staff on a regular basis?
- Are certain patients segregated?
- Do privately paying patients receive the same food as patients on Medicaid?
- Talk with a few patients. What is their feeling about their "home"?
- Do staff members involve residents in their own care?
- Do staff members encourage patients to be dependent, or do they encourage them to make certain decisions for themselves?
- Into what kinds of decisions do residents have some input?
- How stable are staff positions? Is there a high turnover rate?
- Do staff seem to enjoy their work or do you sense a lack of satisfaction and lack of involvement with patients?
- Does each resident have a primary helper or designated staff member? Even though team care is important, patients or residents relate most to people, not to a team.
- Do you feel that the staff work together for the benefit of the patient?

Physical Design

The physical and architectural design is important. The environment should meet the personal needs of the patients as well as foster efficiency of operation. Cheerful, pleasant, and supportive surroundings may be one of the most significant factors to maintain or enhance the comfort of even severely impaired patients.

- Is the lobby attractive? Do patients use it? Do staff use it?
- Are there windows in patients' rooms?
- Is lighting adequate?
- Are there areas for socializing?
- Is there a separate dining room on each floor? Is it attractive?
- Does the physical design allow enough space for the patient?
- Are patients overcrowded?
- Are beds comfortable?
- Is there a call system at every bed? Does it work?
- Are there grab bars and call buttons in bathrooms and showers?
- Are there reading lights for patients' beds?
- Are there sprinklers or fire extinguishers in patients' rooms?
- Is there carpeting? Is it fireproof?
- When was the last fire safety inspection?
- Are exits clearly marked? Are ramps available?
- Are stairways enclosed? Are doors shut?
- When was the last fire drill? How often are fire drills held?
- Is there enough space for a reasonable number of personal belongings?
- Are there opportunities for personal touches—pictures, personal desks, chairs, chests, or bureaus?
- Does the decor make you feel comfortable?
- Are there spacious activity rooms or dayrooms on each floor? Is there a library or quiet room or chapel?
- Are patients lined up in hallways? Are some patients isolated in the corridors or hallways?
- Are colors pleasant and bright?
- Are rooms and areas clearly marked (with color codes or large signs)?
- Are the grounds spacious and attractive? Can patients with walkers or wheelchairs get outdoors easily?
- Is there a closed outdoor area where patients with dementia can use the corridors?
- What is your general impression of the place?

Housekeeping

The cleanliness and attractiveness of the institution have a powerful effect on morale.

- Is the home well kept?
- Is the home comfortable?
- Are these stains on floors or odors (from urine, feces)?
- What is the condition of patients' rooms?
- Is there fresh water at the bedside?
- Is the heating and cooling system effective? Do patients seem comfortable? Ideally, thermostats should be set between 71 and 76 degrees year-round.
- Are burned-out bulbs replaced?
- Does the facility cut back on heat or turn off air conditioners at night?
- Check more than one floor. Sicker patients are usually kept on separate floors.
- Is a barber or hairdresser available?

Food Services

Quality of life depends on many physical and environmental factors—the comfort of home, financial security, family and friends, good times, and good food and drink. Invest time inspecting the kitchen area, visit during mealtime hours, and even ask to taste the food. Eating is not only a biological necessity but also one of life's greatest pleasures.

- Is the kitchen clean? Examine floors, stoves, refrigerator, and storage areas.
- Is there evidence of roaches, ants, or rodents?
- Does the home have an extermination service?
- Evaluate the cleanliness of the people preparing the food. Do they care for patients as well as prepare food?
- Have all kitchen employees had tests for infectious diseases? How is garbage disposed?
- Check the alley where garbage is stored.
- Does the home have a dietician or nutritionist? Who makes up the menu?

- Does the food served conform to what is written on the menu? Are therapeutic diets followed? Examine special-diet meals to make sure.
- Is food appetizing? Is it adequate in quantity and quality?
- Are warm things served warm and cold things cold?
- How many meals are served each day? At what time? Do they allow time for patients to eat? Can people have seconds? Are snacks served between meals and at bedtime?
- Can patients have beer or wine or other alcoholic beverages?
- Who feeds those who cannot feed themselves?
- Are meals made available to appeal to the minority composition of the home?

Community Ties

Nursing homes should be part of the local community. The home should not only be physically attractive but also be seen by the local residents as a desirable place.

- Do children in the community volunteer in the home?
- Do schools have visitation relationships with the home?
- Do local organizations such as the Lions Club or the Rotary hold their meetings in the auditorium?
- Do the police stop by to visit?
- Do older people who live in the neighborhood volunteer?
- Do staff members live in the neighborhood?

Professional Affiliations

Many nursing homes have affiliations with university medical centers or community hospitals. In larger cities they may be fortunate to have ties with large medical centers with specialists in geriatrics and Alzheimer's disease.

- Does the institution have student volunteers from local high schools or schools of podiatry, nursing, and physician's assistants?

- Is there a formal affiliation with a medical center, medical school, nursing school, or other professional training programs?
- Have residents in the nursing home participated in research projects conducted by scientists or professors from neighboring colleges or universities?

Cost of Nursing-Home Care

Ask specific questions about the cost of care provided in the different institutions you visit, and compare prices. Establish in detail exactly what you would be paying for each month, such as room, board, laundry, therapies, drugs, and miscellaneous expenses.

- Contact the local Social Security office to learn about Medicare. Medicare pays only for certain skilled nursing care following hospitalization. Eligibility is strict and limited.
- Contact the local welfare office to learn about Medicaid. Medicaid is a state and federal program, and eligibility varies from state to state. Medicaid is given to people with limited assets.

Preparing the Patient and Making the Move

Our advice is that you get to know everything you can about the place and its people. Put forth the same amount of effort and care as you would if you were buying a new home. If you do not feel good about a facility, try another place. Remember, it is best to plan ahead for placement. Waiting for a final crisis to occur before you decide may deny you the options you need. Excellent facilities exist, but most are full and take time to process new applications. Many will have SCUs or they may have their own rules about patients with dementia. Some will accept only those who are bedridden, and some will want to admit only those patients who are more intact so that they have the capacity to adapt to the facility.

Remember, too, that once the patient is admitted, you will still be a part of the caring process, and you should feel comfortable in your new role. Adaptation to the institution is not always easy. It may even be easier for the patient than for a guilty relative. Sometimes the guilt surrounding institutionalization is so strong that the decision is made much later than it should have been, and after the patient is admitted, the guilt keeps the spouse, children, and other members of the family away because they cannot face the new setting.

When possible, talk with the patient about moving into a nursing home, or allow him or her to sit in on family meetings when the topic is being discussed. Even when it is clear that the person is severely impaired, in most cases the simple act of being present in relevant discussions often reinforces the patient's importance as a person in the family.

Include all family members in the decision-making process. Even when you are the patient's husband or wife, you do not have to do it all.

Carol Reiss had cared for her mother, Patricia Brown, for almost eight years. Mrs. Brown's husband died two years after she had been diagnosed as having dementia, but she had continued to live in the duplex next to her daughter. Carol was able to cook and clean for her mother and to check on her several times during the day, and every day Mrs. Brown joined her daughter's family for supper and the rest of the evening.

This arrangement had worked well until Mrs. Brown began to wander around the neighborhood, sometimes half-dressed. Although their friends were watchful and often gently guided Mrs. Brown back to her home, it was becoming evident that the family would have to consider moving her into a nursing home. Carol could not spend time with her mother during the day. She was divorced and had to work to support herself and her two teenage children.

For the next six months Carol hired a young woman to stay with her mother during the days. Mrs. Brown continued to deteriorate physically as well as mentally, and the young home attendant found the job too demanding. After hiring and firing several more attendants, Carol reached the conclusion that a nursing home would be a safer place for her mother.

Many phone calls later, Carol selected six places to visit. After making the rounds, she eliminated four of them. One was particularly appealing, and she decided that her mother should see it with her.

One evening after cooking a special supper for her mother, Carol and her two daughters, Bess and Evi, sat with her and spoke directly and quietly about looking at a few nursing homes together. Mrs. Brown listened carefully for several minutes before breaking in: "Carol . . . I'm not sure it's a good idea. But . . . we can visit if you like."

The four of them—Mrs. Brown, Carol, Bess, and Evi—visited two nursing homes in their town. The two girls felt it was important to do this with their grandmother to emphasize how important she was to them. For each trip Carol and the girls took the full day off. After visiting the home, they all had lunch and later went shopping.

Mrs. Brown moved easily into the nursing home they chose together. It was Carol, Bess, and Evi who felt upset, sad, and guilty. They had arranged to move Mrs. Brown on a Monday morning so that the family could have a special weekend together. Carol invited close family members and special friends together for a party. Mrs. Brown enjoyed the festivities and the company of those she loved.

The gathering was so successful that Carol almost changed her mind. During the day her mother seemed happy even though she was unable to say very much. However, the nights reinforced the importance of following through on their decision. Mrs. Brown would not sleep, wandered about the house, and even went outdoors several times to roam the streets. Carol had not slept well for months and could no longer bear the worry. She was exhausted and reached the painful decision that she could no longer keep her mother safe and comfortable at home.

The day of the move went smoothly. Their family and friends had agreed to accompany Carol and her mother. Carol later admitted she needed the moral support more than her mother did. All pitched in to help in many different ways. They agreed on an intensive visiting pattern for the first month so that she would have a few visitors each day rather than everyone at the same time. Carol and other members of the family worked out plans in many areas, including decorating Mrs. Brown's room, taking her out for lunch, going on short shopping trips, or taking walks.

As Carol and the girls saw how well Mrs. Brown adapted to her new home, they were able to relax and feel less guilty. Indeed, with time they were able to reflect on recent events and feel very good about everything they had done. Mrs. Brown lived another three years and remained an integral part of her family until she died.

Not every patient and family make the transition so easily. The key factors appear to be the amount of emotional preparation for the move, the insight of family members that they have done everything possible within their financial and human limits, and the availability of acceptable nursing homes.

It is important to recognize when home care ceases to be a viable alternative. Financial matters often make home care impossible. Especially in cases involving other dependents, the main caregiver may find some form of employment necessary for the family's financial security. Bringing home a paycheck while carrying the burden of responsibility for a relative with Alzheimer's disease can be too taxing for the most dedicated and energetic caregivers.

Sometimes it is simply not possible to keep a relative at home if the apartment is too small or if other family members have serious health problems. Even families that care for their relatives at home for years often eventually decide that, for one reason or another, the care the patient is receiving at home is simply not as good as nursing-home care would be.

In many cases caregivers are unable to handle the patient because of his or her violent or unmanageable behavior. Caregivers may be powerless to handle a patient who is bigger than they are, especially if the patient becomes violent or insists on wandering out of the house and into dangerous situations. One woman with severe arthritis who used a walker even tolerated being knocked down by her husband until she was so incapacitated that she could not stand up after an assault. Often a whole family will become tyrannized by a violent patient. Nursing homes are advisable in situations like this, not only for the protection of the family but also for that of the patient.

As this chapter has indicated, there are positive steps you can take when the issue of nursing-home placement becomes a real one. Institutionalization is not a defeat. It is often an important and realistic choice in caring. You need to reframe the issue from thinking that you have failed at home care to an attitude of finding a new home.

The following interview is with Helen Lucho, the sixty-five-year-old wife of a dementia patient. She describes how she coped with her husband and the events surrounding his institutionalization. Her feelings, actions, and thoughts capture much of what we have reviewed in this chapter. Her doctor tries to help her to continue to cope adaptively with the future.

DR.: I understand your husband just moved into a nursing home.

MRS. L.: Yes, in January of this year.

DR.: How was that for you? And how are you doing now?

MRS. L.: Well, it's upset me, to say the least. He was in the hospital three months before he went into a nursing home, and in that time I think I learned to adjust a little.

DR.: So you had some time to get used to the idea.

MRS. L.: Yes, I did, but to have him picked up and taken into the home is the hardest thing I ever did in my life.

DR.: It sounds painful. What led up to this decision?

MRS. L.: He changed a great deal over the past two years. He became very abusive and he struck out at me. And for two years I put up with it. He knew something was happening, and he begged me not to leave him. I told him I would not leave him—that I would take care of him as long as I could. But I couldn't stand much more abuse. Just before he went into the nursing home, I had a feeling I needed help soon or I would fall apart. I went to the medical center, and they helped me.

In January I had him committed. I hate to use the word "committed." Louis was not in his right mind, and this is pretty hard to cope with. At least, I find it so. I know that it isn't his fault, and I love the man.

DR.: It's very painful for you to see all this happening. You were saying it's hard to cope. What kinds of adjustments have you had to make?

MRS. L.: I have had to make all the financial decisions in the last two years. Before the illness he wouldn't let me do anything, and that was fine with me. Gradually I took over, but I had to do it carefully. I would give him a choice: "Do you want me to write a check for the rent, or do you want to do it?" He would accept that. But I have had to do everything because there is no one else. We don't have a family.

DR.: So you have really been alone trying to struggle with these changes.

MRS. L.: Yes, making decisions that I hope are right. I really had no choice when it came down to it. I do have some good friends, and they kept telling me that I should do something before he hurts me badly.

DR.: What was it like for you to hear that?

MRS. L.: I knew they were right, but I was going to put up with it as long as I could.

DR.: Do you find yourself feeling guilty about anything?

MRS. L.: At first I did, but then I remembered how he would take a swing at me when we were alone. I put up with it as long as I could, and I don't feel guilty about that part. I feel I did the best I could.

DR.: It sounds like you have done exactly what you needed to do. Is there anything that bothers you now?

MRS. L.: Yes, financial problems. It's expensive to keep Louis in a nursing home, and I am worried about what might happen to me. I'm not getting any younger. Do I spend all my money on him? And what do I do then? This could go on for years, even after I run out of money. This is a community state. Do I spend his half and save mine for me? I may end up in a nursing home.

DR.: Did you have any financial advisers?

MRS. L.: Well, I did go to the bank to see about a living trust. If something happened to me, he would be taken care of.

DR.: Have most of the nursing-home issues been resolved?

MRS. L.: Well, he's settled down now. He's not happy, but he's there. And I feel as good as I can about it. I feel it's the best for him.

13

Death and Dying

Patients and families are so distressed by the emotional impact of the dementia that only after some time do they grapple with their anxieties and fears about the future and the eventual death of the patient. Patients are often the first to bring the subject up, and it is critical not to overreact when they talk about deterioration and death. The fears and sadness of individual family members often impair communication and lead everyone to withhold information from one another, including the patient. Often we hear, "If I let him find out too much about Alzheimer's disease, I know he will kill himself." Or "If we don't talk about the future, maybe John won't get worse." Unfortunately, families often shrink from discussions with loved ones about the loss of self and death, precisely at the time when they need to talk as an affirmation of caring and life.

Mrs. Proto, the wife of a professor with Alzheimer's disease, shared a story with us:

One afternoon I came home to find my husband in our library looking at an art book. He was staring at Chagall's *Gate to the Cemetery*. When I walked into the room, he showed me the picture and asked when he would join that community of graves. He seemed peaceful, but I was scared. I turned and walked out of the room upset and angry that he should suffer such a cruel disease. I cried in our bedroom for several minutes; I didn't want him to see me cry.

As I sat alone, I realized it was wrong of me to walk away and not respond to his question. I returned to the library ready to talk about death. He was still sitting in the chair with the book closed. I asked him to show me the Chagall picture. He didn't remember the right picture or the book. He asked to go outside for a walk. I felt confused and angry and, even more, sad that I had lost my chance to communicate with him.

This experience and many others were painful for Mrs. Proto. She spoke at great length about how difficult it was to talk with her husband when he wanted to share important issues with her. She was frustrated with his periods of confusion and her inability to communicate with him. At times she also thought that he might kill himself if she allowed him to talk about death.

Mrs. Proto's predicament is one that many families experience. It is natural to avoid the issue of death, but however difficult it may be, beginning to face a relative's death is necessary to be able to live and work effectively with him or her. Eventually Mrs. Proto decided it was important to convey her feelings about death to her husband. She did not share her husband's view that death is a continuation of life. She felt that death, specifically his death, was a cruel waste. She showed him a picture of another work of art that she thought reflected death destroying their lives together even before he actually died. Mrs. Proto described her condition as a restless peace. Although she was taking good care of her husband, her feelings were confused by two deaths—the psychological and the physical.

Family members need to cope with the emotional dilemmas presented by the physical death as well as "the death of the self," which precedes the physical death by many years. The challenge of dealing with the ongoing psychological death of the patient causes profound grief, and the grieving is very much like the reaction to terminal illness, but with one major difference. In the early and middle stages of the illness the patient appears healthy, looks very much like he or she used to look, and is likely to be alive for many years in this peculiar state of physical health and psychological decline. It is not easy to deal with the invisible changes that alter behavior and mood and destroy the husband, wife, patient, or friend whom one has known for years.

The deterioration and death of a relative from Alzheimer's disease are experienced differently by every family member. Many factors contribute to the way each individual feels and acts as the dementia progresses. One's personality, the history of relationships between family members, the ability of people to communicate with the patient, the speed with which the illness progresses, the quickness with which physical death occurs, and the competence of health care professionals with end-of-life care play a role.

Many individuals die feeling emotionally and spiritually alone. Even the most loving relatives may inadvertently isolate patients psychologically and socially. Patients are people who need to feel needed and be treated like responsible human beings even though they have dementia. The unspoken attitudes and behavior of family, friends, and professionals influence how persons with dementia feel and respond.

One patient, Mr. Boyle, told us he felt like someone wandering by himself along the lonely seashore. He knew that everyone in his family loved him, but they did not know what the disease meant to him. He wanted his wife to understand how much it hurt not to be able to care for her and meet her needs: "What makes me so upset is not that I have no one to share my burden. It is that I have only my own burden to bear. I am only a shadow of my former self." Mr. Boyle was finally able to communicate his sadness to his wife and family before the dementia robbed him of his ability to express his feelings. After he died, his wife told us she felt that his death had been a good one and that she had been able to help him retain his sense of identity to the end. She considered herself blessed to have had a husband whose love for her had transcended the dementia.

Grieving is healthy, but with it there emerges a subtle, inevitable change in the way you relate to the person for whom you grieve. This change involves getting closer to him or her initially and then developing a degree of emotional distance. Although you may actually do more for the patient as he or she becomes more dependent, you also begin to regard the patient as the shell of someone you once knew. Emotional separation is helpful in dealing with your psychological pain, but it also affects your ability to relate to the patient and to keep him or her as involved as possible. This distancing needs to be monitored closely and may even require that you talk with a professional or a friend. The greatest danger of distancing is that the patient becomes an object—a flesh-

and-blood container holding memories and deep emotional ties to the past but with no real relationship or humanity in the present.

The following three principles are important guides to interactions with an individual with dementia to maintain both a closeness and separation at the same time.

1. *Do not let emotional ties die too far ahead of the patient.* The changes in dementia are gradual. It is important to engage the individual in meaningful activities consistent with his or her cognitive and behavioral limitations. Nurture the hope to enjoy today and tomorrow for as long as it is possible.

2. *Treat your relative like a human being, with a role and an identity, not like a patient.* Share information as you see him or her ready to receive it. Do not minimize the seriousness of the disease but do not overreact. Goethe wrote, "If we take people as they are, we make them worse. If we treat them as if they are what they ought to be, we might help them to become what they are capable of becoming."

3. *Accept that your relative is a "patient" when you are helping him or her in ways that are burdensome, but call your relative by name and treat him or her as your beloved when you are engaging in pleasurable activities.* Coping effectively with caring is made easier if you can compartmentalize your thoughts, feelings, and activities as a function of your relative's ability to participate in the relationship. When you are enjoying his or her companionship, including the pleasures of eating, walking, and talking, learn to celebrate the human connection. When your relative is acting in ways that are not the person you once knew, give yourself permission to pull back. Do what needs to be done to respond to your relative's needs, but think of him or her as a patient with serious disabilities, not simply as your husband, father, mother, or wife who is totally unimpaired.

Facing the Terminal Stages of Alzheimer's Disease

Living with dementia in the later stages is a struggle for everyone. Family members describe it as a more intense experience of what they have been engaged in since the diagnosis. It is not unusual during this period to wish the patient a speedy and painless death rather than see the on-going destruction of his or her human dignity.

These death wishes stem from deep feelings for the patient as well as from notions of how we ourselves would like to end our lives, yet they provoke upset and guilt. Death would clearly be a release not only for many patients but for the family as well. This then becomes the basis for an internal crisis—"How could I want my husband to die! I am so self-ish." Death then not only comes as a release but often generates pain—provoking guilt and self-doubt.

The emotional turmoil around the patient's decline and death of the mind is extraordinary. The physical presence of the person evokes thoughts and feelings that bind the patient to family members at the same time that the individual's deterioration makes them wish him or her dead. The following excerpt from a letter expresses the impulses we often hear from families.

> Dear Sis,
>
> We visited Mom and Dad again today. Just as old leaves strug-gle hard to hold onto the vine in a strong winter wind, Dad is fighting not to die. He doesn't want to give up, but I wish he wouldn't fight anymore. I wish he would die. Sometimes I find myself thinking about ways to end his suffering.
>
> Last week when Mom was in the hospital, we stayed with Dad. It's rough! He has really gone downhill this winter. He paces up and down all day long, and he doesn't sleep at night. It's impos-sible to get any rest with him wandering around the house. I don't know how Mom puts up with this.
>
> We did find a solution to at least get him to sleep for a few hours. A hot bath at night relaxed him, and once we got him out of the tub and into bed he would sleep three or four hours. One night I found myself staring at the open-face heater by the tub. I know what I felt—lonely and scared. I wanted to place the heater on the edge of the tub. If he accidentally pulled the heater into the water, then it would be God's will . . . and I almost did it!

The wish that the patient be dead is an upsetting feeling, yet it is nat-ural to have these feelings. It is also natural for thoughts of death to be accompanied by guilt. Alzheimer's disease is painful for everyone, and one of the reactions to pain and hurt is to run away from or attempt to eliminate the cause of the pain. As a result, some family members shy away or limit time spent with the patient. As the letter expressed, some people even have the impulse to act in a way that increases the risk of an "accidental" death.

Living with a loved one exacts an enormous emotional toll because you not only see and feel the suffering of the patient, but you also have your own reactions to contend with. The desire for the death of a patient evolves naturally from the desire to end the irreversible suffering of another human being and sometimes—when you identify with the patient—from the fear of being a burden to others. These feelings may emerge soon after the diagnosis or only after a period of time has passed and the losses and changes seem to have become unbearable.

It is important to acknowledge death wishes and to talk about them with family, friends, or clergymen. The process of sharing these difficult thoughts show that you are not sick or cruel and that others also feel helpless and hopeless in the face of Alzheimer's disease. Many people would rather see death come soon rather than watch progressive suffering. If these unspoken wishes are not expressed to someone, they can build up and become more and more troublesome and difficult to manage. These desires coupled with depression and caregiver strain also can lead the caregiver to kill the patient or commit a homicide–suicide, killing the patient and then immediately committing suicide.

Death with Dignity

Strong feelings about dying and death often bring family members into direct conflict with one another. In the turmoil, seemingly forgotten emotions tend to be confused with present feelings toward the patient. Adult children may be upset and torn between the desire to care for a dying parent and anger toward the person who was never a "good" mother or father to them. Old rivalries between children or between children and parents re-emerge, and death becomes the new battleground for old playroom feuds. Raw emotions, which everyone had considered long buried, emerge again.

The family may be torn apart, just at a time when collaboration is essential. Sensitive decisions need to be made about the patient's comfort and well-being, family needs, legacies, sharing of possessions, funeral arrangements, and even the use of the patient's brain for research. At best these can tax even the strongest family. Part of dying "a good death" is that family members (and the patient, as long as it is cognitively possible) derive comfort knowing that they acted together to do what they could, and as much as possible, helped one another. When families work as a unit and do what is right for all concerned, they can face the end with a greater sense of peace. If conflicts are disruptive, families may need a counselor to help them understand their responses or even to serve as a referee to mediate the problem.

Family members have described the long process of watching a loved one die with Alzheimer's disease as a "living funeral." Inevitably, physical death becomes a reality. The moment of death is often painful despite the years of mourning and adjustment during the course of the dementia. With Alzheimer's disease and related dementias the grieving process begins well before death, and while this anticipatory grieving helps family members deal with their emotions, it does not entirely alleviate the pain of the final loss. The period following death is difficult, even though families often feel a sense of relief that the agony is over, both for them and for the patient.

Jacobo Ruiz had suffered with Alzheimer's disease for eight years in Argentina before his daughter, Lucia, moved him to Florida. There he lived with Lucia and her family for another two years until nursing-home placement was necessary because of his heavy care needs. After one month in the nursing home, Mr. Ruiz died of a stroke. Lucia was consumed with guilt and asked a series of questions generated by members of the family: Did her father really have Alzheimer's disease if he died of a stroke? Was there any possibility that his health care was neglected at the home and that had contributed to the stroke? Did the move stress him? Did they kill him by taking him out of their home?

Everyone in the family was relieved that the stroke was a blessing, and he did not linger, but at the same time they were anxious to know everything about Alzheimer's disease and strokes. The lingering quest was to determine whether anyone could have prevented the stroke, while at the same time they were relieved he was no longer suffering. The long litany of questions left Lucia exhausted but content that she and her family had done everything possible.

Wherever death occurs—in a nursing home, an assisted living residence, a hospital, or at home—only a few families are prepared for it. If plans have not been made, a number of decisions must be made about funeral arrangements, including costs, the acceptability or desirability of an autopsy, notification of family and friends, and rearrangement of other commitments.

Modern medical technology also has created new ethical dilemmas for family members and medical caregivers, even before death occurs, regarding decisions to use nutrition, life-support systems, and emergency cardiac resuscitation measures. In the later stages patients may undergo many medical crises or prolonged suffering before they die, and most die in a hospital rather than at home.

The following interview with Geraldine Mason was conducted five months after the death of her husband, James. He had suffered from what was probably a vascular dementia for seven years. The ethical challenges are evident in her description of the last seven days. For many patients the painful dilemmas may last months or years.

A week before my husband died—he died on a Wednesday—we took him to the doctor because he had great difficulty breathing. The doctor said it was bronchitis and prescribed some medicine, but it didn't help, In fact, he became worse.

By Saturday he was so much worse that I took him to the emergency room. The doctors checked him and confirmed that it was bronchitis. They told me he would be fine, but I wanted him to stay in the hospital. I was certain he had pneumonia. The doctors told me he didn't belong in a hospital. What bothers me is the way they treated him or, more accurately, did not treat him. They really did not treat him as a human being. Nor did they examine him carefully, as I found out later. They did not understand that he did not comprehend their questions.

The next day, Sunday, was horrible. He woke up about ten in the morning. He slept sitting in a cuddle sack in the couch because he was unable to breathe lying down. When we tried to help him off the couch, we noticed his lips and fingernails turning blue. We took him to the bedroom and sat him on the bed. I kneeled in front of him and look into his eyes. And then he collapsed on top of me.

I screamed to my daughter, "Call 911!" All I remember thinking was, "Don't die, James. Please don't die!" My daughter gave him artificial respiration until the medic team arrived. One medic ordered me to leave the room until they got him talking. I tried to tell them he would not talk as they pushed me out of the bedroom. I screamed, "He has Alzheimer's disease and does not communicate well with people, especially strangers."

Two medics worked on him for about ten minutes. Finally, one gentleman came out and asked me several questions, something about medications and James's swollen feet. They told me that my husband was in heart failure and had been for several weeks. I was shocked! We had seen two doctors in the last two weeks, and nobody said anything about heart failure!

The medics continued to work on him for a long time. Finally, one of them told us James was breathing again, but that he had suffered a massive coronary. If they were not able to get the heart started within another twenty minutes, they would call the coroner. I remember pleading with them not to stop.

They finally got the heart started again and took him to the hospital. The doctor there talked to us. He was very kind. He wanted to know whether we wanted resuscitation and life support if James had another coronary. The entire family was there, including several friends, and we all agreed, "No." The doctor explained that the coronary was so severe that there was probably very little brain functioning. James was living off machines. We instructed the doctor not to resuscitate him if he had another coronary.

That was Sunday.

On Monday, things were the same. The doctor told us that he wanted someone to check James's brain waves. He also asked us if we wanted the life-support system removed if there were no brain waves. I told Dr. P. that if my husband was not going to be conscious on his own, I did not want the life-maintenance system. James had always thought it was terrible for instruments to be put on people who would probably never recover.

And that was the case. I guess there were no brain waves. He passed away Wednesday afternoon.

Mrs. Mason's story touches on many issues. She and her family were able to make decisions together that reflected the wishes of her husband. The physician at the hospital shared information and alternatives with them, and he asked the family what they wanted him to do.

These are not easy decisions for families, nor indeed are they for professionals. Death with dignity is a humane goal, particularly when life as we know it seems absent from a human body that is functioning marginally and then only because it is attached to machines by wires and tubes. Caring for the dying person, however, confronts the clinician with ethical dilemmas. Physicians are committed to keeping people alive and to the principle "Do no harm." It may be a painful internal struggle to adhere to this mandate and also respond to the need to relieve human suffering. Active euthanasia is an unacceptable medical practice and can be considered murder. Passive euthanasia, the withholding of medical procedures or drugs in order to allow someone to die "when there is irrefutable evidence that biological death is imminent," is sanctioned by many, including church leaders, but these decisions are for the patient and the responsible family to make, not the physician alone.

Families have the right to expect guidance and information from the doctor. Families should seek out someone who will be available to them on an ongoing basis to provide information, advice, and opinions about the alternatives available. If it is at all possible, these discussions should take place during the early phases of the disease, when the patient may be able to discuss the issues and let relatives know his or her desires. It is helpful if the patient's thoughts and feelings can be made as explicit as possible to provide guidelines for family action when the time comes. If the patient cannot or will not participate, it may be desirable for the family to be guided by a trained professional who can listen and answer questions about the rights of patients, family rights, the position of physicians, and the rulings of the legal system.

As of December 1991, all hospitals, nursing homes, hospice programs, and home health care agencies that receive Medicare and Medicaid funding are required by the Patient Self-Determination Act to give all adult patients information on advance directives—how health care should be provided if and when they are incapacitated.

There are several sources to guide discussions about advance directives and end-of-life care. One of the most useful tools is a document called "Five Wishes" distributed by the Florida Commission on Aging with Dignity with support from the Robert Wood Johnson Foundation. The Florida Commission on Aging with Dignity was founded in 1996 in Tallahassee, Florida, to be an advocate for the human dignity of men and women across the country, including the preservation of their dignity when sick or disabled. You can write them (see Appendix 2) and ask for a copy of "Five Wishes." The document is easy to understand and use as you consider how you want to be treated when you cannot speak for yourself. The wishes include (1) the kind of medical treatment you want or do not want, (2) how comfortable you want to be, (3) how you want people to treat you, (4) what you want your loved ones to know, and (5) what person you want to make health care decisions for you when you cannot make them.

Working with Your Physician

Unfortunately, it is likely that the patient's physician has not been adequately trained in end-of-life care in general, let alone in the care of people dying with Alzheimer's disease. Most medical schools, residencies, and fellowships offer almost no training in palliative care for those who are dying. (*Palliative care* refers to the prevention and relief of suffering by carefully managing symptoms and providing responsive support to the emotional, spiritual, and practical needs of patients and families.) The few courses available are usually elective ones, and national medical licensing examinations ask only a few questions in this area. Textbooks in the medical specialties devote about 2 percent of their total pages to end-of-life care. About one-third of textbooks in psychiatry, family medicine, and geriatrics have helpful information, but spiritual, ethical, and family issues as well as the responsibility of physicians after death are not well covered. Although changes are underway to raise the standard for competence in care at the end of life, family members need to be prepared to take several steps to guard against a needlessly bad death for their relatives.

People do not die *from* Alzheimer's disease; they die *with* it. Pneumonia, infections, and strokes or heart attacks are the usual causes of death. You should seek out a geriatric specialist in medicine, psychiatry, psychology, social work, or nursing and ask him or her questions about the symptoms patients may show, given the medical conditions they may have in addition to dementia.

You have the right to expect professionals to care, honor, and respect your dying relative and your family by their words and actions. Physical comfort is a priority, and it includes attention to hygiene, nutrition, skin care, and other physical circumstances. When patients are dying, they are usually unable to move around or care for themselves, and quality daily care (i.e., good nursing care) is essential. The major physical symptoms that require care when people with dementia are dying include anorexia (diminished appetite), cachexia (wasting of muscle mass), dysphagia (difficulty swallowing), bowel incontinence, pressure sores, and mouth problems.

After Death

After the patient's death, the spouse and surviving family members are likely to change their pattern of living. During this period of adaptation, the family will continue to feel great sadness. Usually, a spouse has the most difficult time finding a new personal identity. Grieving takes time, and months may pass before the worst part is over.

The following interview with Ollie Richards, a middle-aged woman, took place approximately eighteen months after her husband's death. She and Albert had been married for twenty-six years and had raised three children. Albert had been diagnosed as having Alzheimer's disease at the age of fifty-two, after perhaps a year of disturbing symptoms. He deteriorated quickly and died at the age of fifty-four. Mrs. Richards kept him at home, involving Albert as much as possible with friends and family up until the end.

DR.: How did Albert die?

MRS. R.: He just died one night after I had put him to bed. He had been incontinent, and I had him in Pampers. I changed him after dinner, put him to bed and kissed him. He was perspiring like crazy, but

I thought he was upset about wetting his pants since we had company. Three other couples had come for dinner that night. They were in the living room when he died. I was preparing tea. I went into Albert's room to see if he was still awake and wanted a cup. When I walked into the room, he wasn't with us anymore.

DR.: What did you do?

MRS. R.: The first thing I did was to tell one of my friends, "Albert is sleeping. I can't wake him."

DR.: Did you know he was dead then?

MRS. R.: In the back of my mind, I think I did. But his eyes were open. And his hands were behind his head, just as he normally slept. One of my friends went into the bedroom, came back, and said he could not wake him either. At that point we called the doctor.

DR.: And how long did it take before the doctor arrived?

MRS. R.: We never reached the doctor. We called Medic 1. I had had a nurse out to the house the Friday before he died. I had called the hospital to say that Albert had not bathed himself for three weeks, nor would he let me do anything for him. They sent a visiting nurse out on Friday, and the nurse said to me, "Should your husband aspirate"—and I really didn't know the meaning of the word *aspirate*—"call Medic 1 immediately, but tell them he is a terminal patient and not to use any life-support equipment on him."

DR.: What did you do when they arrived?

MRS. R.: I told them I didn't want any support equipment used on him. They said they would just test to see if there was a heartbeat, which, of course, there wasn't. From there the police came and next the funeral home. I also called a good friend who came right over and helped me.

DR.: Did you know what to do when Albert died?

MRS. R.: Yes, I did. I had made a list of priorities.

DR.: When did you make that list?

MRS. R.: The day before he died. After I spoke with the visiting nurse, she really brought it home to me that maybe he might die. Up to that time Albert had been very weak. He couldn't get out of the chair or the bed. I had to lift him, drag him to the bedroom, and put him on the bed. He was very weak. But I never—I don't think I ever thought he was going to die.

DR.: How did you feel when you knew he was dead?

MRS. R.: Relieved . . . for him. Because I think he went through hell. Albert had not been able to hold a conversation with me for a year. It was like talking to a child. He would just smile or grin. Every time I tried to make conversation, he would just say "seven four seven" or "spitfire." Airplanes were his life. So I never ever got to talk to Albert in that last year.

DR.: During your marriage did you and he ever discuss what to do when one of you died?

MRS. R.: Yes, we wanted to be cremated. We never wasted our money. We did not feel the lavish funeral was the thing for us. We would spend our money whilst we were living.

DR.: After Albert was diagnosed, did you and he ever have a conversation about his death, at least when it was possible to communicate?

MRS. R.: Albert never accepted the fact he had Alzheimer's disease. He never admitted he was going to die. Albert was a perfectionist. Immediately after the diagnosis, he wanted to go back to England. He thought if he could go back to his earlier days, he would recover and be fine. He never admitted he was sick. The only time we discussed it, I just said, "Well, we'll work it out together." He simply answered, "Okay." We never really talked about it.

DR.: Were your children home when their father died?

MRS. R.: No.

DR.: Were your children helpful to you during the year that you were caring for him?

MRS. R.: My youngest one was very supportive. She was eighteen at the time. She would take Albert out for a drive or walk with him, at least when he was able to walk. I also have a middle daughter—Albert transferred all his aggressions to her, so she moved out about a month before he died. She is the one who is having the hardest time accepting Albert's death. I think she feels bad about leaving when she should have stayed home.

DR.: Have you talked about that since?

MRS. R.: To her? Yes. But she doesn't open up very much either. We are very reserved people. We don't discuss our feelings too much.

DR.: So, after Albert died, you didn't spend too much time discussing your feelings?

MRS. R.: No, no. Because we have all accepted what is. There is nothing we can do to change it, so we must go on from there.

DR.: How did you go on from there? What plans did you make?

MRS. R.: I didn't make any plans. I tended to drift.

DR.: Were your children and friends around you during the period after Albert died?

MRS. R.: Yes. But I am a self-sufficient person. I don't need—I don't
want a lot of sympathy. I never have wanted sympathy, I needed support, yes, and most of my friends were very helpful. But the children
were very good. In fact, too good. They smothered me. They were
always telling me what I should do and what I should not do. I told
them to get on with their lives because that's the way we wanted it.
And they have adjusted quite well.

DR.: What changes do you face now?

MRS. R.: I am engaged to be married now. Albert and I were friends
with another couple for more than twenty-five years. Peter's wife
died of cancer two months before Albert died. We just gravitated together and have gone on from there. . . . And it's marvelous.

DR.: When did you get engaged?

MRS. R.: New Year's Day. About a year after Albert's death. I'm excited now. Things go on, you know. It's no good looking back. You
can't look back.

DR.: How do the children feel about your getting married again?

MRS. R.: They're pleased because it makes me happy. I'm more relaxed
with them, and I don't worry about their lives as much. But they're
not too keen on the choice. But then I don't think they ever would
be.

DR.: But you're happy about the choice!

MRS. R.: I'm happy, yes. And I think it's a relief for them to know
they don't have to worry about me. They can go on with their own
lives.

DR.: And you?

MRS. R.: Oh, I'm very pleased. I'm relieved for Albert that he died
when he did. I'm relieved for me that I didn't have to go through
the experience of finding a nursing home. Everything just worked
out beautifully; it really did. He went quickly. By and large, as I look
back—the longer he's gone . . . you know, you look back and think.

I have a few guilt feelings wishing that I hadn't been so . . . I was mean to him sometimes. He needed constant attention and care. He would follow me around, and I would hide in the closet just to get away from him for five minutes. And I wished I hadn't done that, but you can't change what was. I did the best I could. I pray he is at peace now.

Grief differs from person to person, family to family, and culture to culture. Complex emotions are expressed—sadness, anger, hurt, guilt—and many thoughts and feelings erupt. It is painful to lose someone we love. It is also difficult to lose a spouse or parent when the relationship has been strained, ambivalent, or disrupted. The nature of the relationship we cultivate with someone throughout life greatly influences the way we react when he or she dies.

Getting on with the future does not mean that the sense of loss disappears. Death does not erase the impact of one human life on another. The memories of a relationship will always exist at some level. Indeed, it is not unusual for older men or women to refer to their spouse in daily conversation long after death has occurred. The memories of a long life together are powerful and sustaining. For some individuals they seem to provide the emotional foundation on which to build a new life in the future. However, not all memories are happy ones. Human relationships are very complicated, and over a long lifetime many events occur. Therefore, for some persons death is a release, and the grieving is abbreviated.

Warning Signs for Abnormal Grief Reactions

There is no right way to grieve. The way we grieve is as personal as the way we show our love, anger, or friendship. After the patient has died, many different factors may complicate the process of mourning. The way death occurs may have a major impact on the ability to grieve, especially if there is an accidental death, suicide, homicide, or homicide-suicide. Personality traits of surviving family members that have nothing to do with the patient, such as a depressive personality, may place certain individuals at high risk of long-term complications. The nature of the relationship between the deceased and various family members also has a profound influence on how people deal with their grief. Finally, the inability to express feelings related to the loss is a powerful predictor of problems sometime in the future. Although the individual at highest risk is a surviving spouse, anyone who has been close to the patient can be affected.

Knowing the complicating factors that prolong the grieving process may help family members be watchful for possible problems. "Pathological mourning" occurs when individuals do not deal with their initial reaction to death and do not resolve their feelings of loss. If several months after a death life still seems empty and devoid of meaning, and if there is no enjoyment of any activity, professional attention should be sought.

Pathological mourning is not a disease, but it can lead to a serious depression. Families should not feel embarrassed to seek help if the grief is immobilizing and persists over months. Caring for someone with dementia and dealing with the complex feelings it arouses before and after death takes a toll and is highly stressful. Needing help is not a sign of personal weakness or a character flaw. We are all vulnerable at different times in our lives, and it is an act of courage and character to seek help!

A number of complicating factors that can prolong mourning are related to the psychological makeup of the survivors rather than to their relationship with the deceased patient. Individuals may be particularly susceptible to problems if they have had a lifelong tendency toward depression or difficulties in expressing anger or sadness. Widows or widowers may develop abnormal reactions if they are very old, frail, and chronically ill, have limited finances, or are socially isolated, since all of these factors serve to limit options in changing to a new lifestyle. Individuals who are extremely dependent on others to meet their emotional and social needs may also be at risk. The spouse who has tried to manage a husband's or wife's total care and who experiences excessive guilt about failure to do enough may need help if he or she cannot come to terms with such feelings.

Sometimes the family may create a situation in which a mother or father or child cannot grieve, by consciously or unconsciously blocking the process, by actively insisting that he or she "stop crying" or "carrying on." Abnormal reactions can result when people are not able to express feelings related to loss. There are many potential complications. Some individuals simply may not be able to tolerate the intense pain surrounding the death of a loved one, or they may hide their feelings completely in an effort to protect others around them. It is not uncommon for family members and friends to act in ways that do not acknowledge a person's need to grieve. Families may do great harm if they insist that a spouse or other individual manage grief in very specific ways.

Legal and Financial Steps after Death

Several legal and financial matters involving many immediate as well as longer-range issues must be taken care of soon after death. Hopefully, many of these issues will have been decided long before your relative has died. The information in this section is intended to guide family members who have the responsibility to tend to the deceased's legal affairs. A useful workbook for families is *Last Wishes* by Lucinda and Michael Knox, listed in the references.

- Examine your insurance policies to check whether the deceased was designated as a beneficiary; if so, have the policies changed.
- Individuals often have several insurance policies. When bills arrive in the mail, check whether there is any life insurance coverage of the sort tied to credit cards. It is also a good idea to examine canceled checks for the past two or three years for evidence of payments on insurance premiums.
- Cancel all the deceased's credit cards; when appropriate, arrange for them to be reissued in the spouse's name.
- If the deceased is named in your will, contact your attorney and revise the will.
- It is important to ask a friend, clergyman, or attorney to help you make a checklist of other financial issues important for you to resolve.

Someone in the family should investigate what death benefits the survivors may be eligible to receive in addition to life insurance. The Social Security Administration and the Department of Veterans Affairs offer benefits, as do many business, church, and fraternal organizations. Survivors are often eligible for Social Security benefits if the deceased was employed. These benefits can be paid to the surviving spouse if they were living together at the time of death, or if the spouse is not alive, the money may be given to the person responsible for the burial expenses. When there is no surviving spouse, survivors may request the Social Security Administration to send the maximum allowable payment to the funeral director for burial costs.

The Department of Veterans Affairs provides a qualified veteran with $300 toward funeral expenses. Like the one with the Social Security Administration, the claim must be filed within two years. You must complete special forms, which are available from the department or the mortuary you choose. In addition, veterans' benefits include a plot in the nearest veterans' cemetery or a sum of $150 toward burial in a private cemetery, a memorial marker for the grave, and an American flag for the casket. If the surviving spouse does not remarry, he or she may be buried in an adjoining plot in the veterans cemetery.

Table 3 identifies what documents are needed when filing for Social Security, veterans', and other benefits.

Preparing for the Funeral

Today, most funerals are handled by a licensed funeral service that coordinates all the details. However, there is a range of alternatives, including cooperational groups to reduce the cost of burial, direct removal and burial without a formal ceremony, and cremation. The family decides how ashes are to be disposed. They can be placed in a receptacle for the family to keep, or they can be buried or placed in a solumbarium. The family also may have the ashes scattered where doing so is not prohibited by law. Although cremation is usually handled by the funeral home, various groups will dispose of the body without any ceremonies if the family wishes.

Donation of the body is another alternative. Most medical research institutions require that the donor or survivors make arrangements with the funeral director to embalm the body and transport it to the medical facility. Most medical schools allow time for the family to have a funeral service before the body is delivered to the hospital. Families also may request that the remains of the body be returned to them after they have been studied by the medical school. The body, or the ashes of the body after cremation, may be returned to the family.

Table 3. What You May Need When Filing for Death Benefits

	Social Security Benefits	Veterans' Benefits	Life Insurance	Credit Life Insurance	Casualty Insurance	Railroad Benefits	Teachers' Benefits	Civil Service Benefits	Other Benefits
1. Death certificate or equivalent	x	x	x	x	x	x	x	x	x
2. Birth certificate or proof of age of									
a. Deceased	x	x				x		x	
b. Survivor	x	x				x			
c. Children	x	x				x		x	
3. Social Security number of									
a. Deceased	x	x				x	x	x	
b. Survivor	x	x				x			
c. Children	x								
d. Dependent parents	x								
4. W2 forms and income tax returns for past three years	x	x				x			
5. Marriage license	x	x				x		x	
6. Divorce documents	x	x				x		x	
7. Military records (ID number, hon. discharge, etc.)	x	x				x		x	
8. Adoption documents	x	x				x		x	
9. Evidence of unborn child	x	x				x	x	x	
10. Receipted, itemized funeral bill	x	x							

Note: This information was generously provided by Riverside Memorial Chapels, Bronx, New York.

A memorial service without the body is another alternative. Although the memorial service may meet the needs of the family, the decision should be made carefully. It should not be done because it is convenient or because the family is trying to avoid the reality of what has happened. Funeral practices may evoke strong emotions among family members. This is natural. It is important to have someone who has been with the family throughout the disease—friend, clergyman, or health professional—help plan the funeral.

Many families are prearranging and prefinancing funerals. This is another area in which professional advice is necessary. The payment of money in advance for services is controlled by law in most states. If there are no such laws in your state, the prepaid funeral agreement should provide for a trust fund, and the person making the payment should control the account. The fund should include all money paid in advance for coffins, services, and burial vaults. The prearranged agreement should allow the person controlling the trust to receive interest earned, which may be applied to the principal to offset inflation. Finally, the person should have the right to terminate the contract at any time and receive all funds, including any interest earned.

The Postmortem Examination

The decision to have an autopsy performed can be a difficult and emotional issue. Mrs. Jarvis describes how she changed her mind about a postmortem examination:

> As you know, Jim died this afternoon at two-ten. Shortly after his death the nurses let me sit alone with him to say good-bye. He was so peaceful. He even seemed to smile.
>
> So many memories are with me tonight. We were married fifty-two years this January. Two weeks ago, when I started to leave him at the nursing home, he asked, "Are we married?" When I said yes, he asked, "Why are you leaving me here?" The look in his eyes broke my heart. I told him, "You are very sick and you must be here. I cannot take care of you by myself." He told me, "I am not sick. But go home now. You look very tired." I left

and had a good cry. I will never forget that day as long as I live. Jim was a good husband and a good father. He worked hard all his life. Why should he end up like this? What caused his brain to change?

The doctors wanted to do an autopsy. I was against it for a long time. Jim had lost his ability to do everything for himself. His mind was gone, but his body was pure. And he had suffered too much. I didn't want anybody to touch him.

When I saw Jim dead, I suddenly changed my mind. I thought back to our last sailing trip before Jim became sick. We had decided to take the boat out together. The last night out we lay in the cabin listening to the sounds of the sea. I remember we made love or at least tried. He held me tightly and cried.

"I hate this growing old. Something is very wrong, but I don't know what it is. I wish I knew. Whatever happens I want to give you and the kids everything you deserve. You are what I live and die for. As long as I can move or breathe, I will care for you." After Jim spoke those words, he looked at me in the strangest way for several minutes. He smiled the same smile when we said good-bye for the last time.

I signed the papers for the doctors to study his brain. Jim cared so much for everybody that I know he would want to help others with this awful disease. Jim's self is not lost. He has left a part of himself in all of us.

Donating the brain after death for scientific study is a gift to humanity. Without brain tissue from dementia patients, scientists will be unable to carry out investigations to study the causes of Alzheimer's disease and related disorders. Without this research there can be little hope of curing the disease.

Autopsy Planning

The patient's doctor may ask you to sign papers for an autopsy, or if you are a member of a family support group, you may be approached to enroll patients for autopsies. Scientists may visit your family group to describe the research that can be done when brain tissue is available. Some scientists are doing research to determine what parts of the brain, including receptor sites that bind with certain drugs, are still functioning. To do this work the scientists need to get access to the brain as soon as possible after the person dies. If you are asked to participate in this type of fast autopsy, talk with the investigators involved to clarify what kind of care your relative will get when they are in the phases of dying. In these circumstances it is usual for the patient and the family to be in a caring, attentive hospice setting.

Publications from the national Alzheimer's Association as well as newsletters from the local chapters may contain information about the dementia brain banks that have been established in several medical centers throughout the country. The Alzheimer's Association has helped support the establishment of brain banks on the East Coast, on the West Coast, and in the Midwest to ensure the availability and careful storage of tissue. At the moment, you can find out where university-affiliated brain banks are by calling the Alzheimer's Association or going to the Web site.

When and how do you involve patients themselves in a discussion about their willingness to consent to an autopsy? There is no right way or right time. Since family members usually know the patient far better than the doctors do, a family meeting is often a useful means of airing the thoughts and feelings of everyone involved. Discussions about autopsies are not a kiss of death. They are a healthy way to think about and plan for the future, however distant that future is. Writing a will, buying life insurance, selecting a burial plot or deciding on cremation, and making decisions on several other legal and financial matters require meetings and discussions to anticipate personal and family needs.

Many patients will sign the autopsy consent form as easily as they sign the organ donation statement on the back of a driver's license. Some may refuse to discuss the possibility, while others may have family members who will not allow them to talk about it. A significant number of patients ask many questions, and you may want to involve a doctor, clergyman, or close friend. Still others want to think carefully about the decision, and several meetings and phone conversations may be necessary before patients consent. In certain situations religious law and convictions complicate or prohibit decisions about an autopsy.

If discussions and decisions do not occur early in the disease, at a time when the patient has the ability to participate in the decision making, family members will be in the position of signing consent forms during the late or terminal phases of the dementia. If this occurs, candid discussions with the doctors and a confidant are helpful. Sometimes it is best to have several family members participate in this process; at other times it is appropriate for one family member to assume leadership.

Regardless of the situation, the following points of information will help you know what is involved in autopsy planning as well as what to do at the time of death.

The Cost-Absorbed Autopsy

When you meet with the doctor to sign the consent form, ask him or her to tell you where the autopsy will be performed. Find out whether that hospital or research center will absorb all the costs of the autopsy. Autopsies are expensive, and you should not have to pay for them. Several steps need to be taken ahead of time, so that the necessary information can be given to doctors and nurses in the hospital or nursing home. Patients are often eligible for a cost-absorbed autopsy at a hospital where they have been inpatients.

Most hospitals and medical centers specializing in Alzheimer's research have an arrangement whereby they absorb the total cost of the autopsy. If you live a great distance from an Alzheimer's research center, ask the doctor to help you both to get a cost-absorbed autopsy and to ensure that the brain is sent to the center you designate. A few suggestions may be useful:

Tell the patient's physician the names of the doctors conducting the research in Alzheimer's disease who have asked you and your relative to arrange for an autopsy.

Ask the doctor to place an autopsy request in the patient's medical records that says that your relative has the doctor's consent for autopsy.

Ask the doctor to write two specific items in the written request form: first, that the patient needs a neurological and diagnostic autopsy; second, that your relative has Alzheimer's disease or a related disorder and that you have made or would like to make arrangements with researchers in the field of dementia to have the brain used for special research.

If you or the patient's physician have any questions, call the scientists at the center where your relative's brain will be studied and ask them to speak with your doctor and explain the situation.

Some hospitals have a rule stating that a person must die in the hospital in order to qualify for an autopsy. This means that if your relative dies at home or in a nursing home, he or she will not be eligible for a cost-absorbed postmortem examination. If this is the case, consult your doctor or the national Alzheimer's Association (see Appendix 1) to help you find centers that will cooperate with you.

Mortuaries

Contrary to what some people fear, autopsies do not prohibit an open-casket funeral or any other type of funeral you may wish your relative to have. However, it is important to choose a mortuary that will take your plans into consideration ahead of time so that you will not have to deal with these decisions when death occurs. Some mortuaries will transport the deceased from the place of death to an area where the body can be kept cool until the hospital is ready to do the autopsy. When choosing mortuaries, ask whether they provide such a service and inquire about the cost. If the cost is high or if they do not have the service, ask your doctor for advice. Many researchers also have grants and will pay the costs for you.

Assisted Living Residences and Nursing Homes

If your relative is in an assisted living facility or a nursing home, the medical, administrative, and nursing staffs will probably know what to do at the time of death to ensure that your plans are carried out, but they should know your wishes. The doctor must write a statement in the patient's nursing-home chart to state that an autopsy has been requested and agreed to. Ask your doctor to talk with the nurses so that they will know what to do when death occurs. You may wish to speak personally with the head nurse as well. Indicate which mortuary is to provide transportation from the nursing home to the hospital or other facility until the autopsy can be performed. If this makes you uncomfortable, ask the doctor or administrator to help see to these arrangements.

What to Do at the Time of Death

At the time of death several phone calls need to be made. Survivors will need to contact the minister, priest, or rabbi tending the patient, the doctor or site of the autopsy, and close relatives and friends. Keep a list of important phone numbers in an accessible place. Furthermore, your relative's doctor—that is, the attending physician who made the official medical request for the autopsy—must be called if he or she did not sign the death certificate. If that doctor is unavailable, someone else at the hospital should be covering for him or her. Tell whoever is on call that your relative has died and that you would like to initiate the autopsy arrangements. Finally, the mortuary needs to be called and asked to transport the deceased from the place of death to an appropriate holding area until the autopsying hospital is ready to admit the body.

The hospital may need to complete certain arrangements before it can admit the patient's body for an autopsy. In most situations, the hospital staff will need to call you—you do not have to call them—about the autopsy permit. We suggest, however, that you call them anyway, or have someone else do so, to let them know that the deceased is in the mortuary waiting to be admitted for autopsy. Also inform them of your location and give them your phone number so that they know where to reach you when they are ready to call about the permit. This helps to ensure that the body is handled as carefully and quickly as possible.

When you call or are called to sign the permit, a second member of the hospital staff also will be on the line to witness your permission. At the same time, indicate that there are two very important points you wish to be made clear on the autopsy permit. First, it is to be a neurological and diagnostic autopsy, not a donation of the brain to general science. Second, the patient has Alzheimer's disease, and you wish the brain to be given or sent to scientists conducting research on Alzheimer's disease or dementia.

There are two circumstances in which the autopsy permit may be signed in advance of the patient's death and held until the time comes.

First, if the next of kin has legal guardianship, he or she can sign the autopsy permit in advance of death. The usual legal order of next of kin is spouse, children, parents, siblings, legal guardians, and then closest next of kin. Second, in some states the patient, if legally competent, can sign his or her own permit.

Suicide and Accidental Deaths

Patients speak frequently of the desire to be dead rather than go on living with the disease in a nursing home or be bedridden and incontinent. In this situation, family members and close friends often become fearful that the patient may actually commit suicide. The available evidence suggests that although half or more of patients have suicidal thoughts, 8 to 10 percent of individuals with dementia are at risk for suicide, 5 percent attempt it, but very few take their lives. However, depressive symptoms and depressive illness occur in 30 to 60 percent of patients, so the wish to die should not be ignored. The patient should be evaluated for depression and monitored daily.

We do not know why suicide is so rare in patients with Alzheimer's disease and related disorders. Indeed, we still do not know enough about the social and psychological nature of suicide in the general population, where it ranks among the first ten causes of death in the United States. We can speculate, however, that the very nature of Alzheimer's disease limits the individual's ability to think about and carry out such an action in much the same way that it impairs other abilities. In those situations where individuals have successfully taken their lives, the available evidence suggests that although there was evidence they wanted to die, they did not understand how to kill themselves easily and painlessly. Firearms are the method of choice for most suicides of older persons, but people with dementia use a range of methods—insecticides, rat poison, jumping out of a window, or setting the house on fire—methods that are not pleasant or quick ways to die.

John De Turk's death relays the sad circumstances of his suicide. Mr. De Turk was found in a small body of water in his trailer park, with a gallon jug filled with water tied to his neck. He was eighty-nine years old and had been diagnosed with Alzheimer's disease for five years. Mr.

De Turk also had a history of multiple medical problems, including heart disease, chronic obstructive pulmonary disease, and diabetes. The autopsy confirmed his dementia and multiple areas of atherosclerosis. Mr. De Turk's wife reported that he had been depressed about his cognitive decline, that he had spoken about suicide, and that he threatened he would jump in the lake. The night before his death Mr. De Turk complained about the difficulty of maintaining his diabetic diet, and he defiantly ate three desserts.

Mr. De Turk showed several indications that he wanted to die. His suicide plan involved several specific steps. He found a gallon jug in his house, filled it with water, and tied it around his neck with rope from the garage. He then proceeded to the lake in the trailer park and walked into the water. There were no indications from the postmortem toxicology reports that he used medications or alcohol.

In a number of instances, patients with dementia have accidentally overdosed on their drugs and died. It is important to keep medications out of reach of patients when they can no longer manage their own drugs.

Accidental death or apparent suicide are painful experiences when they occur because so many questions are left unanswered. Professional help, if available, can help surviving family members to deal with their responses to events beyond their control. These are times when it is necessary not only to grieve but also to come to grips with the uncertainty of what happened. Did my wife, my husband, my friend, really take his or her own life? In the absence of a genuine suicide note, this question often lingers.

The following letter was written by an eighty-year-old widow whose husband had dementia for more than ten years. Thomas Bucht was not actually diagnosed until shortly before his death. Although his wife, Erma, suspected that something was wrong, she was afraid to ask for help. For years Mr. Bucht went from doctor to doctor, receiving numerous medications, but the dementia went unrecognized. It was only after an episode during which Mr. Bucht beat her until she was unconscious that Mrs. Bucht telephoned her family for help.

As the events unfolded, it became clear that Mr. Bucht had deteriorated greatly over the last eight months. Mrs. Bucht had struggled to deal with the problem alone and as a result became physically and emotionally exhausted. Mr. Bucht was diagnosed as having Alzheimer's disease after a two-week hospitalization and was then discharged home with twenty-four-hour nursing coverage. Mrs. Bucht sustained a heart attack shortly after her husband was hospitalized, and she too went to the hospital. Mrs. Bucht never saw her husband again. A week after Mr. Bucht left the hospital, he overdosed in a confusional state and died.

Mrs. Bucht recovered with time, and during the year following her husband's death she wrote a series of letters to her doctor. The excerpt below is from one of those letters.

Dear Doctor,

I am writing to let you know that I am doing as well as can be expected. My family is wonderful, and I have some good friends. But I miss Tom, and I think of him all the time. It has been nine months. I still think I might have saved him if I had been home.

You have always told me not to blame myself for his death. I understand that Tom did not really commit suicide, but if I had been home he might not have been so unhappy. I might have kept him from taking all those pills. I know the night nurse was watching him all the time. She heard him get up from bed and go into the bathroom that night. She heard tap water running and opened the door to find Tom swallowing the sleeping pills. He smiled at her and said, "Darling, please get my breakfast. I am late for the office." Poor Tom, he was so sick for many years. His brain was not working right.

I have talked to my pillow all these years. I did not know what else to do. Tom would take so many pills. He took two for his heart, something for his sugar, pills for his nerves, and then there were the sleeping pills. Tom was forever taking pills. There were pills hidden all over the house. He went to so many doctors, and they all gave him pills, pills, pills.

Tom slept all day except for meals. And then at night—the nights were terrible. Tom would kiss me and say it was the last kiss he would ever give me because he was going to die. Each night I would sit in the chair fully dressed, wrapped in a blanket waiting for something to happen. If Tom began to have problems, I wanted to be ready to take him to the hospital. For more than a year I waited for something to happen.

Tom could be so cruel sometimes. I knew he did not know what he was doing. He would scream at me, and once, no, more than that, he struck me. I finally had to call my son one weekend because Tom hit me so hard I could not get up again. I must have passed out and been unconscious for more than an hour. When I came to, I could not walk. My leg was broken, and my hand was throbbing. And more than that, my heart was breaking.

Now that Tom is dead, I think back and try to remember the good times. But it is hard to erase those last years. The doctors should not have given him all those pills. They were not helping him. He was a sick man, and they should have figured out what was wrong.

I also made things worse—I think I hurt us both. I hid everything from the family and worse still, I tried to hide it from myself. I made myself sick, and if I had asked for help earlier, maybe he would still be alive today.

Sometimes I wonder if he killed himself because he thought I had left him. He was my husband for fifty-nine years. But the last ten years he was not himself, and in the last year, he deteriorated rapidly. Forgive me for sounding this way. You and the other doctors have all told me that Tom did not know what he was doing when he took all those pills. His brain disease affected the mind. He was confused. He was not himself. I hope you are right! My heart is breaking. I miss him so.

With time and the support of family and friends, Mrs. Bucht recovered her strength and a sense of the future. She was fortunate to have an attentive family and many friends, mostly widows, who surrounded her during the months following his death. Her family was surprised at the number of other widows who always seemed to be present. This network helped Mrs. Bucht deal with her deep feelings of loss. And as time went by, she moved on with her life. Mrs. Bucht was able to deal with her grief in a healthy way, and she also reached a point when she could review her past objectively.

Although she accepted the results of the psychological autopsy, which indicated that her husband did not commit suicide, she still admitted that there was some doubt in her mind but she could live with it. She had to live with it. A *psychological autopsy* is the process whereby a group of professionals examine all the available evidence to determine the likelihood that a suspicious death was either a suicide, an accident, or homicide. When the results of this deliberation are communicated to the family, they can provide the information needed to deal with the uncertainty about the cause of death. Since many professionals may take part in the psychological autopsy, the outcome reflects a reasonably authoritative opinion. After the decision is made, the family may need to hear the professional analysis several times. The accidental death or apparent suicide disrupts the normal grief process because the notion of suicide may be almost incomprehensible, as Mrs. Bucht expressed in her letter.

If you are concerned about your relative's suicidal behavior or death wishes, seek professional help. Research suggests the following danger signals:

1. Someone with a history of suicide attempt prior to the diagnosis of dementia may be at heightened risk. People who have attempted suicide in the past are more likely to attempt it again.
2. Individuals with a diagnosis of depression have a higher rate of suicide. The presence of a significant depression should not be ignored. Depression is a treatable disease, even in patients with dementia.
3. Individuals who talk about how they are going to kill themselves in some detail are at risk to attempt suicide.
4. A history of suicide or mental hospitalization of other family members is more common in people who have committed suicide, particularly if depression, in any of its forms, was diagnosed.
5. The availability of a handgun or rifle, particularly if easily accessible and kept loaded, increases the risk of suicide.

Homicide

Although 15 to 20 percent of patients living at home or in nursing homes commit violent, aggressive behaviors, including kicking, hitting, biting, or threats with a weapon, homicide is an extremely rare event. The available evidence indicates that when a dementia patient kills someone, the perpetrator is almost always a man and the victims are usually older than the perpetrator. Most homicides occur in nursing homes where a male resident with paranoia kills another male resident, usually by beating him. Firearms are the method of choice when the homicide occurs in the home, and the victims are usually wives.

The perpetrator usually survives and often faces criminal charges or placement in a locked facility. At age eighty-nine Jack Edmund was accused of beating his eighty-eight-year-old wife Lucy to death. Both had Alzheimer's disease, and they lived together in a retirement community with a health aide coming to the home every day. Their son Andy checked in on them daily, and their grandchildren as well as great-grandchildren also visited frequently.

The night of the homicide, the couple had arranged to sleep in the living room instead of the bedroom so they could watch the closing ceremonies of the Olympic games. The aide prepared dinner, did the dishes, and helped open up the sofa bed. When she left at eight o'clock that night, both Jack and Lucy were lying in the sofa bed watching television.

The next morning the same aide found Lucy on the floor next to the sofa bed in a pool of blood, and Mr. Edmund was sitting in the bedroom. The aide called the police and Andy. Mr. Edmund had apparently beaten his wife to death, but he probably did not know it was the woman he had loved for over sixty years. The likely scenario was that Mr. Edmund had awakened in the middle of the night in unfamiliar surroundings, and probably also awakened his wife who may have startled him. Mr. Edmund may have believed she was an intruder and beat her with the phone as well as his cane.

The police obtained an arrest warrant for second-degree murder because there was no evidence the murder was premeditated. Mr. Edmund was moved to a medical facility, and the arrest warrant was never served. He had no memory of killing his wife and no awareness that she was dead. According to the son, family, and friends there were never any arguments or violence between the two, and indeed the last few days before the murder had been happy ones spent with family and friends.

Prosecutors agreed not to charge Mr. Edmund with murder if Andy found a secure nursing-home facility that agreed to keep his father. Andy had to make a difficult decision. He could let his father be charged and risk the state placing him in a mental institution to await trial, or he could go along with the state and lose control of where his father was placed.

Andy chose to let his father stay in the locked facility. Mr. Edmund died six months later, unaware of what he had done and without hurting anyone else in the nursing home before he died.

Homicide-Suicide

Homicide-suicide involves a perpetrator, usually a man, who kills one or more victims, usually a wife or intimate, and then commits suicide, usually immediately. About 25 percent of victims of homicide-suicide involving older persons are wives with Alzheimer's disease being cared for by depressed husbands. Homicide-suicide by older men caring for wives with dementia is not an act of love or altruism. It is an act of desperation and depression.

The motivations for a homicide-suicide when the victim has dementia are complex. The couple usually has been married a long time, and the husband has been the caregiver for a long time. Depression, increasing social isolation, and stressful life events such as the deaths of friends and family are among the many risk factors.

Homicide-suicide is not a spontaneous event. The husband usually has thought about the act for several months or years. The three most common circumstances that precipitate the perpetrator taking action are a change in his health, hospitalization of the wife, or a pending move to a long-term-care institution.

How You Can Help Prevent a Homicide-Suicide

There are common clues to a possible homicide-suicide that must be taken seriously. Knowing and acting on these clues can help you save lives.

- The older couple has been married a long time, and the husband has a dominant personality.
- The husband is a caregiver, and the wife has Alzheimer's disease or a related disorder.
- One or both have multiple medical problems, and the health status of one or both is changing.

- A move to a nursing home or assisted living facility is pending or under discussion.
- The older couple is becoming more socially isolated, withdrawing from family, friends, and social activities.
- The older couple has been arguing or there is talk of divorce or a history of estrangement.

Since the husband is usually the perpetrator, look for the following signs:

- Changes in eating or sleeping
- Crying for no apparent reason
- Inability to feel good about the future
- Talk of feeling helpless or hopeless
- Talk that the future is bleak
- Talk that there is nothing they can do
- Threats to harm the wife
- Loss of interest in activities that used to give pleasure
- Anxiety and agitation
- Giving things away that are important to them
- Making plans to give someone a key to the home

If you are an adult child or relative and you see these changes in a parent, talk to them. Do not ignore these signs.

What to Do If You See Signs

- Do not be afraid to ask if the older person has thought about suicide or homicide-suicide. You will not be giving him or her new ideas.
- Do not act surprised or shocked. This will make the person withdraw from you. Continue talking and ask how you can help.
- Offer hope that alternatives are available. Do not offer glib reassurance. It may make the person believe that you do not understand.
- Get involved. Become available. Show interest and support. If you cannot do this, find someone who can, such as a neighbor or a minister, priest, or rabbi.

- Ask whether there are guns in the house. Ask the person what plans he or she has to die. The more detailed the plan, the higher the risk.
- Remove guns and other methods to kill.
- Do not be sworn to secrecy. Get help from persons or agencies that specialize in crisis intervention.
- Call a crisis hotline in your area or seek the help of a geriatric specialist. Do not try to do things by yourself.

There is help in the community. If you believe there is a risk for homicide-suicide, contact a professional immediately. Call a suicide crisis center, a crisis hotline, a family physician, a psychiatric or medical emergency room, or a community mental health center listed in the yellow pages of your phone book.

What to Do after a Homicide-Suicide

When a homicide-suicide occurs, you are confronted with many tasks— talking with law enforcement officers conducting the investigation; identifying or viewing the bodies of the deceased at the medical examiner's or coroner's office; talking with media; visiting the crime scene; having the crime scene cleaned; preparing for the funeral; and dealing with family, friends, and others who want to help. If the homicide-suicide is not successful, and the perpetrator survives, you may need to deal with the criminal justice system—arrest, jail, bond, finding a lawyer, and perhaps a trial. In addition to your dead family members, you become a co-victim. There is no way to escape the trauma that begins with witnessing or being notified.

Homicide-suicide also has a profound effect on the community where it occurs. Persons other than family members—significant others, neighbors, and friends from church, work, clubs, and other places in the community—are also co-victims. When homicide-suicide occurs in a hospital, nursing home, or assisted living residence, the staff become co-victims.

The families and co-victims we have worked with over the years have taught us how they lived through the ordeal. They have helped us learn about the complex circumstances leading to homicide-suicide, the mourning process, changing family relationships, the long-term impact of homicide-suicide, and the challenge of rebuilding their lives.

There are many things you can do not only to cope with the ordeal but also to prevail and get on with life. Understanding that you are victimized by older relatives who die in a homicide-suicide gives you a framework to think about and deal with the many tasks ahead of you. There are professionals and resources to help you deal with your traumatic grief, mourn your losses, and heal yourself. After a homicide-suicide, your life will never be the same. However, there are things you can do to become a survivor and integrate the experience of the tragedy into a stronger sense of self.

The Emotional Impact of Homicide-Suicide

After a homicide-suicide, there are many natural reactions.

- You keep thinking about the deceased.
- You visualize the bodies and the crime scene, even if you were not a witness.
- You keep thinking about events that occurred after the homicide-suicide, such as visiting the medical examiner's office.
- You wish things were the way they were before the homicide-suicide happened.
- You feel a mixture of anxiety, anger, and sadness.
- You feel numb.
- You withdraw from others.
- You have difficulty with thinking and your memory.
- You have trouble sleeping.
- You feel others do not understand what you are going through.
- You want help, but you feel it is a sign of weakness.
- You may or may not want to talk about your feelings and what happened.

Every conceivable human emotion is provoked by a homicide-suicide—shock, numbness, anger, fear, anxiety, guilt, shame, and pain. When loved ones have died this way, it is natural to be very angry with the perpetrator. Many say they can understand that a father or grandfather would kill himself, but it is unacceptable to kill a wife, sister, or other relative. Some family members describe the anger as so intense and uncontrollable that it scares them because they have never felt this way before. Anger toward the perpetrator can be intense and last a long time. Some family members say that their anger is confusing; it is a combination of anger toward the deceased, anger coupled with guilt because they should have seen it coming, and anger combined with shame that this happened in the family. Some family members fight, often blaming each other for not seeing the signs or not recognizing the depression. This is very common in siblings as well as adult children of the deceased.

Feelings of anger and rage are normal. Co-victims frequently vent their anger on people around them—family, friends, law enforcement officers, and professionals working with the family. Anger is an emotional response to block painful emotions, and getting angry is a way to get rid of the tension, anxiety, guilt, hurt, and frustration.

The grief can be overwhelming. Shock, sadness, and confusion may last for days or weeks or longer. It is not uncommon to cry uncontrollably, to become irritable and angry, and even to scream and rage, to feel helpless and hopeless, and to withdraw from others. The immediate grief is only the beginning of the experience. Homicide-suicides are violent deaths that lead to a traumatic grief. Two or more loved ones are dead, and it is important to get professional help to work through the emotional impact.

Questions every co-victim asks are, "Why did this happen?" and "Why did this happen to me?" and "Why did Dad kill Mom?" There are usually no certain answers to these questions. Even when the deceased perpetrator and victim have had a history of arguments and domestic violence, these same questions arise. With two or more parties deceased, family members obsess about circumstances leading to the homicide-suicide.

Guilt and shame are also common emotions. Guilt, like anger, is a normal reaction, but if it goes on too long, it interferes with mourning. Family members often become obsessed with what they could and should have done or what they did not do. Family and friends may recite a list of "if only's." "If only we hadn't moved away." "If only I had realized what Dad meant when he called and said he couldn't take it any more." "If only . . ." Blaming yourself can be adaptive in the early phases of grief because it allows you to make some sense of what happened. However, there is a time to stop blaming yourself because there is nothing you can do to change what happened. On the other hand, you can focus your energies on healing yourself.

Even the most competent and resourceful individuals can be devastated by the homicide-suicide. It is not a sign of personal weakness to feel a roller coaster of emotions, to be incapacitated by them, and to reach out for help. Homicide-suicide is a traumatic event, and the natural response is to review and judge what happened. Feelings of guilt are universal, and they can be overcome.

When Family Relationships Are Not Loving

Not all family members care about and love each other. If you have been estranged or emotionally distant from older parents and other family members who die in a homicide-suicide, you may not feel grief. You may even feel they deserved it. You may be angry that the homicide-suicide occurred, and you now have to interrupt your life to deal with the investigation, the funeral, the estate, and other issues. You may feel that they are better off dead, or if you were closer to your mother or the victim, you may feel overwhelming rage at the perpetrator.

Family conflict, feuds, and hostility are part of the human condition. These negative feelings and circumstances are real, and they affect the way you act with police officers and medical examiners during the investigation as well as health professionals and others after the homicide-suicide. It is appropriate for you to tell persons you interact with after the homicide-suicide about your negative relationships.

You have at least three options in these situations. One is to ignore the situation. The second is to find someone else to handle what needs to be done if you have the resources. The third is to accept your hostility and do what needs to be done, keeping your emotional distance.

Take Care of Yourself: You Can Get Sick

Any kind of death can have a profound effect on you. The grief can overwhelm you, and the mourning process can be long and difficult. Living in the aftermath of homicide-suicide is akin to living in the aftermath of a rape, assault, accident, or more global events such as a war or a natural or manmade disaster.

Homicide-suicide is traumatic because it is sudden and unanticipated when it occurs. In hindsight, you may try to untangle the chain of events that led up to the event, but no clear answers may emerge. Your lack of control over the sudden and violent occurrence of the homicide-suicide puts you at risk for depression as well as a condition known as posttraumatic stress disorder, or PTSD. Some of the toughest and best-trained military, police, and other specially trained professionals become overwhelmed by homicide-suicide.

Getting Help

It is not a sign of weakness to get help. If you were running a business, you would hire a lawyer or get a consultant to help you with a problem. Getting on with your life after a homicide-suicide will be easier if you can rely on professionals to help you. Others in the family or friendship network also may need help. Children and grandchildren may be affected by the homicide-suicide. Family members may escalate fights, blaming one another for what happened and for not recognizing that something was wrong.

Very few agencies provide services to family survivors of homicide-suicide and homicide. In contrast, there are more resources for co-victims of suicide. This is partly because there has been more research on suicide survivors.

> *Victim Advocates*: Do not be afraid to talk with the victim advocates who work with the police and sheriff's department. The medical examiner's or coroner's office also usually have victim advocates working with them. These professionals will be the ones who are best informed about resources in your community. Most homicide divisions in sheriff's departments and larger police departments will run homicide support groups. The needs of survivors of homicide and homicide-suicide are very similar, because both have had to deal with sudden, unexpected death.
>
> *Mental Health Professionals*: Setting up an appointment with a knowledgeable psychiatrist, psychologist, social worker, or mental health counselor can be one of the best decisions you ever make. The victim advocate who works with you can make a referral. You can

also contact university medical centers, community hospitals, and community mental health centers to ask for a referral. Many communities have crisis centers listed in the yellow pages of the phone book. They will know about qualified professionals in your area. Finding help when you or your family do not speak English can be difficult. Call your local Area Agency on Aging listed in the phone book. The persons who work there will likely know where you can go to get help.

Hospice: Most hospice programs run support groups for family and friends whose loved ones have died. Although these support groups are not tailored to the needs of people who have dealt with sudden, violent deaths, the sessions can help you with your grief through the mourning process. Most of the bereavement groups are time-limited. When they are over, hospice professionals can be very helpful to refer you to a mental health professional.

Preparing for the Future

Death is not a challenge unique to the patient with dementia and the family. However, brain diseases rob victims of their ability to think, act, and participate in the decisions that must be made. At the same time the family members must watch and struggle with their own anguish and relate to a loved one who has changed from a former self. Alzheimer's disease destroys the quality of life that gives meaning to the quality of death.

The key is to discover how to live life with the patient "one day at a time" and cope with changes. There are ways to maximize comfort throughout the illness. Much can be done, even in the final stages when the patient is bedridden, semiconscious, and laboring to live. Karen Russell, aged seventy-eight, sat by her husband's bedside in a nursing home for fifteen weeks as he grew progressively weaker but his body refused to succumb to pneumonia. She watched and tended him from eleven in the morning until eight at night. This constant attendance was a natural and necessary activity for her, since both she and her husband had always spent most of their time together. When the staff sensed his final hours, he went on the critical list, and she was allowed to keep her vigil at any time of the day or night. Mrs. Russell had the support of friends, doctors, staff, her children, and her grandchildren. She lived with her husband emotionally to the end. She visited the hospital several weeks after his death and shared an hour with us. She spoke softly and seemed at peace with herself. "It is hard to put love away," she said. "We spent fifty-four years together. My son and I will not forget him. Jewish writings say that we shall continue to live as long as we are not forgotten and as long as we have loved and have been loved."

There are many ways families can work together to help patients develop a legacy, to maximize comfort and dignity, and to reconstruct family life for the future. Families continually show us the strength and power of their love. In *The Bridge of San Luis Rey*, Thornton Wilder wrote these words of consolation, which ring close to the thoughts of Mrs. Russell: "There is a land of the living and a land of the dead, and the bridge is love; the only survival, the only meaning."

14

What Scientists Know about the Causes of Alzheimer's Disease

I know what caused my wife's dementia. It was voodoo. I am being pun-
ished with her sickness because of the car accident last year. I killed the
Shaman's son when he rode his bike in front of my car. He swerved into
my lane to avoid hitting a dog. There was nothing I could do.

K ern Eustace tearfully and reluctantly spoke these words several hours into a family interview. His oldest daughter, Zoe, had answered most of the questions during the interview. After her father's words, she faced us and asked, "Doctor, do you believe in voodoo?" Our response was, "We're not sure. Tell us about it." And she and the rest of the family spoke at great length, relieved that we accepted their beliefs in voodoo.

Joyce Eustace reportedly began showing personality changes and serious memory problems about two months following her husband's car accident. Kern and the children, daughters Zoe and Ali, took her for a diagnostic evaluation a year later because she was screaming at the family and neighbors as well as refusing to cook and take care of the house.

Kern had asked his daughters to leave college and help him care for his wife at home. However, none of them could deal effectively with her behavioral outbursts. Kern refused to get help from the Haitian community and over time became increasingly isolated from his friends. One evening Joyce fell and screamed for over an hour. Fearful that she would be killed by voodoo, Kern took her to the emergency room, where she was treated for a broken wrist and released. After the wrist healed, the screaming continued, eventually precipitating the clinic visit for a diagnostic evaluation.

Voodoo does not cause Alzheimer's disease. Nor does an evil life, bad blood, the devil's curse, or even age per se. Indeed, there are many cultures around the world that view memory problems as part of aging. The unfortunate consequence of this belief system is that affected individuals and their family members do not seek medical help, either because dementia is not seen as a disease and they have a cultural explanation or because they are distrustful of a predominately white medical care system.

Alzheimer's disease and related dementias are diseases of the brain. Aging by itself does not cause Alzheimer's disease or other dementias. These brain disorders are caused by specific pathological processes. In the absence of disease, the human brain and mind continue to function well into old age. However, there are some who still believe that if you live long enough, you will get Alzheimer's disease. This chapter is written in response to the many questions asked by individuals who want specific details about the causes of Alzheimer's disease and vascular dementias. What starts the disease process in the first place, and what contributes to the ongoing development of the disease? Why does the prevalence increase with advancing age? Are there several types of Alzheimer's disease?

Alzheimer's disease develops as the result of a complex series of events that occur in the brain over time. Scientists do not yet understand what causes the disease, but they know that a cascade or "domino effect" involving a set of steps occurs. This means that the disease can be triggered by any number of small changes in this cascade, and these events may occur and interact differently in different individuals. This chapter is more technical than the rest of the book because it describes the exciting scientific advances in our growing knowledge about the causes of Alzheimer's disease. The material has been simplified to make it comprehensible to a lay audience without sacrificing scientific accuracy. However, the story of possible causes is more complicated in the details, and the interested reader may consult references in the selected readings or other available sources through the Alzheimer's Disease Information

Clearinghouse at the National Institute on Aging (see Alzheimer's Disease Education and Referral (ADEAR) Center in Appendix 1).

Changes in the Alzheimer's Brain

The size and weight of the brain are significantly reduced in Alzheimer's disease as a result of the death and loss of brain cells. Although this loss occurs throughout the brain, certain areas are more affected than others. Significant cell loss occurs throughout the outer mantle of the brain, known as the *cerebral cortex*. The normal brain has a rugged, almost mountain-like appearance. It is full of grooves known technically as *fissures* or *sulci*. The elevated parts between these fissures are called *gyri*. In Alzheimer's disease the mountains appear more rugged, the gyri are narrowed, and the fissures or grooves are widened as a result of cell loss.

These gross brain changes, which are obvious to the naked eye, in and of themselves do not prove that the deceased patient had Alzheimer's disease. The diagnosis rests on the results of the microscopic examination of brain tissue that has been chemically treated to stain a number of anatomical structures. The diagnosis is established when a large number of anatomical lesions known as *tangles* and *plaques* are found. These structural changes are also found to some degree in the brains of older persons without dementia, but they are far more numerous in Alzheimer's disease. The density of these tangles and plaques is used to arrive at a definitive diagnosis.

The tangles, technically called *neurofibrillary tangles*, are made up of insoluble, twisted fibers that accumulate inside the nerve cell. They resemble hairlike hooks or teardrop-like structures when they are stained and photographed under a powerful microscope. If we observe these tangles using the very high magnification of the electron microscope, we can see that they are composed of many bundles of little hairlike structures called *filaments*. These filaments may occur alone or in pairs. When they are paired, they are wrapped around each other in a helix, and not surprisingly they are called *paired helical filaments of the Alzheimer type*. They are structurally different from any other filaments in normal brain cells.

The plaques, called *neuritic plaques* or *senile plaques*, are spherical structures composed of an insoluble (cannot be dissolved) protein called *amy-*

loid. Plaques accumulate outside and around nerve cells. They are most often seen in the cerebral cortex but also develop in other areas of the brain. Although a small number of plaques are seen in the brains of most older people, what distinguishes Alzheimer's brains from others is the extraordinary number of plaques per volume of brain tissue examined. The presence of a few plaques in the brain is not unusual, but the presence of many is abnormal.

The cortex, the most highly evolved part of the brain, is responsible for what are called higher brain functions—thinking, judgment, reasoning, speech, and language. Different locations in the cortex also have specialized functions that affect such behaviors as mood and sexual expression as well as language and thinking. Therefore, as more and more of the brain cells are destroyed in Alzheimer's disease, all aspects of intellectual functioning become worse, and normal behavior disintegrates.

Underneath the many thick layers of the cerebral cortex is a part of the brain known as the *limbic system*, which contains a number of different structures. One of these structures is a small group of cells shaped somewhat like a sea horse; hence it is given the name *hippocampus*. Autopsy studies have shown that in Alzheimer's disease the plaques and tangles are very dense in the hippocampus, especially in the bottom half. This widespread destruction of hippocampal cells significantly disrupts attention and memory. Damage in the hippocampus and other parts of the limbic system also affects the way emotions are expressed. Ferocious rage and extraordinary irritability, or their opposite, apathy and docility, may occur. The loss of cells in the limbic system probably accounts for many of the changes in emotional control and personality that occur with Alzheimer's disease.

Certain cells in the hippocampus undergo another change characteristic of Alzheimer's disease. By the use of special dyes to stain the hippocampal cells, we can reveal what is called *granulovacuolar degeneration*. The cells of the hippocampus are pyramid shaped, and they contain small spherical vacuoles, or holes, with a small granule in the center of the hole. Alzheimer's disease is distinguished by the high density of these vacuoles. This granulovacuolar degeneration is quite rare in persons under the age of sixty but is seen with increasing frequency in the aging brain after the age of sixty. By the age of eighty, more than three-quarters of all brains show some amount of granulovacuolar degeneration. However, a high density of such change is indicative of Alzheimer's disease, regardless of age.

Autopsy studies have shown degeneration in other parts of the brain. The spinal cord connects with the base of the brain and runs into the brain stem, which looks like a flattened part of the spinal cord. Groups of cells in the brain stem regulate many critical functions including breathing and the beating of the heart. Thus, damage to the brain stem is usually quite dangerous. The brain stem contains several structures, including a group of nerve cells named the *locus coeruleus*. Many of these cells are destroyed in Alzheimer's disease. *Locus coeruleus* means "blue place," and if the brain is cut and the locus coeruleus examined, it actually appears to be blue. This region is the site of a large number of nerves, some of which continue up into the cerebral cortex and some of which run into an area in the brain called the *cerebellum*. The cerebellum appears to sit on the back of the brain, and it looks very much like a small head of cauliflower. It is responsible for coordinating the many muscle movements that allow us to walk, bend, and move about. The destruction of the locus coeruleus probably contributes to changes in awareness, emotional outbursts, and perhaps the motor coordination problems observed in Alzheimer's disease.

Nerves from the brain stem ascend into the brain and join the cortex in a structure called the *hypothalamus*, which also is affected in Alzheimer's disease. The hypothalamus controls the functions of many of the body's internal organs. It regulates the pituitary gland and can stimulate this "master gland" to release into the bloodstream many of the hormones essential for life and growth. These hormones in turn affect other glands, causing them to secrete other essential hormones. Like the hippocampus, the hypothalamus also has special centers of activity involved in the ability to control emotions and in the experience of such emotions as pleasure, hunger, and satiety, the sensation of fullness one gets after enjoying a meal.

Causes of Alzheimer's Disease

The structural changes in the brain described here and in the earlier chapter on diagnosis do not cause Alzheimer's disease. They are the end result of pathological processes, and the challenge is to discover what causes the degeneration in the first place. Understanding how brain cells lose the ability to communicate with each other and why some brain cells die is at the heart of the mystery of Alzheimer's disease.

Amyloid Plaques

Amyloid plaques appear to develop first in the parts of the brain involved with memory and other cognitive processes. They are known to develop even before neurofibrillary tangles. Plaques are composed of the deposits of several substances. The most common is a protein called *beta-amyloid*, which is a protein segment literally snipped from a larger protein known as *amyloid precursor protein* (APP). The other components of the plaques include pieces of nerve cells, cells called *astrocytes* that help support the functioning neuron, and other non-neuronal cells such as microglia. The *microglia* are part of the brain's immune system. They converge around damaged cells or foreign substances, cause an inflammatory reaction, and then digest the cells.

We do not know whether these plaques cause Alzheimer's disease or whether they are end-products of the Alzheimer process or even both. However, it is known that changes in the APP can cause Alzheimer's disease because one inherited form is caused by mutations in the APP gene. This is discussed in the genetics section later in this chapter.

APP is produced in the brain. After it is made, APP attaches itself to the cell membrane surrounding the nerve cell. When we observe APP on the membrane, it looks like a needle in a swatch of fabric. Given its placement, APP plays an important role in the growth and maintenance of nerve cells. It also helps damaged nerve cells repair themselves and to grow after they have been injured.

However, because APP sticks out of the membrane, it is vulnerable to being cut into pieces. Each tiny piece released from each snipped APP is called *alpha-beta*, and it leaves the cell and accumulates outside the membrane. The enzymes that snip the APP are known as *proteases*, and they cut it in two specific places. One protease, known as *beta-secretase*, cuts APP to form the beta-amyloid protein (BAP). Another protease, known as *alpha-secretase*, snips the APP at another site, so it does not form BAP. The BAP created when APP is cleaved has two lengths. The shorter BAP is soluble and aggregates slowly. The longer BAP, known as *sticky BAP*, forms insoluble clumps very quickly.

Over time the clumps of sticky BAP grow and evolve into long filaments outside the nerve cell membrane. These insoluble BAP filaments are called *diffuse* or *preamyloid plaques*. They are considered precursor lesions because they lack the pieces of dead and dying neurons, as well as the microglia and astrocytes, that form the amyloid plaques characteristic of Alzheimer's disease. These precursor lesions are analogous to the early fat deposits in the heart and blood vessels that are the beginning of atherosclerosis. Precursor lesions as well as pieces of alpha-beta are produced naturally in the brain in people without Alzheimer's disease, and as a result they accumulate with age in persons who do not show cognitive impairment. Many researchers are analyzing the proteases that cause BAP to be formed, as well as the process of how BAP aggregates to form the precursor lesions and plaques that grow in large numbers in specific parts of the brain.

Although scientists once believed that more plaques were formed as the disease progressed, gradually affecting more parts of the brain, this does not appear to be the case. The amount of BAP appears to be relatively constant over time. Using a special laser scanning microscope to see the plaque in three dimensions, scientists discovered that the plaques are not solid but have very small holes through them. Therefore, it is possible that the beta-amyloid is assembling and breaking up in a dynamic process of equilibrium. This line of research has fueled optimism that it may be possible to find ways to break down the insoluble plaques after they have formed.

A number of researchers believe that beta-amyloid is harmful to brain cells in several ways. BAP may cause inflammation or create free radicals. Free radicals are formed when oxygen is metabolized into molecules that react with other molecules, causing cellular damage. BAP also may cause nerve cells to be more vulnerable to damage caused by poor blood flow, known as *ischemia*. BAP deposits may interfere with connections between nerve cells in the area around the plaques. This may affect the ability of blood vessels in the brain to dilate in response to the decreased blood flow. Finally, BAP may be toxic to brain cells by increasing the amount of calcium in the cells. Calcium helps brain cells with many functions, and one of the most important is the transmission of nerve impulses. However, too much calcium inside brain cells kills them.

Neurofibrillary Tangles

The major component of the neurofibrillary tangles is one form of a family of proteins called *tau*. Tau proteins play a critical role holding together the microtubules inside the nerve cell. These microtubules are a major component of the cell's internal support system or skeleton. Microtubules form structures analogous to train tracks in healthy nerve cells, and they move molecules through the nerve cells to the end of the cells known as *end branches*. The end branches are where neurotransmitters are released so cells can communicate with each other, a process described in the next section.

The railroad system of microtubules collapses in cells affected by Alzheimer's disease. In healthy nerve cells, the tau protein forms what looks like "railroad ties," connecting pieces that stabilize the microtubule system. In Alzheimer's disease, tau is chemically changed so it cannot hold the tubules together. A protein called *p25* is believed to initiate the molecular changes that destabilize tau. The destruction of the nerve's transport system may first affect the ability of the nerve cell to transmit impulses, which disrupts cell communication and later leads to cell death. The chemically changed tau in Alzheimer's disease twists into paired helical filaments, which means that two pieces of tau wrap around each other. These filaments are the primary component of the neurofibrillary tangles, as described earlier. As the number of tangles formed increases, more neurons die over the course of the disease.

Cell Functioning and Death

The brain damage in Alzheimer's disease involves changes in three processes—communication among nerve cells, metabolism, and cell repair. Healthy brain functioning requires the coordination and integration of many biological processes to facilitate communication between neurons, maintain cell metabolism, and repair damaged cells and tissues. Neuronal communication depends on a healthy neuron, its many connections, and the ability to produce neurotransmitters. Losses, dysfunction, or the absence of any one of these interferes with normal brain functioning.

Changes in the brain's cell-to-cell communication interfere with behavior. The overuse of alcohol leading to slowness, slurred speech, and other behavioral changes is a good example of disrupted cell communication throughout the brain. Neurons use many different chemicals to communicate with each other, including neurotransmitters, hormonal peptides, and metal ions. As discussed later in this chapter, changes in the neurotransmitter acetylcholine, neuroendocrine peptides, and metals interact in the pathology of Alzheimer's disease.

Metabolism refers to the pathways whereby molecules break down chemicals to produce energy, which is necessary for healthy cell functioning. Healthy metabolic processes require good blood circulation to provide neurons with oxygen and glucose, and neurons die within minutes when the brain is deprived of oxygen and glucose. Metabolism is altered in Alzheimer's disease, vascular dementias, as well as other dementias. The use of positron emission tomography, described in Chapter 2, has shown that certain parts of the brain in living Alzheimer's patients are not able to metabolize the sugar glucose normally. The reasons for this are not well understood, but these cells are under the chronic metabolic distress of being undernourished.

Although the human brain accounts for only about 2 percent of body weight, it accounts for 20 percent of the oxygen used. Therefore, the brain is the most oxidative tissue in the body. Several biological processes are involved in oxidative metabolism to create the energy necessary for the brain to function. Disruptions in any of these processes can lead to neural dysfunction, and substantial evidence exists for oxidative metabolic impairments in Alzheimer's disease as well as vascular dementia.

In contrast to many other cells in the body, such as in the skin and liver, brain cells live a long time, and the vast majority do not replicate. Therefore, brain cells are affected by toxic substances in a different way than other cells. When brain cells die from disease or injury, they usually do not replace themselves. However, certain nerve cells in specific parts of the brain can replace themselves. Repair of injured neurons is essential to prevent death, and if the biological processes that clean up, maintain, or repair the cells slow down or stop, the nerve cell will not function. However, it is not clear why and when nerve cells die, as well as when nerve cell communication is obliterated in Alzheimer's disease.

Many toxic substances cause selective damage to different cell groups in the brain. Toxins used in animal studies selectively damage parts of the brain called the *substantia nigra*, the *cerebellum*, and the *hippocampus*.

Whether toxins produced in the brain play a role in Alzheimer's disease and other chronic neurodegenerative conditions is controversial.

In Alzheimer's disease, certain cells in the hippocampus and cortex, called *pyramidal neurons*, show significant pathology, as described earlier. These neurons use a neurotransmitter called *glutamate*, which also occurs in other parts of the brain. Glutamate operates with four sets of receptors, but in the hippocampus of Alzheimer's patients one of the receptors, called *NMDA*, is decreased, consistent with cell death. However, the affected cells in the cerebral cortex have significantly more NMDA receptors.

When activated, NMDA causes the neuronal membranes to depolarize the cell membrane, making it permeable to calcium, which means calcium passes in and out of the neuron through the cell membrane. (Depolarization is described in the next section.) Calcium transport is particularly important because too much calcium leads to cell death. The neurotransmitter glutamate is highly sensitive to the chronic lack of glucose. The altered glucose metabolism seen in Alzheimer's disease can change glutamate into a toxic killer of nerve cells. The toxicity of glutamate in turn is affected by the high amounts of calcium in the neuron.

One of the most exciting scientific discoveries in brain research is evidence that some nerves in the adult human brain do have the ability to replicate throughout life. It may soon be possible to find new approaches to stimulate brain mechanisms to replace neurons and glial cells lost through Alzheimer's disease, other diseases, stroke, and trauma.

Neurotransmitter Changes: The Cholinergic System

As we described in the chapters on medications (see Chapters 5 and 6), the brain contains chemicals known as *neurotransmitters*, and although several of these neurotransmitters are affected in Alzheimer's disease, one—acetylcholine—is significantly altered. In order to understand what these chemical changes mean, it is useful first to review how neurotransmitters play a role in the way the brain works. There are more than 10^{10} nerve cells or neurons in the brain—that means more than 10,000,000,000 cells. Nerve cells form many interconnections allowing them to communicate with each other through a combination of chemical and biological events.

Each neuron has a cell body, an axon, and many dendrites in tree-like formations. The entire neuron is enclosed in a cell membrane. Every neuron also has a nucleus inside the cell, which contains genes composed of DNA—deoxyribonucleic acid—which controls how the cell functions. The axon is a long thin part of the nerve that extends away from the cell body, and it is a bridge for communication to other neurons. Groups of dendrites branch off the cell body, and they receive messages from the axons of other nerve cells using special receptor sites. The neurons also are surrounded by glial cells whose role is to support and provide nutrients the neurons need to survive.

Neurons communicate with each other by producing, releasing, and deactivating neurotransmitter chemicals. As neurons receive these chemical messages from other neurons, an electrical charge, or nerve impulse, develops inside the cells. This electrical impulse travels along the length of the nerve to the end of the axon, much the way an electrical impulse is carried by a wire. At the end branches of the axon, it triggers the release of neurotransmitters to continue to send the message or to initiate messages in other areas of the brain.

Neurotransmitters are discharged from the nerve endings into an area between the nerves, which is called the *synapse*. When these chemical substances reach the nerve on the other side of the synapse, they cause the next cell(s) in the sequence to become excited and carry on the impulse. A typical brain cell has up to 15,000 synapses. Since so many neurons are clustered at each synapse, entire groups of nerve cells may become excited. Thus, different groups of nerves become activated when we smell the aroma of a freshly baked pizza, hear the sounds of a jazz band, watch a ball game, read a novel, write a letter, or try to solve a problem. Entirely different parts of the brain are active when we sleep and when we are awake. Thus, the neurotransmitters of the brain are essential for learning, memory, and all the thoughts, behaviors, and actions that make us human.

After crossing the synapse, neurotransmitters bind to very specific receptor sites on the dendrites. These receptor sites are proteins in the cell membrane that recognize and react to specific neurotransmitters. When the receptors are activated after binding to a neurotransmitter, they set up a series of processes in the cell membrane. These events in turn effect the interior of the cell and determine what the receiving neuron will do. Some neurotransmitters stimulate nerve cells to become active and send a nerve impulse, while other neurotransmitters inhibit nerve cells so they do not send an impulse down their axon. Thus, millions of signals are being sent throughout the brain at any one time as cells communicate with each other.

Most individual nerve cells use or respond to only one type of neurotransmitter. However, there are hundreds of substances that can act as neurotransmitters in the brain. This area of science, known as *neurochemistry*, is growing rapidly and giving us profound insights into the way the brain works.

Neurons that contain acetylcholine are known as *cholinergic neurons*, and many of these are bunched together into clearly defined bundles of cells called *brain tracts*. The cholinergic tracts radiate throughout the entire brain. A large group of cholinergic nerves come together deep in the brain in a region called the *nucleus basalis of Meynert*, which may be one of the first parts of the brain affected in Alzheimer's disease. Autopsy examinations show that not all, but a significant number, of the nerve cells in this nucleus as well as other cholinergic tracts throughout the entire brain are destroyed.

From autopsy and laboratory studies we know that several chemical changes occur in the cholinergic nerves before they die. It is clear that the ability of these affected cells to produce acetylcholine is altered in several ways. Two substances, choline and acetyl coenzyme A, are joined together by an enzyme called *choline acetyltransferase* (CAT) to form acetylcholine. There is a dramatic reduction in the amount of CAT in the brains of Alzheimer's patients. Furthermore, this reduction is greatest in the areas of the brain where the well-recognized plaques and neurofibrillary tangles occur in the greatest numbers.

A decrease in CAT activity is not the only change observed in the cholinergic system. The synthesis or formation of acetylcholine also has been measured directly in brain material taken from patients using a brain biopsy procedure. Brain samples containing plaques and tangles show more than a 50 percent reduction in the production of acetylcholine. However, brain samples without plaques and tangles retain their ability to synthesize acetylcholine.

These early findings are exciting and important. They suggest that not all cholinergic nerve cells lose their ability to produce acetylcholine in

Alzheimer's disease. The existence of healthy tissue provides a basis for hope. They also have focused researchers on understanding how to chemically stabilize or improve cholinergic functioning in the brain. Once the production of acetylcholine within many of the cholinergic nerves has fallen off greatly, much less is available to be discharged into the synaptic cleft. However, if ways are found to increase the amount of acetylcholine secreted into the synapse, a nerve impulse should be generated. This is theoretically possible because the receiving apparatus of the cholinergic neurons and their capacity to fire a nerve impulse are not affected, at least not in the early stages of Alzheimer's disease.

Other significant changes occur in the cholinergic system. Acetylcholinesterase and butylcholinesterase are two important enzymes whose activity is changed in Alzheimer's disease. Acetylcholinesterase levels are reduced but not as great as the reduction observed for the CAT enzyme. However, butylcholinesterase levels increase, especially in the later stages of dementia. The function of both enzymes is to break down acetylcholine after it has been secreted into the synaptic cleft. Altering a neurotransmitter after it has done its job is essential. The human body needs a mechanism to remove or chemically change neurotransmitters in the synapse so that stimulation of the nerve ceases, to prepare for the next transmission.

Three drugs that prevent the deactivation of acetylcholine, tacrine (Cognex), donepezil (Aricept), and rivastigmine (Exelon), are currently being used to treat individuals with Alzheimer's disease. These are described in Chapter 5. Although specific changes in certain cholinergic neurons are well established, it is not possible to say at this time that cholinergic changes cause Alzheimer's disease. It seems more likely that the destruction of these cells is a later stage of the pathological process, but the cholinergic changes account for many of the cognitive changes.

It is not clear whether the loss of cholinergic functioning occurs before, after, or commensurate with mild, early cognitive deficits. It appears that patients in the early stages of Alzheimer's disease, showing memory deficits as well as plaques and tangles in the brain, have normal levels of the enzymes that regulate acetylcholine. In contrast, patients with severe dementia have significantly reduced levels of these enzymes. Therefore, lower levels of the enzymes regulating acetylcholine may not be an early sign of the disease. However, it is possible that overall acetylcholine levels are lower or the deficits are in certain cells in the cholinergic tracts. The success of Aricept and Exelon in mild to moderately impaired patients may be due to their ability to increase normal levels of acetylcholine rather than merely maintain falling levels.

Immune System Changes

Proteins that affect the immune system may play a role in the initiation of Alzheimer's disease. A substance called the *amyloid beta peptide*, which is a component of the sticky deposits of amyloid plaques, sets off a process that damages brain cells. Amyloid beta peptides use a cell receptor called *CD40*, and it usually facilitates cells in the immune system to communicate with each other. However, when amyloid beta peptide activates the CD40 receptor, it sends signals to microglia, the immune cells in the brain, to cause inflammation in the brain, which can damage brain cells as well as the brain's vascular system. The microglia are activated to produce a substance called *tumor necrosis factor-alpha* (TNFα), which kills neurons. Therefore, it appears that the activation of the CD40 receptor causes a chemical imbalance that causes the microglia to attack the very neurons they usually protect from infection and disease. It is as if the brain is fighting ghost microbes that are not really there.

Research using mice as a model for Alzheimer's disease shows that the peptides begin to activate the CD40 receptors long before symptoms of the disease appear or amyloid plaques begin to accumulate. It is not known why this long-term chronic inflammatory response causes more damage to cholinergic neurons than the other nerve tracts. The bad news is that the disease may begin very early in life, but the good news is that drugs that block the activation of CD40 might prevent symptoms from developing. The discovery of compounds that block amyloid beta peptides from activating the CD40 receptors to stimulate microglia could someday lead to effective drugs to treat Alzheimer's disease.

Hundreds of clinical studies and basic research studies provide evidence that inflammatory processes play a role in Alzheimer's disease. Neuroinflammation research is focusing on mediators of inflammation, inflammatory cells, animal models of inflammation, as well as therapies, including new drugs and vaccinations.

Neuroinflammation coupled with oxidative stress in the Alzheimer's brain plays a role in cell death. Oxidative stress occurs when oxygen, one of the brain's most important fuels, is metabolized and free radicals are formed in the process, killing nerve cells. Free radicals are oxygen- or nitric oxide–containing molecules with an unpaired electron that makes them very reactive. They react with sites on fats, carbohydrates, proteins, RNA (ribonucleic acid), and DNA in the brain. RNA is more vulnerable than DNA to oxidative stress. RNA plays a critical role in the synthesis of protein; thus, the damaged RNA will produce a malfunctioning protein that can cause neurons to die. Although the body has natural repair mechanisms, if the production of free radicals is too high, the repair mechanisms cannot keep up and damage accumulates in the cell. In brain cells as well as muscle, the impact of free radical damage is significant because the cells are not replaced as in blood or skin.

Accumulation of Trace Elements

The toxic effects of trace elements in Alzheimer's disease have been detected for many years. The elements that have received the most research attention are aluminum, zinc, iron, and mercury. The lethal effect of these elements can occur at least two ways. High accumulations of these elements can be toxic to neurons, or the high concentrations can displace other essential elements for healthy nerve functions.

Aluminum

Excess aluminum in the brain has received the most attention. It is unlikely that it has a primary causal effect, but aluminum is neurotoxic and could speed cell death in already damaged neurons. Several investigators reported that higher concentrations of aluminum are present in the brains of patients with Alzheimer's disease than in those of healthy older persons without dementia. Other investigators reported elevated concentrations in the brains both of healthy older persons and of Alzheimer's patients. They also found that the amount of aluminum in the brain varies with geography. In some parts of the country, where the soil or drinking water contains more aluminum, everyone has higher aluminum levels, but there is no evidence of a greater prevalence of Alzheimer's disease.

Using special techniques, scientists have been able to measure the actual concentration of aluminum in different parts of the nerve cell. Nerves containing a high density of tangles appear to be richer in aluminum compared with cells without tangles. High concentrations of aluminum also have been found in the brains of patients with other types of dementias. Therefore, the uptake of aluminum is probably not specific to Alzheimer's disease. It may be that aluminum and other chemicals surrounding the neurons may be taken into damaged or partially impaired cells.

Aluminum may be associated with other forms of dementia. Patients with kidney disease who must use dialysis for many years can develop a condition called *dialysis dementia.* They show intellectual deterioration, muscle tremors, and seizures. Autopsy studies demonstrated a heavy accumulation of aluminum in the cortex of their brains, which probably comes from solutions used in the dialysis treatments. What is significant is that the brains of these dialysis patients do not show the rich concentration of plaques and tangles seen in Alzheimer's disease. Furthermore, the aluminum does not seem to accumulate inside the nucleus of the nerve cells of dialysis patients, as it does in persons with Alzheimer's disease.

In sum, it appears unlikely that aluminum accumulation by itself causes Alzheimer's disease. On the other hand, if the patient has Alzheimer's disease, aluminum is probably taken into the already defective neurons and may cause further damage. Aluminum may also form a chemical bond with the protein filaments manufactured by the brain. This complex of aluminum-protein material could then interfere with the normal assembly of microfilaments in the brain. The result might then be the obstruction of the normal functions of the nerve cell involved. Since aluminum is the most abundant metal in our environment, composing 8 percent of the earth's crust, its presence in the brain is not surprising. The selective deposit of aluminum inside nerve cells with tangles that has been observed in different forms of dementia is a mystery that remains to be solved.

Zinc, Iron, and Mercury

Zinc may play a role in Alzheimer's disease. Studies done using cell cultures show that zinc causes the BAP to form clumps resembling the plaques in Alzheimer's disease. A few studies demonstrated that patients given zinc supplements showed worsened cognitive functioning.

Iron is another of the most common elements in the earth's crust, and it is essential for both animal and plant life. Iron could mediate the disease process in several ways. A number of studies indicated that iron metabolism is disrupted in Alzheimer's disease. Iron concentrations are increased in the gray matter of the cortex, the amygdala in the limbic system, and the olfactory pathway (to the nose). Iron also accumulates in high concentrations in the neurofibrillary tangles and plays a role in free radical formation. An active form of iron known as a *free ion* catalyzes the formation of free radicals.

Mercury is another prevalent element and has long been known to be poisonous. The most common source of mercury is in dental fillings, but it also occurs in drugs as well as food, plastic, paint, and cosmetics. Exposure to mercury in seafood is one of the most common exposures for people.

Studies of the brains of Alzheimer's patients showed that mercury concentrations are high in the cerebral cortex and other deeper structures including the nucleus basalis of Meynert. Mercury is toxic to neurons in many ways. In Alzheimer's disease, mercury interferes with the construction of microtubules or neurofilaments and therefore may play a role in the collapse of the neurofilaments that lead to the formation of neurofibrillary tangles.

Genetic Factors

Genes play a complex role in Alzheimer's disease. Genes can be thought of as recipes that give instructions about how to make something in the body. However, the environment such as what we eat, drink, and breathe, as well as the biological processes in the body, also affect what ingredients are used as well as their form and quantity.

Genes need to be activated by something to exert their effort. They are housed in the cell's nucleus and wait until other molecules come along to read their messages. The instructions or messages the genes carry are used to build proteins, and they can build proteins correctly or incorrectly depending on the DNA instructions. Genes build proteins incorrectly when they have defects or mutations in the DNA, and these proteins can lead to changes that cause cells to function improperly, diseases, and death.

Alzheimer's disease is not caused by a single gene like cystic fibrosis and Huntington's disease are. More than one gene can cause Alzheimer's disease, and genes on several chromosomes are involved. Furthermore, in most cases genes alone are not sufficient to cause the disease.

There are two types of Alzheimer's disease—familial Alzheimer's disease (FAD), where families show a pattern of inheritance, and sporadic Alzheimer's disease, where there is no obvious pattern of inheritance. Alzheimer's disease is also described as early onset, occurring before age sixty-five, and late onset, occurring at age sixty-five or later.

Early-onset Alzheimer's is relatively rare, occurring in about 10 percent of all persons with Alzheimer's disease. Familial Alzheimer's disease has an early onset, and about half of all familial cases are known to be caused by mutations or defects in three genes on three chromosomes. These include mutations in the gene associated with the production of the APP on chromosome 21, mutations in a gene called *presenilin 1* on chromosome 14, and mutations in a gene called *presenilin 2* on chromosome 1. If one of these three mutations is present on only one of the two genes inherited from one of the parents, that person would develop that form of early-onset Alzheimer's disease. None of these mutations are known to have a major role in the more common sporadic Alzheimer's disease.

The mutation in the gene associated with APP production on chromosome 21 was the first to be discovered. It appears that mutations on the APP gene increase the likelihood that beta-amyloid will be snipped from the APP, causing more of the sticky form of beta-amyloid to be made. The presenilin mutations may cause the death of neurons in several ways. They may affect the production of beta-amyloid. Most patients with presenilin 1 and 2 mutations have more of the sticky beta-amyloid than do patients with sporadic Alzheimer's disease. The presenilin mutations also could cause neurons to die more directly. Some research suggests that mutations in presenilin 1 and 2 accelerate the process of apoptosis or programmed cell death.

At least one gene on chromosome 19 increases the susceptibility to Alzheimer's disease. The apolipoprotein-E (APOE) gene does not cause Alzheimer's disease as do the APP, presenilin 1, and presenilin 2 gene mutations. The APOE gene controls a protein produced in the liver and brain. This protein helps carry blood cholesterol and performs other functions. It is found in neurons and glial cells in healthy nerve cells. Of special significance, increased amounts of the protein are associated with the occurrence of amyloid plaques.

The APOE gene has three different forms known as alleles: E2, E3, and E4. The APOE genes occur in pairs like all other genes, and people may have one, two, or none of these. The E2 form seems to decrease the risk of Alzheimer's disease, and E4 increases the risk. About 40 percent of patients with Alzheimer's disease have at least one E4 gene. Also, the E4 gene is found in people with and those without a family history of Alzheimer's disease. E3 is the most common form in the population and may play a neutral role in Alzheimer's disease.

APOE E4 has been associated with both sporadic and late-onset familial Alzheimer's disease. People with two E4 genes are eight times more likely than those with two E3 genes to develop Alzheimer's disease. However, it is possible to have one or two copies of the APOE E4 gene and not develop Alzheimer's disease. It is also possible to have no E4 genes and still develop Alzheimer's disease. The ways E4 increases risk are not known, but it is thought that it facilitates the accumulation of beta-amyloid.

The presence of an E4 gene only means that the risk for Alzheimer's disease is increased. It does not predict the disease in a person who does not have any symptoms of Alzheimer's disease. Some research suggests that most people with one E3 gene and one E4 gene will not get the disease, and that as many as 50 percent of people with two E4 genes will not develop the disease. The association of E4 and Alzheimer's disease is weak in very old people, where the risk of Alzheimer's disease is very high because of advanced age. E4 may have a greater impact on risk in whites compared to Hispanic Americans or African Americans, but these minority groups may have a higher overall risk of Alzheimer's disease.

A blood test can reveal which forms of the APOE gene a person carries. However, a consensus statement issued by the American College of Medical Genetics and the American Society of Human Genetics, and approved by the American Academy of Neurology, the American Psychiatric Association, and the National Institutes of Health, states that APOE testing is not recommended for clinical diagnosis and should not be used for predictive testing. Research findings of the risk estimate are based on populations, not on individuals. This means that the results are only estimated risks, which do not reflect an individual's risk. Further, because Alzheimer's disease develops when E4 is not present, and many people with E4 do not develop Alzheimer's disease, genetic testing is not recommended.

Research Studies on the Genetics of Alzheimer's Disease

If you are asked to participate in a research study on the genetics of Alzheimer's disease, the investigators will give you a consent form before you enter the study. The consent form will contain information about the reasons for the study and the possible benefits and risks involved in your participation. The purpose of the research study is to gather more information about the genetics of Alzheimer's disease.

Any questions you have about the research must be answered before you sign the consent form. You have the right to ask questions and have them answered. You are free to decide not to participate in the research. All information is kept confidential.

You will be told that one important condition of consent is that you will not learn the results of the testing. Several scientists and medical groups reached this consensus because it is not known what individual test results mean about the risk of developing Alzheimer's disease. Scientists are beginning to examine the ethical, psychological, and legal implications of genetic research. It is important to understand these issues in the event that predictive tests and diagnostic genetics tests prove reliable and become available in the future.

The scientists will need a small amount (about 4 tablespoons) of blood or a saliva sample, or both. These samples will be used to analyze your genes. They will also ask you about your medical history and the medical history of your family that pertains to Alzheimer's disease. They may ask for records from the doctors involved in your care and in other family members' care.

The testing should be performed with strict confidentiality. Samples will be given a code number, and information with the code number and your name will not be kept together. No information will be released to anyone, including other members of your family.

The Role of Viruses

Individuals with Alzheimer's disease as well as other brain diseases, including prion diseases, Parkinson's disease, Huntington's disease, and frontotemporal dementia, have deposits of abnormal proteins in the brain. Dr. Stanley Prusiner won the Nobel Prize for his discovery of prions, an infectious type of protein. Prion diseases, such as Creutzfeldt-Jakob disease and kuru in humans, bovine spongiform encephalopathy or "mad cow disease," and spongiform encephalopathy in other animals such as sheep, cause dementia and death. All forms show insoluble amyloid in the brain but the amyloid fibrils are different from those seen in Alzheimer's disease. Mad cow disease was discussed in Chapter 2.

Kuru is the name of a brain disease that has been observed in a group of people living in Papua New Guinea. Although individuals may carry the "kuru agent" for a long period without symptoms, once the disease appears, it progresses fairly rapidly and causes death in six to twenty-four months. As the illness worsens, individuals have severe dementia and a number of other neuromuscular signs, such as uncontrolled muscle twitches, tremors, and problems in walking. Dr. D. Carleton Gajdusek received a Nobel Prize for discovering that kuru is caused by a virus-like particle, transmitted probably through food and primarily to women and children who participate in cannibalistic rituals. Men also can get kuru, but they usually are excluded from consuming the infected brains of the deceased in funeral rites. Women and children are entitled to the brains as reward for preparing the bodies.

Creutzfeldt-Jakob disease is named after the two people who described the neuropathological changes in the brains of patients with this dementia. Unlike kuru, it occurs throughout the world, but it is relatively rare, compared with Alzheimer's disease. To date there is no evidence that Alzheimer's disease can be transmitted directly from human to human or from human to animal. However, there are clinical similarities between Alzheimer's disease and Creutzfeldt-Jakob disease, and some scientists have used these similarities as a rationale for looking for a possible viral cause for Alzheimer's disease.

There have been a few reports of Creutzfeldt-Jakob and Alzheimer's diseases occurring together in the same individual. Furthermore, Creutzfeldt-Jakob and Alzheimer's diseases have occurred in the same family. Both of these observations have been used as evidence for the view that these two brain disorders are related.

Overlap of Alzheimer's Disease with Vascular Dementia

A number of cerebrovascular diseases cause vascular lesions that impair cognitive functioning, and affected persons are diagnosed with vascular dementia or multi-infarct dementia. Vascular dementia is not a specific disease but a syndrome with many clinical symptoms and many causes. About 15 to 20 percent of all dementias in the older population are caused by vascular dementia, although the proportion is higher in other parts of the world. For example, in Sweden it accounts for over 45 percent of all dementias.

Another 15 percent of patients have what is called a *mixed dementia*, that is, a combination of Alzheimer's disease and a vascular dementia. As people are living longer with Alzheimer's disease, a certain group is at risk for developing vascular dementia as well. This suggests that there is some interplay between the pathological process for primary neuronal degenerative and cerebrovascular pathology.

Vascular Dementia

The principal cause of vascular dementia is a stroke that occurs when blood cannot get to the brain. A blood clot or fat deposits can block the vessels that bring blood to the brain. Strokes also occur when a blood vessel in the brain bursts. The major causes of stroke are untreated high blood pressure, diabetes, heart disease, and high blood cholesterol levels. Strokes are the second major cause of death in the United States and a leading cause of death throughout the world. Strokes do not always kill. They often cripple individuals and affect their ability to walk, talk, and carry out many activities of daily life. They also can cause dementia.

It may be helpful for our discussion to divide vascular dementia into three clinical groups. The first group includes dementia due to one or more strokes caused by the blockage of large- or medium-sized blood vessels in the brain. Large multiple infarcts do not occur as frequently as they did in the 1960s because of the success of antihypertensive drugs in preventing strokes. The second clinical group involves dementia in which the small arteries are affected, resulting in lacunar strokes. *Lacunae* is the Latin word for "holes." Lacunae are very small areas of tissue loss in the brain. In patients with multi-infarct dementia, these lacunae or infarcts are seen at autopsy. Something clogs or blocks a small artery in the brain, causing a loss of circulation beyond the blocked area. When the blood supply is cut off for a long enough time, the cells die. Individuals with a history of arrhythmias, irregular heart rhythms, may be particularly vulnerable to this type of problem.

The third form of multi-infarct disease affects the smallest blood vessels in the brain and is called microinfarct dementia. It is difficult to distinguish this disease from Alzheimer's disease. Patients are not necessarily hypertensive, they may not have heart disease or irregular heart rhythms, and their blood vessels do not show clear evidence of arteriosclerosis.

We do not fully understand the pathogenesis of vascular dementia. There are patients who can have a single major infarct and develop a progressive dementia without any other infarcts, as well as other patients who have multiple infarcts and develop dementia secondary to these infarcts. Furthermore, the amyloid angiopathy in Alzheimer's disease can lead to infarcts, especially in patients who have high blood pressure.

Although the exact cause for cerebrovascular disease is not understood, we do know a great deal about risk factors. A famous study in Framingham, Massachusetts, has helped us understand the risk factors for stroke, which are high blood pressure, impaired cardiac functioning, diabetes, high levels of cholesterol in the blood, and cigarette smoking. High blood pressure is a major culprit, found in about half of all individuals who have a stroke. The risk for stroke also increases when several cardiovascular abnormalities are present in the same individual.

Well-identified large blood vessels and many small tributaries circulate the blood throughout the brain. The pattern of these arteries and the territory of the brain that each supplies are fairly similar, though not identical, in all people. If the blood flow is interrupted in a specific artery, it usually will cause similar deficits in most individuals. Therefore, the symptoms a patient displays can indicate what part of the brain has been affected by the blockage of a particular vessel. For example, in patients with problems in speech or the use of the right hand or leg, physicians can localize the stroke to the left side of the brain and identify the areas involved, and then implicate the arteries that feed blood to those areas.

The major blood vessels, which connect the heart to the brain, are the vertebral and the carotid arteries. They emanate from the major arteries leaving the heart and travel into the neck, where they feed into the base of the brain. Many different arteries branch out from these major vessels to ensure that the blood circulates to all parts of the brain. Some arteries branch deep into the interior of the brain as well as to the outside of the brain. Arteriosclerosis, or the narrowing of the arteries, is one of the most conspicuous changes in the blood vessels of the brain. The vessels may be blocked because of the buildup of foreign material or fat droplets. If the arteriosclerosis is severe, the artery will even have a yellow color.

Aneurysms are another cause of cerebrovascular disease. Aneurysms appear as small balloons or blisters in the blood vessels where the vascular wall has become thinned. If they break, blood flows into the brain, damaging brain tissue and sometimes even causing death. Such a bursting also interrupts the flow of blood beyond the rupture and leads to starvation of the affected brain tissue. Aneurysms are often fatal.

The blood supply can be interrupted permanently when a stroke occurs. When the artery is blocked, the area of the brain that the artery usually supplies becomes impaired and surrounding areas also become swollen. Strokes usually occur rapidly and are generally painless. Many happen during sleep. Some occur over several days and may be accompanied by a headache. If the individual survives, the worst deficits are seen between the third and tenth days after a stroke because the brain swelling is worst at this time. Most people with strokes recover some lost functioning, because with time the swelling subsides and circulation from other vessels supplies some of the areas affected. However, the areas of dead tissue remain as scars, and their functions are lost.

Transient Ischemic Attacks

Several other forms of cerebrovascular disease may be early warning signs of an impending stroke. The word *ischemia* means "without blood," and *transient ischemic attacks*, sometimes called *TIAs* by physicians, are conditions in which the blood supply in the brain is interrupted briefly. They are a sign that there may be arteriosclerosis in the brain's blood vessels. Sometimes these attacks can be caused by a change in the heart rhythm or by a brief drop in blood pressure. During a TIA, persons temporarily lose their ability to function. They may even lose consciousness and often do not remember what happened. After several minutes they usually can function again but may not feel quite like themselves for another day. Over time these attacks may become more frequent. Without treatment about 25 percent of all people with TIAs develop a serious stroke within a year.

The Future

The new millennium promises to be a period of revolutionary scientific advances in many areas, including the brain sciences. Some day scientists from many disciplines will discover the genetic, molecular, and cellular mechanisms that lead to Alzheimer's disease and related disorders. It also follows that these discoveries will lead to the development of new drugs and new drug combinations to treat and prevent the dementias of later life. We can hope for new drugs that can replace neurotransmitters as well as drugs that are neuroprotective agents, such as antioxidants, anti-inflammatory drugs, antiamyloid agents, glutamatergic agents, calcium channel blockers, and nerve growth factors.

Research into the causes of Alzheimer's disease can be enhanced significantly by the use of the specialized methods of a science called *epidemiology* to study the occurrence of the disease, the exposure of affected persons to specific risk factors, and clinical patterns. The epidemiological approach was a powerful tool in the study of smoking as a risk factor for cancer and heart disease. The process of identifying risk factors as well as specific variables and conditions associated with heightened risk to a disease creates new ways of thinking about the biological basis of the disease as well as intervention and prevention strategies.

A number of risk factors are implicated in the cause(s) of Alzheimer's disease. Age and genetic background are the strongest putative factors. Considerable evidence suggests that the following are important risk factors, but not all scientists agree: a high-fat meat diet, smoking, a sedentary lifestyle, head trauma, advanced age of mother, cardiovascular disease, depression, and the infrequent use of nonsteroidal anti-inflammatory drugs. Controversial risk factors include low educational attainment, poor linguistic ability, head circumference, and seizure history. With continuing research we are likely to improve our predictive models and discover new insights.

15

The Cost of Caring

Caring is expensive financially as well as emotionally over the course of the illness. Persons with Alzheimer's disease have the same physical health problems as others of their age, but because of the progressive cognitive impairment, they have a range of special needs, including comprehensive diagnostic services, expensive medications, and a range of community-based long-term-care programs. Many home and community services are not always available, and they are usually expensive if not supported by the community publicly or through private agencies. Assisted living facilities, with very rare exceptions, must be paid for by the patient or family, at a cost of $2,000 to $6,000 a month, and nursing-home care can cost $3,500 to $6,500 a month.

Families caring for relatives with dementia often find that the out-of-pocket costs cut into family savings, reduce resources allocated for future plans, and ultimately erode financial security and quality of life. Managing financially is a daunting challenge for those on limited incomes who cannot afford necessities, let alone health care, drugs, day care, home care, as well as assisted living and nursing-home care. However, you can take a number of steps to plan for your estate, for long-term-care needs, and for incapacity, a time when the dementia will compromise personal, financial, and health care decisions.

The cost of caring for dementia patients has to be placed in the context of a larger economic and social picture. The total amount spent on health care in this country, as well as in many other countries in the world, has been increasing steadily and significantly. For example, in the United States health care expenditures on the older population have consistently surpassed the gross domestic product by 4 percent per year, and the costs continue to rise. Thus, our country will continue to be challenged by the affordability of medical care in the future, and the political choices we make will affect our quality of life and productivity.

Medicare and Medicaid have become the largest expenditures in federal and state budgets, respectively. And despite government efforts to limit cost escalations, these expenditures continue to increase as a result of an escalation in technology, expensive medications, the growth of an older, sicker population, the increased hospital costs and salaries of health care workers, and other factors. In this era of escalating health costs, the responsibility for patients with dementia places a special financial burden on the family. Government programs and private insurance together typically do not cover the types of care these patients need, and many managed care organizations have been particularly unfriendly to patients trying to get examinations and treatment for dementia.

As new approaches to health care financing and delivery are proposed in the future, families need to become educated advocates for policy changes to meet their health needs. Widespread pressure for limits on health expenditures and cutbacks in health care may further jeopardize the already restricted availability of health care for dementia victims. Indeed, recent cuts in federal support have been associated with a burgeoning number of bankruptcies of long-term-care facilities as well as refusals by many health maintenance organizations (HMOs) to take Medicare–eligible patients into their programs.

Overview of the Economics of Health Care: Why Dementia Care Is Not Covered

A brief overview of relevant health financing issues and the history of health insurance in the United States may help explain why dementia patients have been excluded. For every complicated problem, H. L. Mencken once remarked, there is a simple solution, and that solution is invariably wrong. The financing of health care is very complicated. However, at the risk of oversimplification, we will try to explain it as clearly as possible.

Payment systems for health care in the United States can be divided into four categories: (1) care of the aged, (2) care of the poor, (3) care of the worker, and (4) care of everyone else. This simply means that we do not have one but several financing strategies for the country, and financing of health care services for older persons and the poor is different from that for the rest of the population. Prior to 1965 health insurance was a private matter between the patient and health care provider. Many patients and families had health insurance, usually related to their jobs, and therefore the unemployed were typically uninsured. To address the problem of the uninsured, nonwealthy retired, and other unemployed individuals, Medicare was established in 1965 to pay for certain medical services for persons sixty-five years and older. Soon thereafter Medicaid was introduced to pay for the needs of the poor and disabled.

The concept of public health insurance was first introduced in Germany in 1883 to meet the needs of a population whose major problems arose from childbirth complications, accidents, trauma, tuberculosis, and other infectious diseases, but public pressure for health insurance coverage did not build in the United States until the 1900s. While there were repeated efforts in Congress to introduce some form of national health insurance, there was strong opposition from organized provider groups that feared this would lead to the socialization of medicine under federal control.

In this context, private health insurance soon became very popular. The introduction of Blue Cross in 1929 to cover hospital bills, and later of Blue Shield to pay physician fees, made health insurance available to younger people through their jobs. Work-related group plans became widespread largely as a result of the demands of labor unions for more and better benefits. In 1945 some 25 percent of the U.S. population was covered, and after World War II private insurance companies aggressively followed Blue Cross's lead to market primarily union or employer-sponsored plans as well as coverage for those wealthy enough to buy individual insurance. It was clear that private health insurance was available to the middle and upper working classes and not to those who were poor, unable to work, and old.

A wide variety of work-related health care plans became available and still exist today. The employer usually pays a major part of the health policy premium and receives substantial tax benefits for doing so. In many instances employees have options about the kind of plan they can purchase. Benefits and costs vary in different policies. In addition to Blue Cross, Blue Shield, and similar indemnity plans, the choice of health care coverage now includes participation in HMOs. These are group plans in which premiums are prepaid to the provider, who then provides services at no cost or for a nominal copayment to doctors and hospitals. Indemnity plans typically pay the provider of care for the services actually rendered.

Health insurance plans provide different levels of financial coverage for outpatient visits to a doctor's office or clinic as well as for inpatient or in-hospital care. With few exceptions, insurance plans cover the major portion of the cost of acute care. Acute care is an important concept, referring to medical services for sudden and relatively short-term illnesses or operations. Insurance plans make a clear distinction between acute-care conditions and long-term-care or chronic conditions.

The benefit schedule in some plans may exclude conditions and diseases that existed before the policy was purchased, whereas in others a higher premium is imposed. Most plans accept all new employees and their dependents as part of the group coverage. Regardless of the medical plan, the insurance pays the doctor, the hospital, or the patient for expenses associated with acute illnesses of relatively brief durations.

Some policies offer what is known as a *catastrophic illness supplement* for a small surcharge, or individuals may purchase a separate catastrophic insurance policy and add it to their regular medical coverage. Catastrophic insurance pays for specific conditions like cancer and stroke that may require long periods of expensive care with special nursing and rehabilitation programs. Unfortunately, most of these programs do not provide the type of care needed by patients with dementia, and none that we know of assist the family in the day-to-day problems of managing the patient.

In recent years commercial companies have introduced long-term-care insurance. This pays for nursing-home care and in many instances for home-based care, if the patient would qualify for a nursing home but the family prefers to care for the patient at home with outside help. These policies may have high deductibles and a waiting period after they are purchased before the policy will pay benefits. Such plans are worth examining but typically need to be bought prior to the diagnosis and with a clear understanding of the coverage. With the expectation that one in four or five persons over age sixty-five will need some nursing-home care during their lifetime, it would be prudent to evaluate this option. A number of insurance companies have long-term-care insurance products, and the AARP provides resource materials to judge the value of the different long-term-care insurance products available.

Medicaid

Medicaid is a public assistance program in which the federal government contributes funds to match state dollars for medical assistance to individuals otherwise unable to afford such care. Although the Medicaid program is quite large, limitations on eligibility have kept many poor people from receiving Medicaid benefits. Estimates are that perhaps up to two-thirds of the nation's poor are ineligible because of the way state requirements are worded. The federal government established only basic guidelines for the implementation of the program by defining who was "categorically needy." The original intent was to make it possible for even the poorest states to offer medical assistance through the matching program.

Medicaid policies vary from state to state as do eligibility and benefits. The best place to find up-to-date information is to consult an elder law attorney in your area (see Appendix 2 for information on the National Academy of Elder Law Attorneys, Inc. or consult your yellow pages). Eligibility for Medicaid is determined by a means test—a ceiling is placed on the maximum earnings and other assets that individuals and certain dependents may have in order to qualify for assistance. Eligibility levels vary according to the size of family, the number of dependents in the household, benefits available from other sources (such as the Department of Veterans Affairs, union or pension funds, and unemployment insurance), and the income of one's spouse or in some states, the income of children living in the state.

Benefits refer to the type of help and services available under a health insurance plan. A key feature of Medicaid, important for the family caring for a relative with dementia, is the nursing-home benefit. Medicaid,

394 The Loss of Self

not Medicare, pays for long-term skilled nursing care. In some states Medicaid even pays for home- and community-based services for patients who are medically certified for home care, since they would otherwise be in a hospital or skilled nursing home. Because Medicaid is means-tested, long-term benefits are paid for those who are medically indigent, while those with resources have to pay out-of-pocket for their care.

Two tests must be passed to establish eligibility in most states: medical need with disabilities and financial need. *Medical need* refers to impaired personal functioning such that the person requires twenty-four-hour skilled nursing care, assessment, care planning, and monitoring by a registered nurse; care is needed daily; and care needs are not normally provided by a hospital. Determination of financial need is complicated and depends on state laws. Some states use a cap on income to determine eligibility, and others use the monthly income to compute the amount of the benefit. You should consult with attorneys in your state.

Since an individual's assets include savings, certain insurance benefits, and home and property equity (after the primary residence of a spouse is excluded), many families with even small or modest incomes may find that they initially are not eligible for nursing-home Medicaid benefits. A person's monthly gross income must not exceed a cap (which was $1,500 in 1999). Medicare Part B premium deductions from Social Security or withholdings from pensions for taxes are not considered. Furthermore, the income of the spouse is not considered. A nursing-home patient with a gross monthly income over the cap and who owns certain assets can qualify for nursing-home care by using an attorney to establish an irrevocable qualified income trust. The trust consists of only the individual's income in excess of the monthly cap as well as the earnings on the income.

Medicaid was intended to allow the poor and the poor aged to receive health care from the same medical care system as the population with higher incomes. However, many providers discriminate against Medicaid patients. Although benefits are paid directly to hospitals and doctors, the payments are usually less than the usual or "customary" private rates for the same services. These payment rates are determined by states in accordance with local and regional economics. The current trend in most states is to tighten up eligibility and reduce the scope of benefits whenever possible. This comes with increased administrative and regulatory costs, and providers respond accordingly by reducing amenities, cutting personal costs, and overscheduling patients.

Medicaid also was intended primarily to carry the burden of paying for the acute medical care of the poor younger patient. However, because of the way Medicare was structured, to meet only the acute-care needs of the aged, and because of the paucity of private insurance for long-term care in the United States at that time, Medicaid has become the principal payer for long-term institutional care in the United States. Approximately half of the cost of nursing-home care is paid by Medicaid. Only 2 percent is paid by Medicare and about 1 percent by private insurance. About half of long-term-care costs are still being paid by families who often spend their assets to become eligible for Medicaid, which will pay the long-term-care benefit at a reduced rate.

An attorney's counsel is essential in the analysis of your assets and planning. Transferring assets to others to become eligible for Medicaid can be a problem. Legislation makes it a crime only if there is a period of ineligibility in your state. An example of an ineligiblity period is a provision that assets cannot be transferred within thirty-six months of entering a nursing home. If you plan appropriately with your lawyer and do not apply for benefits during an ineligibility period, you will be working within the law.

While it seems cruel for individuals entering long-term-care institutions to pay private rates until they have "spent down" to a level of indigency that makes them eligible for Medicaid support, it is important to remember that the Medicaid program was specifically designed to provide care for those who were poor. Federal legislation creating Medicare Part C programs of long-term-care benefits, largely eliminating the need to spend one's assets, has been proposed but never enacted by Congress.

The average cost of nursing-home care is now between $3,500 and $6,500 per month or more. When personal funds run out, the patient and spouse may apply to the state welfare department to receive Medicaid. This is a complicated procedure and a substantial number of patients need Medicaid. As a result, it often takes a long time to process the application.

Since Medicaid was created to provide a range of health benefits for the poor, it covers a wider range of problems than Medicare does. However, it was never envisioned to be so heavily involved in long-term care.

The result is that the majority of Medicaid funds in many states are paid out in long-term-care benefits, creating competition in funding for children, families, persons with disabilities, as well as the spectrum of out-patient and acute hospital care. Although matching funds are available from the federal government, states control their costs by limiting the state contribution. And even though they pay only half of the cost, the economic and political pressures for competitive use of state dollars is high.

Patients without financial means have a difficult time getting admitted into nursing homes. Some lower-middle-class families are particularly vulnerable. In many states, nursing-home beds are not readily available because the state also controls the number of nursing-home beds, a mechanism to reduce access and save money. Since Medicaid pays less than the private rate for care, and since Medicaid rates are often lower than the actual cost of the care provided by the facility, individuals who own or run nursing homes argue that they can provide quality care only by "averaging out" the income derived from a balance of private and Medicaid patients.

Medicare

Congress enacted Medicare legislation in 1965 to make older Americans eligible for health care benefits. It is not widely known that Medicare was designed to reduce the financial burden of older persons on their families by paying the cost of needed acute and expensive medical or hospital care, including surgery. Congress clearly intended to avoid dealing with the financial burden of long-term care, and therefore Medicare was never designed to cover long-term care. Medicare was modeled after health care plans for middle-aged workers and therefore only provided very limited nursing-home benefits. There was also great concern about the open-ended nature of long-term care and a precise definition of what custodial or medical benefits would be expected. As a result, benefits for two types of illnesses associated with chronic care, tuberculosis and mental illness, were severely limited. Benefits were also defined in such a way as to apply only to episodes or "bouts" of acute illness, not chronic disease or long-term institutional care.

As a result of remarkable medical advances, tuberculosis has largely been eliminated as a major problem requiring long-term care in sanatoriums, and these institutions have faded from the scene. Mental health care has been more complex. Medications like the antipsychotic drugs have been remarkably successful in reducing the state hospital population because patients can be treated in the community. Since community outpatient care is often not available to the chronically mentally ill, many become homeless or live in nursing homes or shelters. These costs also are paid largely by Medicaid or not at all.

With Medicare as with most private insurance coverage, the patient or family has to pay certain costs. These out-of-pocket costs are called *deductibles*. Medicare also pays for in-hospital care for up to 60 days in a semiprivate room. After 60 days, however, another deductible payment is charged to the patient. There is a provision that after 90 days one may draw against a lifetime allotment of 60 days. During this period a larger deductible is levied. Although such a long hospital stay may be rare, it can happen. Finally, after 150 days Medicare pays nothing. And if a person must go into a long-term-care facility, Medicare will pay only for certain types of skilled nursing care, not for management or custodial care. Therefore, it predictably pays only 2 percent of the long-term-care bills in the United States per year.

Part A of Medicare pays for hospital benefits; physicians' services are covered by a separate Medicare provision, Part B. However, Part B requires the payment of a small monthly premium. After an initial deductible, Medicare pays 80 percent of the amount determined to be reasonable by Medicare authorities. If the doctor accepts this assignment, the patient may still need to pay 20 percent of the bill. However, some doctors do not accept assignment because they feel that the long delay in payment, the amount and complexity of the paperwork involved, the low fee schedule, and the intrusion into patient records make assignment a poor strategy. The federal government, on the other hand, regards assignment as a mechanism to ensure access to care as well as to monitor costs to detect fraud, abuse, and unnecessary procedures.

If the doctor does not accept assignment, you may bill Medicare for the Part B payment on the basis of proof of payment or billing to the doctor, but you will still have to cover out-of-pocket the difference between the physician's actual fee and that deemed reasonable by Medicare.

Although there is increasing governmental pressure on physicians and hospitals to control rates and generate universal agreement to accept assignment, it is important to find out early whether your physician does or does not accept assignment.

The complex pattern of Medicare deductibles and Part A/Part B costs has given rise to new private insurance policies, coinsurance, to pay for the deductible portions of Part A and/or Part B. These policies have also come to be known as *Medigap insurance* because they can play a valuable role in filling "gaps" in the insurance coverage for the aged. While this is worth examining, the buyer must be very cautious. Unfortunately, some individuals and companies promote Medigap insurance that is worthless. The language disguises the fact that the coverage it offers duplicates that of Medicare. These policies are often sold by a high-pressure salesperson who frightens older persons or their families into believing that multiple insurance policies are needed. Medigap fraud has been estimated to deprive older persons of billions of dollars per year in premiums for worthless policies.

Although acute episodes of illness in the older patient with dementia are often covered, long-term care and family services are not reimbursed under current Medicare guidelines. Furthermore, Medicare does not pay for special diets, eyeglasses, dentures, hearing aids, or medications. To inquire about Medicare benefits and to apply, call or write your local Social Security office. Each region also has a private contractor like Blue Cross or another private insurance company that acts as the local intermediary for the federal government in handling claims. If you are homebound, you may complete the application over the telephone or send a representative to the office. Once you have qualified for Medicare and visit the doctor, it is important that you and the doctor fill out the Medicare forms correctly. Before you receive a treatment from your doctor, ask what she or he charges. Since Medicare pays only a certain amount of the charges, individuals may be responsible for the additional costs.

Several Medicare terms are important to understand. A *beneficiary* is a person who receives Medicare. The *deductible* is the money you must pay before you can be covered by Medicare. *Premiums* are monthly payments that you must make in order to receive Medicare if you do not qualify for Social Security. *Copayment* is the payment necessary to receive service under Medicare Part B. *Carriers* are organizations that process the claims for physicians' fees and services under Part B. Finally, the *Medicare-approved* amounts are the charges determined by the Medicare carrier in each local area. Each July 1, new approved fee levels are established. The maximum amount Medicare will pay is 80 percent of the approved fee.

Medicare Supplemental Policies

If you can afford to do so, you should supplement your Medicare coverage because it pays less than half of the average bill. There are several places you can contact for information on Medicare supplemental insurance. Two federal publications are updated every year. *Your Medicare Handbook* is published by the Health Care Financing Administration (HCFA) and the Social Security Administration (SSA). The second, titled *Guide to Health Insurance for People with Medicare*, is published by the HCFA and the National Association of Insurance Commissioners (NAIC). You can obtain both of these from your local Social Security office or your state insurance department. The guidebook *How to Use Private Health Insurance with Medicare* is available from the Health Insurance Association of America (1850 K Street, N.W., Washington, DC 20006). Finally, since many state insurance departments have their own guidebook, you can write them for a copy. The address should be included in the state listings in the phone book. Not only will they probably have the most up-to-date information, but also some state insurance departments will tell you which companies have had complaints filed against them.

There are a series of specific questions you can ask as you compare supplemental policies. In addition to going through the checklist below, you should consult *Best's Insurance Reports*, a highly regarded reference work available in most libraries that rates the financial solvency of most insurance companies from A+ to C. You should consider only companies with an A or A+ rating. Blue Cross and Blue Shield plans are not rated but would qualify for an A rating.

- What is the annual premium you must pay? You must be the judge of the quality of the policies and decide what you can afford.
- Does the premium increase as you get older? Some policies have a

single premium regardless of age, whereas others automatically charge
more as you get older.

- Does the policy repay the initial deductible of Part A?
- Does it repay Part A copayments for days 61 to 90 and reserve days?
- Are there Part A benefits beyond 150 days?
- Does it repay Part A copayments for nursing-care days 21 to 100?
- Does it repay Part A copayments for nursing-care days 101 to 365?
- Does the policy repay the Part B deductible?
- What percentage of the provider's charge is paid?
- Does the policy provide benefits that cover the actual cost or only
  the Medicare-approved charge?
- What is the maximum benefit from Part B charges? What is the pol-
  icy's deductible?
- Does the policy cover expenses for pre-existing medical conditions?
  The maximum period a company can make you wait for coverage to
  begin is six months, but many policies have shorter waiting periods.
- What are the conditions for renewal of the policy? The best desig-
  nation is "guaranteed renewable," which means that the company
  cannot cancel your policy if you pay your premiums. Although this
  is not an option with most Blue Cross and Blue Shield plans, officials
  of Blue Cross and Blue Shield have said they would never cancel
  Medicare supplemental policies.
- What items covered by the policy are *not covered* by Medicare?
- Can you get a rider for optional coverage?

If you do not have Medicare supplemental insurance, you should evaluate your ability to purchase a policy, but only one. Examine the policies carefully, using our checklist of questions, and weigh your options
carefully. Even when you have only small medical expenses, the difference between policies in payments for benefits may be hundreds of dollars. When you have large medical bills, the difference in payments may
be substantial, in the thousands of dollars. Many of the best plans have
been issued by Blue Cross and Blue Shield organizations. Although they
may not be the ideal plans in all regions, it is useful to use them as a
standard to judge other policies.

What are the alternatives to a Medicare supplemental policy? Alternatives include Medicaid, continuation of your work group coverage in-

stead of an individual policy, major medical insurance, and HMOs. If you qualify for Medicaid, do not buy Medicare supplemental policies. Long before your retirement you should investigate whether your work group insurance plan continues benefits after age sixty-five and whether the premium changes. Check with your benefits department. If your group policy can be converted to an individual one, compare it with the supplemental policies, using the checklist.

Major medical insurance is intended to cover large medical bills. In many parts of the United States it is almost impossible for individuals sixty-five and older to acquire major medical insurance. If it is available, the premium may be very high. It also may not cover the Medicare deductibles and copayments. If it does, the premium may be even higher. If major medical insurance is available, examine the costs and benefits very carefully. You may wish to purchase only catastrophic coverage for major bills, an option that may keep the premium low.

Health Maintenance Organizations (Medicare HMOs)

The federal government now supports the provision of Medicare benefits for eligible persons who agree to sign over their Medicare benefits to the HMO. The rate given the HMO is based on the average cost of benefits the federal government would expect to pay for the Medicare population, discounted for volume. Once signed up, the Medicare HMO member is subject to the rules of the HMO that will manage the health care service. Your choice of physicians may be limited, as well as your access to specialists and laboratory, imaging, or other diagnostic studies and the facilities used for full or partial hospitalization. Treatment approaches may also be controlled. Physicians may be required to substitute certain medications for less expensive alternatives, and surgeries may be reviewed before approval is given or denied. In short, the HMO plan in question will determine all aspects of health care for which money is required.

HMOs need to be evaluated with great care. They may provide preventive services such as free flu shots, but some may deny important benefits for the care of the patient with dementia, including diagnostic procedures, access to specialists for the treatment and management of dementia, and the use of newer medications. Copayments may be lower or eliminated entirely. Our advice is to examine the HMO option but make your choices carefully! Check out the performance of the HMO, its reputation, state data on violations, and other resources you can access. Discuss this with your physicians. Ask them if they are on the HMO roster, and if not, why not.

Once you assign your Medicare rights to an HMO, it may be a year before you can return to the regular Medicare program. Talk with neighbors and friends. Remember too, the nice person going door-to-door even with a white coat and stethoscope, the friendly individual staffing a table at a shopping mall, and the celebrity on television are there to sell you a product, and as in all sales *caveat emptor*—let the buyer beware!

Legal and Financial Issues Confronting the Family

Complex legal and financial issues face patients and their families. A great deal can be done to help individuals make wise decisions about their personal well-being, property, and other assets, but it is important to begin planning as soon as possible after the diagnosis of Alzheimer's disease is made. In addition to giving families adequate time for deliberate discussions, beginning early will help ensure that individuals suffering from dementia will not be deprived of the right to determine what will happen to them or their assets.

Most people are resistant to planning for when they might be incapacitated by injury or illness, and this is even more difficult for families dealing with dementia. It is too easy to procrastinate and not deal with an unpleasant future of deterioration and ultimately death. It is probably the last thing anyone in the family wants to do. However, the planning can make a great difference, and a failure to plan is a plan for failure.

We review six alternatives in this section: (1) assistance with no legal responsibility, (2) power of attorney, (3) durable power of attorney, (4) living trust, (5) health care surrogate, and (6) nomination of a guardian or conservator. The information presented here is intended to help you understand the various options available, but it is not to be considered a substitute for sound legal advice. Laws vary from state to state, and only lawyers knowledgeable about elder law issues such as asset protection, estate planning, and Medicaid benefits are aware of the legal alternatives in your area. Furthermore, legal arrangements need to be tailored to the individual's specific circumstances. However, regardless of the legal mechanisms used, some amount of control over the patient's assets should be given to someone who is trusted—a family member, a friend, or an institution.

Financial and Personal Assistance without Legal Responsibility

Early in the illness, family members may help the patient manage money and assets without assuming legal power. This usually works well when the individual is minimally impaired. At least once a month, sit down with your relative to go over bills, pay them, and balance the checkbook. It may be necessary to meet on other occasions to review more complicated issues, such as Internal Revenue Service (IRS) forms, financial portfolios, and investments.

Monthly sessions provide the mechanism for discussing longer-term solutions when the patient becomes more incapacitated. This approach gives everyone time to consider options. It also acknowledges your respect for the patient and your desire to involve him or her in preparations for the future. The transition to other legal solutions may be managed more easily if the patient is involved in these discussions over time. However, this may not always be possible if you wait too long and your relative develops significant cognitive deficits.

Power of Attorney

Power of attorney is one recourse for relatives when the patient is becoming too impaired to handle many of his or her financial tasks. It allows the individual to delegate certain powers to someone else, called the *attorney-in-fact*. In this situation the individual patient, called the *principal*, is stating in essence that although he or she could handle his or her own financial affairs, it is more convenient to let someone else handle them. The document must exactly specify what legal and financial responsibilities are being transferred. In reality, the attorney-in-fact may have very limited or very broad control over the patient's assets.

Power of attorney may be a valuable mechanism for assuming more control as needed over the patient's assets. It is a way for the individual to gradually relinquish control over an area he or she has managed successfully for many years. It leaves the patient the dignity of deciding what control he or she wishes to delegate to others. However, the general power of attorney has a serious flaw when planning for incapacity at some future time. The law considers that a power of attorney is automatically withdrawn when an individual is incapacitated. The durable power of attorney, described next, continues to function despite the incapacity of the person who granted it.

Durable Power of Attorney

In some states the patient can sign a document for durable power of attorney. A durable power of attorney is more restrictive than a power of attorney document. In order for a durable power of attorney to be legal, the patient must sign the document while he or she still has substantial mental capacity and must also designate who is the holder of the durable power of attorney. The person who holds a durable power of attorney stands in for and acts for the patient. Said person can write a check and sign his or her name to draw money from accounts as well as buy or sell property or stocks on the patient's behalf. In essence, the person who holds the durable power of attorney can legally do anything the patient can do.

The patient may give the power to two or more people and require that they act together as coholders. This has some protective value if the patient does not entirely trust one person. The holder or coholders control the patient's resources, but the papers can be written so that the holders must follow specific guidelines set forth by the patient. The papers can designate that the holder(s) get(s) the power of durable attorney immediately or only when two or more people, such as family members, clergy, or physician, say in writing that the individual has lost mental capacity.

The legal holder can make decisions about the patient's financial assets and living arrangements, including the right to sign checks or legal documents. Initially, the durable power of attorney document should specify exactly what the holder can do, from being able to open a safe-deposit box to managing stocks and bonds. If the holder goes not handle the individual's assets properly, a court may revoke the power if a trusted party objects.

There are several types of durable powers of attorney—a *durable power of attorney for persons* and a *durable power of attorney for property management.* Durable power of attorney for property does not give the holder legal rights over persons. Therefore, if a patient refuses to go to a nursing home and is not manageable at home, the holder cannot place him or her in an institution against his or her will. This requires what is technically called a *durable power of attorney for health care*, which allows the holder to make many health care decisions for the patient. This document can be written so that the holder can consent to diagnostic and treatment services, make decisions to halt the use of life-support machines when necessary, and decide whether to donate the patient's brain or other organs to research.

The holder of durable power of attorney for health care has the legal obligation to follow whatever wishes or preferences the patient made known before he or she lost mental capacity. Thus, the patient's preferences for medical treatment and placement can be written into the durable power of attorney document. The same individual may be the holder of durable power of attorney for person, property management, and health care. It is important for the patient to also identify who should become the holder if the original designee dies or cannot function in that capacity.

Living Trust

In certain situations, living trusts are set up to handle assets in an acceptable way that avoids estate taxes after an individual dies. A living trust is similar in some ways to a durable power of attorney. The patient signs a document known as a *trust instrument* or *trust agreement*, prepared by an attorney to specify the patient's wishes about how his or her property is to be used during the patient's life as well as after death. The patient usually chooses a family member, a trusted friend, or an institution such as a bank to be the "trustee." The patient should also designate a backup, in the event the first trustee dies or cannot continue.

In creating a living trust, the patient signs a paper that gives the trustee title to the patient's assets. This means that the trustee is the "technical" owner of the assets, while the patient remains the "real" owner of the assets and their benefits. The document reflects exactly how the patient's assets are to be used. Trustees risk a lawsuit and penalties if they do not respect the patient's wishes.

A trust can be written in such a way that the patient can revoke it at any time, or it can be written so that it is revocable only until the patient loses mental capacity. The trustee does not have any control over the patient's "person." Therefore, the trustee will not be able to institutionalize the patient unless he or she agrees to go into a nursing home. This is true even if the patient has lost the capacity to know what he or she is doing.

Health Care Surrogate

A health care surrogate is similar to a durable power of attorney for health care. However, a durable power of attorney becomes effective upon signing the document. A health care surrogate designation only becomes effective when the patient cannot express his or her wishes for treatment. Early in the disease the patient should be able to determine what choices he or she wishes, including end-of-life care. Various states have laws that suggest a hierarchy of persons who can make decisions for the patient.

Guardianship or Conservatorship

A guardianship or conservatorship is a serious step for families to take. Although state regulations differ, it always involves a legal procedure. The results of medical tests must be presented in court, and on the basis of the evidence, the court will decide whether a guardian or conservator will be appointed. A family member or close friend must file a petition with the court requesting a hearing. The judge reads and hears evidence to determine whether a guardianship or conservatorship is necessary. Close family members are notified about the hearing, and they may support or object to the petition.

Generally, a guardianship or conservatorship of estate is designed to control and manage all the patient's finances. However, under new laws the patient may retain control over certain financial matters, such as an allowance or the right to make a will deemed valid by the court. The guardian or conservator controls the patient's assets and must use them for the patient's benefit. A guardian or conservator of the state is appointed if the patient is shown to be unable to manage his or her finances or if the patient requests one and demonstrates a good cause, such as Alzheimer's disease. More than one person or an agency can be appointed to serve as "co-conservators" of the patient.

The conservator is expected to protect the patient's assets and usually must file an account of all financial transactions with the court at the end of the first year of the conservatorship and every two years thereafter. The report must show the patient's assets and document all transactions made by the conservator on behalf of the patient.

A conservator of the patient's person could be appointed if the patient becomes unmanageable and abusive at home and must be placed in a nursing home. Even if the patient wants to be released, the nursing home can legally keep him or her if the patient's conservator placed him or her in the home. However, the patient retains the right to maintain state residence, to marry, and to give medical consent in non-life-threatening emergencies unless the court decides otherwise. The courts usually appoint the same individual as conservator of the estate and person. A conservator of person is appointed only when the individual is unable to provide for his or her personal needs.

Get Legal Help

Remember, laws governing these various protective services differ among the states. Legal advice is necessary. When you do not have an attorney, check the phone book for listings of elder law attorneys or contact your local area agency or commission on aging. Most have a legal office or can refer you to knowledgeable attorneys in your community.

Health Policy Issues Confronting the Family

As the disease progresses, the cost of medical care, home health attendants, and other supportive services can become prohibitive. If and when assisted living placement or institutionalization occurs, the costs may reach well over $40,000 a year. Until a time when long-term-care health insurance is widely available at affordable premiums, the health care costs for patients with dementia will continue to threaten all but the wealthiest of families. One of the greatest challenges facing our country and others around the world is to find ways to provide and pay for the long-term health care needs of the impaired aged. While we have focused on the U.S. health care scene, the growth of an aging population and their care needs is a global problem. Many countries are addressing health care for the aged, including those with dementia, in different ways. All are grappling with a greater proportion of persons with dementia and other chronic conditions than we have ever seen in the history of humankind.

Patients with dementia rely much more on their families than on formal medical services. Indeed, families carry this enormous burden with little help from anyone. At the moment, many areas of the country do not have the community- or hospital-based services that families need to help them care for the patient at home (see Chapter 8). And where these programs are available, families normally must pay the costs out-of-pocket since Medicare does not reimburse for them.

Families usually care for their relatives at home until their emotional and financial resources are exhausted. Although relatives will swear they will never surrender a loved one to an assisted living residence or nursing home, sickness, desperation, inability to manage, and exhaustion often force the decision. Many, unfortunately, regard the move as a defeat rather than as an appropriate decision to provide the best care for the patient as the patient's needs increase. When family members place relatives in a nursing home, they become involuntary members of a large group of Americans. In 1996 there were over 1.6 million nursing-home beds in the United States, and that number is expected to grow every year. Of the 1.6 million nursing-home patients it is estimated that at least half have Alzheimer's disease, and perhaps another 300,000 have dementia caused by strokes or other brain disorders.

Why has Medicare failed to provide for older persons who need long-term care? The answer is simple. Our health care system was developed primarily to meet the needs of our young and middle-aged population with acute illnesses and disorders that can be diagnosed, treated, and cured in a short period of time. However, recent changes in the age structure of our population have led to the emergence of a different disease pattern. The aged are now the fastest-growing segment of the population, and chronic illnesses are much more common among the older old.

Chronic diseases are by definition not curable, although they are treatable and manageable, and Medicare does not pay for most of the services involved in treating chronic illness. For patients with Alzheimer's disease, much of the care needed is not primarily medical. Usually, a combination of physical and social assistance, emotional support, cognitive-rehabilitation efforts, family support, and occasional medical intervention are helpful. Except for the last, such services are disallowed by Medicare.

Until recently, policy makers have not even invested in studies on the benefits of alternatives to nursing homes such as home care, day care, respite care, and other programs. The treatment of dementia also suffers from the stigma associated with mental illness, the prevalent mythology of "senility" if you live long enough, and the belief that families have the responsibility for providing necessary care. The increasing numbers of older persons in nursing homes, many of whom have dementia, and the economic problems we face in the high cost of health care are finally forcing government officials and health care professionals alike to examine the need for reform in long-term care.

First, Medicare has enjoyed great success. If anything, the problem is that it is suffering from the success of its promise to make health care available to everyone in this country over age sixty-five without regard to age or ability to pay. Statistics all confirm that we are living longer and in better health. The problem is that we are now looking at the cost of that commitment and recognizing that we cannot or do not wish to do business in the same old way.

Although most Americans would agree that older persons should get the care they need, the changing age structure of the population, the significant health needs of the aged, and the economics of providing health services all tend to increase the need for services and associated costs. Can we afford to care for the aged? The answer is yes, but we must find a better way than the one we have at the moment.

The Challenge to the Family

Families of patients with Alzheimer's disease have a special responsibility to understand proposals for health policy changes so that they can become advocates for policies that help provide appropriate care. Initiatives are needed to examine the possible role of catastrophic insurance for Alzheimer's disease. Alternative forms of group coverage may also be possible. Special legislation should be passed to support families, through tax relief, who care for patients at home as an alternative to institution-alization. Since family care is far and away the most cost-effective way of helping patients, it should be supported and encouraged.

Social and community services as a component of a health insurance program—or prepaid group plans—should be more available to help maintain the patient at home. Such services can be preventive in nature and can help keep patients out of costly institutions. Investments in these services could lead to important savings as well as an improved quality of life for the family. Respite care (in which families caring for patients can have relief for one or two weeks with needed vacations), hospice care as an alternative to dying in isolated, high-technology hospital set-tings, trained geriatric social workers working as a team with doctors and nurses to help provide care at home, day-care centers, sheltered hous-ing, and similar social and environmental supports have all been success-ful in keeping patients out of nursing homes. Eventually, a plan to organize such community and medical services will have to be under-taken. This linking of social services and preventive care will do much to alleviate the burdens of cost and of caring. It demands only that we take on these initiatives.

Families need to be aggressive advocates to make their feelings known and to indicate where legislative and government investment is needed. Financial aid and support services to the family at home are a means of preventing illness in caregivers, and compelling evidence described else-where in this book clearly shows the stressful burden of caring.

We need to recognize that a new and special effort is required if more and more Americans are not to be pauperized or made ill while trying to care for their loved ones. Sadly, though not surprisingly, it is the families themselves who need to place these issues before the decision makers.

Selected Readings and Internet Resources

These recent references and materials have been chosen for their overall usefulness to family members and caregivers. Since there are many other excellent books available and many new ones are published each year, check with the Alzheimer's Association, your local bookstores, and the Web sites listed. In addition to information on dementia and caregiving, these references contain information about medical care, health care, nutrition, exercise regimens, and devices and appliances to compensate for impairments.

General Readings

Alzheimer's Disease Education & Referral Center. *Alzheimer's Disease: A Guide to Federal Programs*. NIH Publication No. 93-3635. Washington, DC: NIH, 1993.

Bell, Virginia, and Troxel, David. *A Best Friend's Approach to Alzheimer's Care*. Baltimore: Health Professions Press, 1997.

Castleman, Michael, Gallagher-Thompson, Dolores, and Naythons, Matthew. *There's Still a Person in There*. New York: Putnam, 2000.

Coughland, Patricia. *Facing Alzheimer's: Family Caregivers Speak*. Westminster, MD: Random House, 1993.

Davidson, Ann. *Alzheimer's: A Love Story*. New York: Birch Lane Press, 1997.

Davies, Helen, and Jensen, Michael. *Alzheimer's: The Answers You Need*. Forest Knolls, CA: Elder Books, 1998.

Dyer, Joyce. *In a Tangled Wood: An Alzheimer's Journey.* Dallas, TX: Southern Methodist University Press, 1996.

Edwards, Allen. *When Memory Fails: Helping the Alzheimer's and Dementia Patient.* New York: Putnam Press, 1994.

Hauge, John. *Heavy Snow: My Father's Disappearance into Alzheimer's.* Deerfield Beach, FL: Health Communication, 1999.

Kuhn, Daniel. *Alzheimer's Early Stages.* Alameda, CA: Hunter House Publications, 1999.

Mace, Nancy, Rabins, Peter, and McHugh, Paul. *The Thirty-Six Hour Day.* Baltimore: John Hopkins University Press, 1999.

Raymond, Florian. *Surviving Alzheimer's: A Guide for Families.* Forest Knoll, CA: Elder Books, 1994.

Rose, Larry. *Show Me the Way to Go Home.* Forest Knolls, CA: Elder Books, 1996.

Rozelle, Ron. *Into That Good Night.* New York: Farrar, Straus, and Giroux, 1998.

Sacks, Oliver. *Awakenings.* New York: E. P. Dutton, 1983.

Shanks, Lela. *Your Name Is Aujhes Hannibal Shanks: A Caregiver's Guide to Alzheimer's.* Lincoln, NE: University of Nebraska Press, 1996.

Alzheimers.com—Community message board for patients and families to interact. www.alzheimers.com

Alzheimer List and Alzheimer Digest—The list is an e-mail discussion group, and the digest sends you one message every other day with postings from previous two days. www.biostant.wust1.edu/alzheimers

Alzheimer's books and videos

www.nbn.com/people/elder/alzheimer.html

www.hicom.net/~lakesolitude/index.html

www.amazon.com

www.wellnessbooks.com

American Medical Association:

www.ama-assn.org/insight/spec_con/alzheim/alzheim.htm

Alzheimer's Disease Information: For the Patient

Just for You. Toronto, Ontario: Alzheimer's Society of Canada.

Perspectives: A Newsletter for Individuals Diagnosed with Alzheimer's Disease. La Jolla, CA: University of California–San Diego Alzheimer's Research Center.

Snyder, L. *Speaking Our Minds: Personal Reflections from Individuals with Alzheimer's*. New York: W. H. Freeman, 1999.

Activities

Cohen, Jane, and Wannamaker, Marilyn. *Expressive Arts for the Very Disabled and Handicapped for All Ages*. Springfield, IL: Charle C Thomas, 1996.

Thorsheim, Howard, and Roberts, Bruu. *I Remember When: Activity Ideas to Help People Reminisce*. Forest Knolls, CA: Elder Books, 2000.

Bibliotherapy

Bellow, Saul. *Mr. Sammler's Planet*. Greenwich, CT: Fawcett, 1971.

Coyle, Beverly. *In Troubled Waters*. New York: Penguin, 1993.

Ehrlich, Elizabeth. *Miriam's Kitchen*. New York: Penguin, 1997.

Heard, Alex. *Apocalypse Pretty Soon*. New York: W. W. Norton, 1999.

Leibovitz, Maury, and Solomon, Linda. *Legacies*. New York: Harper Perennial, 1994.

Morrison, Toni. *The Big Box*. New York: Hyperion, 1999.

Sarton, May. *Plant Dreaming Deep*. New York: W. W. Norton, 1968.

Silvermate, Sue. *Tales from My Teachers in the Alzheimer's Unit*. Milwaukee, WI: Families International, 1996.

Sparks, Nicholas. *The Notebook*. New York: Warner Vision, 1996.

Caregivers

Batuik, Tom. *Safe Return: An Inspirational Book for Caregivers of Alzheimer's*. Kansas City, MO: Andrews McMeel Publications, 1998.

Baurys, Florence. *A Time for Alzheimers*. Houston, TX: Emerald Ink Publications, 1998.

Berman, Claire. *Caring for Yourself and Caring for Your Aging Parents*. New York: Holt, 1997.

Cohen, Donna, and Eisdorfer, Carl. *Caring for Your Aging Parents: A Planning and Acting Guide*. New York: Tarcher Putnam, 1993. (Also published in Spanish by Paidos in Barcelona, 1997.)

Granet, Roger, and Falcon, E. *Is It Alzheimer's?: What to Do When Loved Ones Can't Remember What They Should Do*. New York: Avon, 1998.

Jones, Moyra, *Gentlecare: Changing the Experience of Alzheimer's Disease in a Positive Way*. Point Roberts, WA: Hartley and Marks, 1998.

Levin, Nora Jean. *How to Care for Your Parents*. New York: W. W. Norton, 1997.

McLeod, Beth Witrogen. *Caregiving: The Spiritual Journey of Love, Loss, and Renewal*. New York: John Wiley and Sons, 1999.

Roth, Philip. *Patrimony*. New York: Simon and Schuster, 1991.

Smith, Kerri. *Caring for Your Aging Parents*. Lakewood, CO: American Source Books, 1992.

Comprehensive Information and Resources for Caregivers
www.careguide.com
www.caregiving.com
www.caregiverzone.com

Eldercare Resources
www.elderweb.com

Family and Medical Leave Act Home Page
www.dol.gov/dol.esa/fmla.html

Senior Care
www.senior.com

Cognitive Training

Scogin, Forrest, and Prohaska, Mark. *Aiding Older Adults with Memory Complaints*. Sarasota, FL: Practitioner's Resource Series, 1993.

Couples Therapy

http://depts.washington.edu/ccrstaff/ictlist.html

Death

Akner, Lois. *How to Survive the Loss of a Parent: A Guide for Adults*. New York: William Morrow, 1992.

de Vries, Brian (Ed.). *End of Life Illness*. New York: Springer, 1999.

Field, Marilyn, and Cassel, Christine (Eds.). *Approaching Death*. Washington, DC: Institute of Medicine, 1999.

Knox, Michael, and Knox, Lucinda. *Last Wishes*. Chicago: Ulysses Press, 1995.

Nuland, Sherwin. *How We Die*. New York: Knopf, 1994.

Saunders, Dame Cicely, and Kastenbaum, Robert. *Hospice Care on the International Scene*. New York: Springer, 1997.

———

Americans for Better Care of the Dying—Information to deal with serious illness.

www.abcd-caring.org

Partnership for Caring—Consumer information.

www.partnershipforcaring.org

U.S. Administration on Aging—Hospice directories and other resources.

www.aoa.dhhs.gov/aoa/webres/hospice.htm

Depression

Epstein, Laura, and Amador, Xavier Francisco. *When Someone You Love is Depressed*. New York: Free Press, 1996.

Real, Terrance. *I Don't Want to Talk about It: Overcoming the Secret Legacy of Male Depression*. New York: Scribner, 1997.

Styron, William. *Darkness Visible*. New York: Random House, 1996.

Doctors

Blau, Sheldon, and Skimberg, Elaine. *How to Get out of the Hospital Alive: A Guide to Patient Power*. New York: Macmillan, 1997.

Scribnick, Richard, and Scribnick, Wayne. *Smart Patient, Good Medicine: Working with Your Doctor to Get the Best Medical Care*. New York: Walken, 1994.

Elder Abuse

American Psychological Association. *Elder Abuse and Neglect*. Washington, DC: American Psychological Association Press, 1999.

———

Administration on Aging

www.aoa.dhhs.gov/abuse/report/degault.htm

Financial Planning

Quinn, Jane. *Making the Most of Your Money*. New York: Simon and Schuster, 1997.

Walker, David. *Retirement Security: Understanding and Planning for Your Financial Future*. New York: Wiley, 1997.

Weigold, Frederick. *The Wall Street Journal Lifetime Guide to Money: Everything You Need to Know about Managing Your Finances for Every Stage of Life*. New York: Hyperion, 1997.

Home Environmental Modification

Brawley, Elizabeth. *Designing for Alzheimer's Disease: Strategies for Better Care Environments*. New York: John Wiley and Sons, 1997.

Warner, Mark. *The Complete Guide to Alzheimer's—Proofing Your Home*. West Lafayette, IN: Purdue University Press, 1998.

Environmental Coping Strategies for Alzheimer Caregivers
www.usc.edu/dept/gero/hmap/carhom/toc.htm

Homicide and Suicide

Benson, Herbert, and Ellen M. Stuart. *The Wellness Book: The Comprehensive Guide to Maintaining Health and Treating Stress-Related Illness*. New York: Fireside/Simon and Schuster, 1993.

Rico, Gabriel. *Pain and Possibility: Writing Your Way through Personal Crisis*. New York: Tarcher/Putnam, 1991.

Rosenbloom, Dena, Watkins, Barbara E., and Williams, Mary Beth. *Life after Trauma*. New York: Guilford Press, 1999.

Sims, Darcie D., and Williams, Sherry L. *Holiday Help: A Guide for Hope and Healing*. Lexington, KY: Accord, 1996.

Information and Resources for Family Members
www.fmhi.usf.edu/amh/homicide-suicide/index.html

Legal Issues

Morgan, Rebecca (Ed.). *Nursing Home Litigation*. St. Petersburg, FL: Stetson University College of Law, 1999.

Strauss, Peter, and Lederman, Nancy. *The Elder Law Handbook: A Legal and Financial Survival Guide for Caregivers and Seniors*. New York: Facts on File, 1996.

Managed Care Advocacy

Spragins, Ellyn. *Choosing and Using an HMO.* New York: Bloomberg, 1997.

Medical Information—Internet

All of these major sites provide important information about many health problems for consumers.

Access America for Seniors
www.senior.gov

Dr. Koop
www.drkoop.com

Healthfinder—a gateway consumer health information Web site.
www.healthfinder.gov

onhealth
www.onhealth.com

WEBMD
www.webmd.com

Nursing Homes

Amarnick, Claude. *Don't Put Me in a Nursing Home!* Deerfield Beach, FL: Garrett Publishing, 1996.

Hassler, Jon. *Simon's Night.* New York: Ballantine, 1979.

Warren, Athena. *Into the Lives of Others.* New York: Tiresias Press, 1994.

Parkinson's Disease

Cram, David. *Understanding Parkinson's Disease.* Omaha, NE: Addicus Books, 1999.

Duvoisin, Roger. *Parkinson's Disease: A Guide for Patient and Family.* Philadelphia: Lippincott-Raven, 1966.

Landau, Elaine. *Parkinson's Disease.* New York: F. Watts, 1999.

Lieberman, Abraham, and Williams, Frank. *Parkinson's Disease: The Complete Guide for Patients and Caregivers.* New York: Fireside, 1993.

These sites represent the federal government and major national organizations for Parkinson's disease.

American Parkinson Disease Association
www.apdaparkinson.com

Healing Well (book reviews message board)
Members.aol.com/healwell/parkinsons.html

National Parkinson's Association
www.parkinson.org

Parkinson's Alliance
www.parkinsonalliance.net

Parkinson's—National Institute of Neurologic Disorders and Stroke
www.ninds.nih.gov

Products to Overcome Disabilities

Warner, Mark. *The Complete Guide to Alzheimer's—Proofing Your Home.* West Layfayette, IN: Purdue University Press, 1998.

———

A comprehensive resource for disability products is
www.disabilityresource.com

Special Care Units and Settings

Kuhn, Daniel, Ortigara, Anna, and Lindeman, David. *The Growing Challenges of Alzheimer's Disease in Residential Settings.* Chicago, IL: Rush Alzheimer's Disease Center, 1999.

Lyman, Karen. *Day in, Day out with Alzheimer's Stress in Caregiving Relationships.* Philadelphia: Temple University Press, 1993.

Appendix 1

National and International Alzheimer Organizations

Alzheimer's Association

919 North Michigan Avenue, Suite 1100

Chicago, IL 60611-1676

(800) 272-3900, or (312) 335-8700

www.alz.org

The Alzheimer's Association was founded as a national organization in 1980 by a number of family groups from around the country as well as many professionals and scientists. It has become the leading organization in the field dedicated to research, education, formation of a nationwide family support network, advocacy for government support, and service to patients and families.

Alzheimer's Association local chapters can be found at www.alz.org/chapters/index.html. The list of Alzheimer's centers can be found at www.alzheimer's.org/pubs/adcdir.html.

Alzheimer Society of Canada

20 Eglinton Avenue West, Suite 1200

Toronto, Ontario M4R 1K8

(416) 488-8772, or from Canada (800) 616-8816

www.alzheimer.ca

This national organization in Canada provides information about affiliates in every province.

Alzheimer's Disease Education and Referral (ADEAR) Center
P.O. Box 8250
Silver Spring, MD 20907-8250
(800) 438-4380, or (301) 495-3311
www.alzheimers.org
ADEAR is a national clearinghouse for information about Alzheimer's disease. It is sponsored by the National Institute on Aging (NIA).

Alzheimer's Disease International (ADI)
45/46 Lower Marsh
London SE1 7RG
United Kingdom
+44 20 7620 3011
Helpline +44 845 300 0336
Fax: +44 20 7401 7351
www.alz.co.uk
ADI is the umbrella nonprofit organization for over fifty national Alzheimer organizations. It was registered in 1984 in the United States and has official ties with the World Health Organization.

Alzheimer's Society
Gordon House
10 Greencoat Place
London SW1P 1PH
United Kingdom
+44 20 7306 0606
Fax +44 20 7306 0808
www.alzheimers.org.uk

Family Caregiver Alliance
690 Market Street, Suite 600
San Francisco, CA 94104
(415) 434-3388
In California: (800) 445-8106
www.caregiver.org
The Alliance is a national nonprofit organization that provides resources, advocacy, education, and support for caregivers of relatives with memory loss from Alzheimer's disease and related disorders.

Safe Return

Box A-3956

Chicago, IL 60690

(800) 572-1122 to report a lost person with Alzheimer's disease

Safe return is a joint venture of the Alzheimer's Association and the National Center for Missing Persons.

Appendix 2

National Organizations on Aging

U.S. GOVERNMENT AGENCIES

Center for Mental Health Services Knowledge Exchange Network
P.O. Box 42490
Washington, DC 20015
(800) 789-CMHS (2647)

Department of Education
400 Maryland Avenue, S.W.
Washington, DC 20202-0498
(800) USA-LEARN
www.ed.gov

Department of Health and Human Services Agencies
Office of the Secretary
200 Independence Avenue, S.W.
Washington, DC 20201
(202) 690-7000
www.hhs.gov/progorg.ospage.html

Department of Housing and Urban Development
541 Seventh Street, S.W.
Washington, DC 20410
(202) 401-0388
www.hud.gov

Food and Drug Administration Center for Drugs, Evaluation and Safety
5600 Fishers Lane, RM 12B-31
Rockville, MD 20857
(888) INFO-FDA
www.fda.gov

Health Care Financing Administration
500 Security Boulevard
Baltimore, MD 21244
(410) 786-3000
www.hcfa.gov

**National Clearinghouse
for Alcohol and Drug
Information (NCADI)**
P.O. Box 2345
Rockville, MD 20847-2345
(800) 729-6686, or
  (301) 468-2600
www.health.org

**National Institute on
Alcohol Abuse and
Alcoholism/NIH**
Office of Scientific
  Communication
6000 Executive Boulevard
Suite 409
Bethesda, MD 20892-7003
(301) 443-3860
www.niaaa.nih.gov

**National Institute on Drug
Abuse/NIH**
6001 Executive Boulevard,
  Room 5213
Bethesda, MD 20892-9561
(301) 443-1124
www.drugabuse.gov

**National Institute of Mental
Health**
Office of Communications and
  Public Liaison
6001 Executive Boulevard
Room 8184, MSC 9663
Bethesda, MD 20892-9663
(301) 443-4513
www.nimh.nih.gov

**National Institute of
Neurological Disorders
and Stroke/NIH**
Office of Communications and
  Public Liaison
P.O. Box 5801
Bethesda, MD 20824
(301) 496-5751
www.ninds.nih.gov

**Office of the U.S. Surgeon
General**
5600 Fishers Lane
Rockville, MD 20857
(301) 443-4000
Fax: (301) 443-3574
www.surgeongeneral.gov

**Rehabilitation Services
Administration**
U.S. Department of Education
330 C Street, S.W., Room 3211
Washington, DC
(202) 205-5474
www.ed.gov/offices/OSERS/
  RSA

**Social Security
Administration**
Office of Public Inquiries
6401 Security Boulevard,
  Room 4-C-5 Annex
Baltimore, MD 21235-6401
(800) 772-1213
TTY: (800) 325-0778
Fax: (410) 965-0696
www.ssa.gov

Substance Abuse and
  Mental Health Services
  Administration
Room 12-105, Parklawn Building
5600 Fishers Lane
Rockville, MD 20857
www.samhsa.gov
  Center for Substance Abuse
    Treatment
  www.samhsa.gov/csat
  Center for Substance Abuse
    Prevention
  www.samhsa.gov/csap

Veterans Health
  Administration
1120 Vermont Avenue, N.W.
Washington, DC 20421
(800) 827-1000
www.va.gov/health/index.htm

NATIONAL ORGANIZATIONS
  AND ASSOCIATIONS

AARP
601 E. Street, N.W.
Washington, DC 20049
(800) 424-3410
www.aarp.org

American Academy of
  Family Physicians
11400 Tomahawk Creek
  Parkway
Leawood, KS 66211-2672
(913) 906-6000
www.aafp.org

American Association of
  Homes and Services for
  the Aging (AAHSA)
901 E. Street, N.W., Suite 500
Washington, DC 20004-2011
(202) 783-2242
www.aahsa.org

American Association of
  Suicidology
4201 Connecticut Avenue, N.W.
Suite 310
Washington, DC 20008
(202) 237-2280
www.suicidology.org

American Bar Association
Commission on Legal Problems
  of the Elderly
740 15th Street, N.W.
Washington, DC 20005-1022
(202) 662-8690

American Cancer Society
There is no national address.
  Local and regional offices
  are available from the 800
  number or the Web site.
(800) ACS-2345
www.cancer.org

American College of Sports
  Medicine
401 W. Michigan Street
Indianapolis, IN 46206-3233
(317) 637-9200
www.acsm.org

American Council of the
  Blind
1155 15th Street, N.W.,
  Suite 1004
Washington, DC 20005
(202) 467-5081
(800) 424-8666
www.acb.org/index.html

American Council on
  Exercise
5820 Oberlin Drive, Suite 102
San Diego, CA 92121-3787
(800) 825-3636
(858) 535-8227
www.acefitness.org

American Dental Association
211 East Chicago Avenue
Chicago, IL 60611
(312) 440-2500
www.ada.org

American Diabetes
  Association
1701 N. Beauregard Street
Alexandria, VA 22311
(800) DIABETES (800-342-
  2383)
www.diabetes.org

American Health Care
  Association (AHCA)
1201 L Street, N.W.
Washington, DC 20005
(202) 842-4444
www.ahca.org

American Heart Association
7272 Greenville Avenue
Dallas, TX 75231-4596
(800) AHA-USA1
www.americanheart.org

American Parkinson's
  Disease Association
1250 Hylan Boulevard, Suite 4B
Staten Island, NY 10305-1946
(718) 981-8001
(800) 223-2732
www.apdaparkinson.com

American Psychiatric
  Association
1440 K Street, N.W.
Washington, DC 20005
(202) 682-6237
www.psych.org

American Psychological
  Association
750 First Street, N.E.
Washington, DC 20002
(202) 336-5500
www.apa.org

American Society for
  Geriatric Dentistry
Contact: Federation of Special
  Care Organizations in
  Dentistry
211 E. Chicago Avenue, Suite 948
Chicago, IL 60611
(312) 440-2660
www.foscod.org/asgd.htm

American Society of
  Consultant Pharmacists
1321 Duke Street
Arlington, VA 22314-3563
(703) 739-1300
www.ascpfoundation.org

American Society on Aging
  (ASA)
833 Market Street, Suite 511
San Francisco, CA 94103
(415) 974-9600
www.asaging.org

American Speech-Language-
  Hearing Association
10801 Rockville Pike
Rockville, MD 20852
(800) 498-2071
24-hour automated line: (888)
  321-ASHA
www.asha.org

Asociacion Nacional pro
  Personas Mayores
  (National Association
  for Hispanic Elderly)
1452 West Temple Street,
  Suite 100
Los Angeles, CA 90026-1724
(213) 487-1922
In California: (800) 953-8553

Assisted Living Federation of
  America
10300 Eaton Place, Suite 400
Fairfax, VA 22030

(703) 691-8100
www.alfa.org

Children of Aging Parents
1609 Woodbourne Road,
  Suite 302A
Levittown, PA 19057-1511
(800) 227-7294
www.careguide.net/careguide.
  cgi/caps/capshome.html

Consultant Dietitians in
  Health Care Facilities
2219 Cardinal Drive
Waterloo, IA 50701
(319) 235-0991
www.cdhfc.org

Dietary Managers
  Association
406 Surrey Woods Drive
St. Charles, IL 50174
(800) 323-1908
www.dmaonline.org

Eldercare Locator
1112 16th Street, N.W.,
  Suite 100
Washington, DC 20036
(800) 677-1116

Family Caregiver Alliance
425 Bush Street, Suite 500
San Francisco, CA 94108
(415) 434-3388
In California: (800) 445-8106
www.caregiver.org

Florida Commission on
Aging with Dignity
P.O. Box 1661
Tallahassee, FL 32302-1661
(850) 681-2010
www.agingwithdignity.org

Help for Incontinent People
P.O. Box 544
Union, SC 29379
(800) 252-3337

International Psychogeriatric
Association
550 Frontage Road
Suite 2820
Northfield, IL 60093
(846) 784-1701
www.ipa-online.org

Joint Commission on
Accreditation of Health-
care Organizations
One Renaissance Boulevard
Oakbrook Terrace, IL 60181
(630) 792-5000
www.jcaho.org

National Academy of Elder
Law Attorneys, Inc.
1604 North Country Club
Road
Tucson, AZ 85716
(520) 881-4005
www.naela.com

National Aging Resource
Center on Elder Abuse
810 First Street, N.E., Suite 500
Washington, DC 20002
(202) 682-2470

National Association for
Continence
P.O. Box 8310
Spartanburg, SC 29305-8310
(800) BLADDER (800-252-
3337)
www.nafc.org

National Association of
Home Care
228 7th Street, S.E.
Washington, DC 20003
(202) 547-7424
www.nahc.org

National Center for Home
Equity Conversion
360 N. Robert, #403
St. Paul, MN 55101
(651) 222-6775
www.reverse.org/info.nchec.htm

National Citizens' Coalition
for Nursing Home
Reform
1424 16th Street, N.W.,
Suite 202
Washington, DC 20002
(202) 332-2275
www.nccnhr.org

National Family Caregivers
  Association
10400 Connecticut Avenue,
  #500
Kensington, MD 20895-3944
(800) 896-3650
www.nfcacares.org

National Hospice
  Organization
1901 N. Moore Street,
  Suite 901
Arlington, VA 22209
(800) 658-8898

National Institute on Adult
  Day Care
409 3rd Street, S.W., 2nd Floor
Washington, DC 20024
(202) 479-6682

National Stroke Association
8480 East Orchard Road,
  Suite 1000
Englewood, CO 80111-5015
(800) 367-1990
www.stroke.org

NIMH Depression
  Awareness, Recognition &
  Treatment Program
5600 Fishers Lane, Room 7C02
Rockville, MD 20857
(800) 421-4211

Sex Information &
  Education Council
  of the United States
130 West 42nd Street,
  Suite 2500
New York, NY 10036
(212) 819-9770

Suicide Information and
  Education Centre
201-1615-10th Avenue, S.W.
Calgary, Alberta
Canada T3C 0J7
(403) 245-3900
www.siec.ca

Visiting Nurse Associations
  of America
11 Beacon Street, Suite 910
Boston, MA 02108
(617) 523-4042
www.vnaa.org

Administration on Aging and State Agencies on Aging

National Aging Information Center
Administration on Aging
330 Independence Avenue, S.W.
Room 4656
Washington, DC 20201
(202) 619-7501
www.aoa.gov/naic

The Administration on Aging is the principal government agency for implementing the programs of the Older Americans Act. The National Aging Information Center is a valuable source of information on Alzheimer's disease and other dementias, caregiver resources, and minority organizations.

Many state agencies on aging provide free information about state, county, and city services for older people. They also often have information about private agencies. The addresses and phone numbers for each state agency on aging is listed below. Updates will be posted on the Web site for the Administration on Aging (www.aoa.gov/aoa/pages/state.html).

Key sections of the Administration on Aging Web site for caregivers are as follows:

Information about Services in Your Community
www.aoa.gov/elderpage/locator.html

Information for Older Persons and Their Families
www.aoa.gov/elderpage.html

Resource Directory for Older Persons
www.aoa.gov/aoa/resource.html

Administration on Aging Fact Sheets
www.aoa.gov/factsheets

Elder Action
www.aoa.gov/elderpage.html#ea

Alabama

Region IV
Melissa M. Galvin, Executive
　Director
**Alabama Commission on
　Aging**
RSA Plaza, Suite 470
770 Washington Avenue
Montgomery, AL 36130-1851
(334) 242-5743
Fax: (334) 242-5594

Alaska

Region X
Jane Demmert, Director
Alaska Commission on Aging
Division of Senior Services

Department of Administration
Juneau, AK 99811-0209
(907) 465-3250
Fax: (907) 465-4716

American Samoa

Region IX
Lualemaga E. Faoa, Director
**Territorial Administration
　on Aging**
Government of American Samoa
Pago Pago, American Samoa
　96799
011-684-633-2207
Fax: 011-864-633-2533 or
　633-7723

Arizona

Region IX
Henry Blanco, Program Director
Aging and Adult Administration
Department of Economic Security
1789 West Jefferson Street, #950A
Phoenix, AZ 85007
(602) 542-4446
Fax: (602) 542-6575

Arkansas

Region VI
Herb Sanderson, Director
Division of Aging and Adult Services
Arkansas Department of Human Services
P.O. Box 1437, Slot 1412
1417 Donaghey Plaza South
Little Rock, AR 72203-1437
(501) 682-2441
Fax: (501) 682-8155

California

Region IX
Lynda Terry, Director
California Department of Aging
1600 K Street

Sacramento, CA 95814
(916) 322-5290
Fax: (916) 324-1903

Colorado

Region VIII
Rita Barreras, Director
Aging and Adult Services
Department of Social Services
110 16th Street, Suite 200
Denver, CO 80202-4147
(303) 620-4147
Fax: (303) 620-4191

Connecticut

Region I
Christine M. Lewis, Director of Community Services
Division of Elderly Services
25 Sigourney Street, 10th Floor
Hartford, CT 06106-5033
(860) 424-5277
Fax: (860) 424-4966

Delaware

Region III
Eleanor Cain, Director
Delaware Division of Services for Aging and Adults with Physical Disabilities

Department of Health and
 Social Services
1901 North DuPont Highway
New Castle, DE 19720
(302) 577-4791
Fax: (302) 577-4793

District of Columbia

Region III
E. Veronica Pace, Director
**District of Columbia Office
 on Aging**
One Judiciary Square, 9th Floor
441 Fourth Street, N.W.
Washington, DC 20001
(202) 724-5622
Fax: (202) 724-4979

Florida

Region IV
Gema G. Hernandez, Secretary
Department of Elder Affairs
Building B, Suite 152
4040 Esplanade Way
Tallahassee, FL 32399-7000
(904) 414-2000
Fax: (904) 414-2004

Georgia

Region IV
Jeff Minor, Acting Director

Division of Aging Services
Department of Human
 Resources
2 Peachtree Street, N.E.,
 36th Floor
Atlanta, GA 30303-3176
(404) 657-5258
Fax: (404) 657-5285

Guam

Region IX
Arthur U. San Augstin,
 Administrator
Division of Senior Citizens
Department of Public Health
 and Social Services
P.O. Box 2816
Agana, Guam 96910
(671) 475-0263
Fax: (671) 477-2930

Hawaii

Region IX
Marilyn Seely, Director
**Hawaii Executive Office
 on Aging**
250 South Hotel Street,
 Suite 109
Honolulu, HI 96813-2831
(808) 586-0100
Fax: (808) 586-0185

Idaho

Region X
Lupe Wissel, Director
Idaho Commission on Aging
P.O. Box 83720
Boise, ID 83720-0007
(208) 334-3833
Fax: (208) 334-3033

Illinois

Region V
Margo E. Schreiber, Director
Illinois Department on Aging
421 East Capitol Avenue,
Suite 100
Springfield, IL 62701-1789
(217) 785-2870
Chicago office: (312) 814-2916
Fax: (217) 785-4477

Indiana

Region V
Geneva Shedd, Director
Bureau of Aging and In-Home Services
Division of Disability, Aging
and Rehabilitative Services
Family and Social Services
Administration
402 W. Washington Street,
#W454

P.O. Box 7083
Indianapolis, IN 46207-7083
(317) 232-7020
Fax: (317) 232-7867

Iowa

Region VII
Dr. Judy Conlint, Executive
Director
Iowa Department of Elder Affairs
Clemens Building, 3rd Floor
200 Tenth Street
Des Moines, IA 50309-3609
(515) 281-4646
Fax: (515) 281-4036

Kansas

Region VII
Connie L. Hubbell, Secretary
Department on Aging
New England Building
503 S. Kansas Avenue
Topeka, KS 66603-3404
(785) 296-4986
Fax: (785) 296-0256

Kentucky

Region IV
Jerry Whitley, Director

Office of Aging Services
Cabinet for Families and
  Children
Commonwealth of Kentucky
275 East Main Street
Frankfort, KY 40621
(502) 564-6930
Fax: (502) 564-4595

Louisiana

Region VI
Paul "Pete" F. Arcineaux, Jr.,
  Director
**Governor's Office of
  Elderly Affairs**
P.O. Box 80374
Baton Rouge, LA 70898-0374
(504) 342-7100
Fax: (504) 342-7133

Maine

Region I
Christine Gianopoulos,
  Director
**Bureau of Elder and
  Adult Services**
Department of Human Services
35 Anthony Avenue
State House, Station #11
Augusta, ME 04333
(207) 624-5335
Fax: (207) 624-5361

Maryland

Region III
Sue Fryer Ward, Secretary
**Maryland Department
  of Aging**
State Office Building, Room
  1007
301 West Preston Street
Baltimore, MD 20201-2374
(410) 767-1100
Fax: (410) 333-7943
E-mail:
  sfw@mail.ooa.state.md.us

Massachusetts

Region I
Lillian Glickman, Secretary
**Massachusetts Executive
  Office of Elder Affairs**
One Ashburton Place, 5th Floor
Boston, MA 02108
(617) 727-7750
Fax: (617) 727-9368

Michigan

Region V
Lynn Alexander, Director
**Michigan Office of Services
  to the Aging**
611 W. Ottawa, N. Ottawa
  Tower, 3rd Floor
P.O. Box 30676

Lansing, MI 48909
(517) 373-8230
Fax: (517) 373-4092

Minnesota

Region V
James G. Varpness, Executive
  Secretary
Minnesota Board on Aging
444 Lafayette Road
St. Paul, MN 55155-3843
(651) 296-1531 or (800) 882-
  6262
TTY: (800) 627-3529
Fax: (651) 297-7855

Mississippi

Region IV
Eddie Anderson, Director
**Division of Aging and
  Adult Services**
750 N. State Street
Jackson, MS 39202
(601) 359-4925
Fax: (601) 359-4370
E-mail:
  ELANDERSON@msdh.
  state.ms.us

Missouri

Region VII
Andrea Routh, Director

Division on Aging
Department of Social Services
P.O. Box 1337
615 Howerton Court
Jefferson City, MO 65102-1337
(573) 751-3082
Fax: (573) 751-8687

Montana

Region VIII
Charles Rehbein, State Aging
  Coordinator
**Senior and Long Term
  Care Division**
Department of Public Health
  and Human Services
P.O. Box 4210
111 Sanders, Room 211
Helena, MT 59620
(406) 444-7788
Fax: (406) 444-7743

Nebraska

Region VII
Mark Intermill, Administrator
Division on Aging
Department of Health and
  Human Services
P.O. Box 95044
1343 M Street
Lincoln, NE 68509-5044
(402) 471-2307
Fax: (402) 471-4619

Nevada

Region IX
Mary Liveratti, Administrator
**Nevada Division for Aging
Services**
Department of Human
  Resources
State Mail Room Complex
3416 Goni Road, Building D
Carson City, NV 89706
(775) 687-4210
Fax: (775) 687-4264

New Hampshire

Region I
Catherine A. Keane, Director
**Division of Elderly and
  Adult Services**
State Office Park South
129 Pleasant Street, Brown
  Building #1
Concord, NH 03301
(603) 271-4680
Fax: (603) 271-4643

New Jersey

Region II
Eileen Bonilla O'Connor,
  Acting Assistant
  Commissioner
**New Jersey Division of
  Senior Affairs**

Department of Health and
  Senior Services
P.O. Box 807
Trenton, NJ 08625-0807
1-800-792-8820
(609) 588-3141
Fax: (609) 588-3601

New Mexico

Region VI
Michelle Lujan Grisham,
  Director
State Agency on Aging
La Villa Rivera Building,
  Ground Floor
228 East Palace Avenue
Santa Fe, NM 87501
(505) 827-7640
Fax: (505) 827-7649

New York

Region II
Walter G. Hoefer, Executive
  Director
**New York State Office
  for the Aging**
2 Empire State Plaza
Albany, NY 12223-1251
1-800-342-9871
(518) 474-5731
Fax: (518) 474-0608

North Carolina

Region IV
Karen E. Gottovi, Director
Division of Aging
Department of Health and
   Human Services
2101 Mail Service Center
Raleigh, NC 27699-2101
(919) 733-3983
Fax: (919) 733-0443

North Dakota

Region VIII
Linda Wright, Director
Aging Services Division
Department of Human Services
600 South 2nd Street, Suite 1C
Bismarck, ND 58504
(701) 328-8910
Fax: (701) 328-8989

North Mariana Islands

Region IX
Ana DLG. Flores, Administrator,
   Director
CNMI Office on Aging
P.O. Box 2178
Commonwealth of the Northern
   Mariana Islands
Saipan, MP 96950
(670) 233-1320/1321
Fax: (670) 233-1327/0369

Ohio

Region V
Joan W. Lawrence, Director
Ohio Department of Aging
50 West Broad Street,
   9th Floor
Columbus, OH 43215-5928
(614) 466-5500
Fax: (614) 466-5741

Oklahoma

Region VI
Roy R. Keen, Division
   Administrator
Aging Services Division
Department of Human Services
P.O. Box 25352
312 N.E. 28th Street
Oklahoma City, OK 73125
(405) 521-2281 or 521-2327
Fax: (405) 521-2086

Oregon

Region X
Roger Auerbach, Administrator
**Senior and Disabled Services
   Division**
500 Summer Street, N.E., 2nd
   Floor
Salem, OR 97310-1015
(503) 945-5811
Fax: (503) 373-7823

Palau

Region X
Lillian Nakamura, Director
State Agency on Aging
Republic of Palau
Koror, PW 96940
9-10-288-011-680-488-2736
Fax: 9-10-288-680-488-1662 or
  1597

Pennsylvania

Region III
Richard Browdie, Secretary
**Pennsylvania Department of
  Aging**
Commonwealth of Pennsylvania
555 Walnut Street, 5th Floor
Harrisburg, PA 17101-1919
(717) 783-1550
Fax: (717) 772-3382

Puerto Rico

Region II
Ruby Rodriguez Ramirez,
  M.H.S.A., Executive Director
Commonwealth of Puerto Rico
**Governor's Office of Elderly
  Affairs**
Call Box 50063
Old San Juan Station, PR 00902
(787) 721-5710, 721-4560, 721-
  6121

Fax: (787) 721-6510
E-mail: rubyrodz@prtc.net

Rhode Island

Region I
Barbara A. Raynor, Director
**Department of Elderly
  Affairs**
160 Pine Street
Providence, RI 02903-3708
(401) 277-2858
Fax: (401) 277-2130

South Carolina

Region IV
Elizabeth Fuller, Deputy Direc-
  tor
**Office of Senior and Long
  Term Care Services**
Department of Health and Hu-
  man Services
P.O. Box 8206
Columbia, SC 29202-8206
(803) 898-2501
Fax: (803) 898-4515
E-mail:
  FullerB@DHHS.State.sc.us

South Dakota

Region VIII
Gail Ferris, Administrator

Office of Adult Services
and Aging
Richard F. Kneip Building
700 Governors Drive
Pierre, SD 57501-2291
(605) 773-3656
Fax: (605) 773-6834

Tennessee

Region IV
James S. Whaley, Executive
Director
Commission on Aging
Andrew Jackson Building,
9th Floor
500 Deaderick Street
Nashville, TN 37243-0860
(615) 741-2056
Fax: (615) 741-3309

Texas

Region VI
Mary Sapp, Executive Director
Texas Department on Aging
4900 North Lamar, 4th Floor
Austin, TX 78751-2316
(512) 424-6840
Fax: (512) 424-6890

Utah

Region VIII
Helen Goddard, Director

Division of Aging and Adult
Services
Box 45500
120 North 200 West
Salt Lake City, UT 84145-0500
(801) 538-3910
Fax: (801) 538-4395

Vermont

Region I
David Yavocone, Commissioner
Vermont Department of
Aging and Disabilities
Waterbury Complex
103 South Main Street
Waterbury, VT 05671-2301
(802) 241-2400
Fax: (802) 241-2325
E-mail: dyaco@dad.state.vt.us

Virginia

Region III
Ann Magee, Commissioner
Virginia Department for
the Aging
1600 Forest Avenue, Suite 102
Richmond, VA 23229
(804) 662-9333
Fax: (804) 662-9354

Virgin Islands

Region II
Sedonie Halbert, Commissioner

Senior Citizen Affairs
Virgin Islands Department of
    Human Services
Knud Hansen Complex, B
    uilding A
1303 Hospital Ground
Charlotte Amalie, VI 00802
(340) 774-0930
Fax: (340) 774-3466

Washington

Region X
Ralph W. Smith, Assistant
    Secretary
**Aging and Adult Services
    Administration**
Department of Social and
    Health Services
P.O. Box 45050
Olympia, WA 98504-5050
(360) 493-2500
Fax: (360) 438-8633

West Virginia

Region III
Gaylene A. Miller,
    Commissioner
**West Virginia Bureau of
    Senior Services**

Holly Grove, Building 10
1900 Kanawha Boulevard East
Charleston, WV 25305
(304) 558-3317
Fax: (304) 558-0004

Wisconsin

Region V
Donna McDowell, Director
**Bureau of Aging and Long
    Term Care Resources**
Department of Health and
    Family Services
P.O. Box 7851
Madison, WI 53707
(608) 266-2536
Fax: (608) 267-3203

Wyoming

Region VIII
Wayne Milton, Administrator
Office on Aging
Department of Health
117 Hathaway Building,
    Room 139
Cheyenne, WY 82002-0710
(307) 777-7986
Fax: (307) 777-5340

Index